Current Review of
Sports
Medicine

second edition

EDITED BY

Robert J. Johnson, MD

Professor of Orthopaedic Surgery
Head, Division of Sports Medicine
Department of Orthopaedics & Rehabilitation
University of Vermont College of Medicine
Burlington, Vermont

John Lombardo, MD

Professor and Chairman
Department of Family Medicine
Ohio State University College of Medicine;
Ohio State University Sports Medicine Center
Columbus, Ohio

WITH 30 CONTRIBUTORS

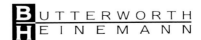

DEVELOPED BY CURRENT MEDICINE, INC.
PHILADELPHIA

Current Medicine, Inc. 400 Market Street   Suite 700   Philadelphia, PA 19106

Managing editor: **Lori J. Bainbridge**
Developmental editor: **Scott Thomas Hurd**
Editorial assistant: **Deborah Singer**
Art director: **Paul Fennessy**
Cover design: **Jerilyn Bockorick**
Design and layout: **Jeff Brown**
Illustration director: **Ann Saydlowski**
Illustrator: **Beth Starkey**
Typesetting: **Ryan Walsh**
Production: **Lori Holland and Sally Nicholson**
Indexer: **Holly Lukens**

ISBN: 1-7506-9965-5
ISSN: 1069-5842

Printed in The United States by Edward Brothers
5 4 3 2 1

Every effort has been made to ensure that the drug dosage schedules within this text are accurate
and conform to standards at the time of publication. However, as treatment recommendations vary
in the light of continuing research and clinical experience, the reader is advised to verify drug
dosage schedules herein with information found on product information sheets. This is especially
true in cases of new or infrequently used drugs.

Joseph A. Abate III, MD
Clinical Assistant Professor
Department of Orthopaedics and Rehabilitation
McClure Musculoskeletal Research Center
University of Vermont College of Medicine
Burlington, Vermont;
Fletcher Allen Health Care
Colchester, Vermont

James R. Andrews, MD
Clinical Professor of Orthopaedic Surgery
Department of Orthopaedics
University of Alabama at Birmingham;
Orthopaedic Surgeon
Alabama Sports Medicine and Orthopaedic
  Center
Birmingham, Alabama

Jack T. Andrish, MD
Professor of Surgery
Ohio State University
Columbus Ohio;
Cleveland Clinic Foundation
Cleveland, Ohio

Joseph A. Buckwalter, MD
Professor
Department of Orthopaedic Surgery
University of Iowa
Iowa City, Iowa

Chris Carr, PhD
Clinical Assistant Professor
Department of Family Medicine
Ohio State University Sports Medicine Center
Ohio State University
Columbus, Ohio

Pierre A. d'Hemecourt, MD
Lecturer
Department of Orthopedics
Division of Sports Medicine
Harvard Medical School;
Sports Medicine
Boston Children's Hospital
Boston, Massachusetts

Harry H. Dinsmore, MD
Fellow
Department of Orthopaedics
Division of Sports Medicine and Hand Surgery
University of Virginia
Charlottesville, Virginia

Jon Divine, MD
Assistant Professor
Department of Family & Community Medicine
Baylor College of Medicine;
Baylor/Methodist Primary Care Associates
Baylor Sports Medicine Institute
Houston, Texas

Paul A. Dowdy, MD, FRCSC
Attending Orthopedic Surgeon
Central Florida Sports Medicine Institute
Davenport, Florida

Cyril B. Frank, MD, FRCSC
Professor
Department of Surgery
McCaig Centre for Joint Injury and Arthritis
  Research
University of Calgary
Calgary, Alberta, Canada

Freddie H. Fu, MD
Blue Cross Professor of Orthopaedic Surgery
Executive Vice-Chairman and Professor
Department of Orthopaedic Surgery
University of Pittsburgh;
Medical Director, Center for Sports Medicine
University of Pittsburgh Medical Center
Pittsburgh, Pennsylvania

Kevin A. Hildebrand, MD, FRCSC
Clinical Fellow
Hand and Upper Limb Centre
University of Western Ontario
London, Ontario, Canada

Ernst B. Hunziker, MD
Professor
M.E. Müller Institute for Biomechanics
University of Berne
Berne, Switzerland

Douglas W. Jackson, MD
Director
Southern California Center for Sports Medicine
Long Beach, California

Todd Kays, MD
Psychology Fellow
Department of Family Medicine
Ohio State University
Columbus, Ohio

David L. Kowalk, MD
Chief Resident
Department of Orthopaedic Surgery
University of Virginia
Charlottesville, Virginia

Frank C. McCue III, MD
Alfred R. Shands Professor of Orthopaedic
  Surgery and Plastic Surgery of the Hand
Department of Orthopaedic Surgery
University of Virginia
Charlottesville, Virginia

Lyle J. Micheli, MD
Director
Division of Sports Medicine
The Children's Hospital;
Associate Clinical Professor of Orthopaedic
 Surgery
Harvard Medical School
Boston, Massachusetts

Mark D. Miller, MD
Clinical Associate Professor
Department of Orthopaedics
USAF Academy
Colorado

Matthew J. Mitten, JD
Professor of Law
South Texas College of Law
Houston, Texas

Claude E. Nichols III, MD
Assistant Professor
Department of Orthopaedics & Rehabilitation
McClure Musculoskeletal Research Center
University of Vermont College of Medicine
Burlington, Vermont

Michael J. Pagnani, MD
Orthopaedic Surgeon
The Lipscomb Clinic
Nashville, Tennessee

Dipak V. Patel, MD
Sports Medicine Fellow
The Hospital for Special Surgery
New York City, New York

Margot Putukian, MD, FACSM
Assistant Professor
Department of Internal Medicine, Orthopedics,
 and Rehabilitation
Hershey–Geisinger Medical Center;
Team Physician, Penn State University
Penn State Center for Sports Medicine
University Park, Pennsylvania

Yvonne E. Satterwhite, MD
Orthopaedic Surgeon
Kentucky Sports Medicine Clinic
Lexington, Kentucky

Stephen F. Schaal, MD
Professor of Medicine
Division of Cardiology
Ohio State University College of Medicine
Columbus, Ohio

Paul J. Schreck, MD
Metropolitan Orthopaedic Associates
St. Clair, Michigan

R. Trent Sickles, MD
Associate Professor of Clinical and Family
 Medicine
Department of Family Medicine
Ohio State University College of Medicine,
Ohio State University Sports Medicine Center
Columbus, Ohio

Russell F. Warren, MD
Surgeon-in-Chief
The Hospital for Special Surgery
New York City, New York

Robert D. Whitehead, MD
Clinical Professor
Department of Family Medicine
Ohio State University College of Medicine
Columbus, Ohio

Contents

CHAPTER 1 1
SPINE AND CHEST WALL
Lyle J. Micheli
Pierre d'Hemecourt

CHAPTER 2 19
SURGICAL MANAGEMENT OF SHOULDER
AND UPPER ARM INJURIES
Claude E. Nichols III

CHAPTER 3 25
ELBOW AND FOREARM TRAUMA
James R. Andrews
Yvonne E. Satterwhite

CHAPTER 4 43
ATHLETIC INJURIES TO THE HAND
AND WRIST
Frank C. McCue III
Harry H. Dinsmore
David L. Kowalk

CHAPTER 5 55
HIP AND THIGH INJURIES
Joseph A. Abate III
Jack T. Andrish

CHAPTER 6 69
KNEE LIGAMENT PROBLEMS
Paul J. Schreck
Douglas W. Jackson

CHAPTER 7 85
OTHER KNEE PROBLEMS AND INJURIES
Dipak V. Patel
Michael J. Pagnani
Russell F. Warren

CHAPTER 8 103
ANKLE AND FOOT
Paul A. Dowdy
Mark D. Miller
Freddie H. Fu

CHAPTER 9 121
BIOLOGY OF LIGAMENT INJURY
AND REPAIR
Kevin A. Hildebrand
Cyril B. Frank

CHAPTER 10 133
ARTICULAR CARTILAGE BIOLOGY
AND HEALING
Joseph A. Buckwalter
Ernst B. Hunziker

CHAPTER 11 151
CARDIOPULMONARY PROBLEMS IN
THE ATHLETE
R. Trent Sickles
Stephen F. Schaal

CHAPTER 12 163
DRUGS IN SPORTS
Robert D. Whitehead

CHAPTER 13 175
PERFORMANCE PSYCHOLOGY
Chris Carr
Todd Kays

CHAPTER 14 187
OPTIMIZING TRAINING AND
CONDITIONING
Jon Divine

CHAPTER 15 207
WOMEN IN SPORTS
Margot Putukian

CHAPTER 16 231
MEDICOLEGAL ISSUES
Matthew J. Mitten

INDEX...237

SPINE AND CHEST WALL

Lyle J. Micheli and
Pierre A. d'Hemecourt

Athletic injuries to the spine and chest wall are relatively rare. The potential for catastrophic injury or chronic limiting injuries, however, make this an area of special concern for sports physicians. For the sake of convenience, the discussion of the management of these problems in athletes is divided into cervical spine, thoracic spine and chest wall, and low back and lumbar spine. The discussion is addressed not only to the clinical management of such injuries but also to their potential prevention. Rehabilitation after injury and discussion of criteria for return to play, which are special concerns of sports medicine clinicians, are also emphasized. Every effort has been made to integrate the advances documented in the current literature.

CERVICAL SPINE

Preparticipation evaluation and training

After treatment for a cervical spine injury, preparticipation evaluation of a young athlete is important whether it is part of the initial examination or is related to the question of a return to sports activity, particularly to contact sports. The history of the athlete contains important information for identifying who may be at increased risk for cervical injury. Careful questioning regarding previous episodes of neck pain, transient paresthesias of one or both arms, or periods of limitation of motion is extremely important. The history of other congenital problems, such as abnormalities of the ears, fasciae, oropharynx, heart, or kidneys, should also be noted.

The physical examination of youngsters preparing for sports is extremely helpful. Pizzutillo [1••] has noted that limitations of lateral bending and rotation are the most significant findings for undetected on unsuspected congenital or acquired abnormalities. In particular, the physician should be alert to asymmetry of rotation (Fig. 1.1). In a young athlete with a history of previous injury or cervical dysfunction plain-film radiographs, including anteroposterior (AP), lateral, and open-mouth views are indicated. If these radiographs are abnormal, further assessment is indicated, including lateral flexion-extension views to determine cervical spine stability in this axis and magnetic resonance imaging (MRI) to assess the relative capacity of the neuroforamina and their relationship to the spinal cord.

The preparticipation examination may reveal relatively little cervical strength. In such cases cervical spine exercises to increase the strength and muscle bulk of the related musculature are indicated. Traditional techniques for cervical spine strengthening have included isometric setting of the paravertebral muscles. Customarily these exercises use an isometric hold. They involve flexion and extension, lateral bending to the left and right, or rotation to the left and right for 5 seconds followed by a relaxation period of 10 seconds, with the exercise repeated 5 to 10 times. One of 3 sets are performed 2 to 4 times per day [3•].

Dynamic exercises for improving or restoring cervical range of motion and strength also include simple movements of the head and neck through the full range of neck excursion. The head is used as the resistive force, which can be supplemented with sling-supported weights or spring-loaded head halters. The concern is that there are no simple parameters for normative values of strength. In some instances the spring-loaded or machine techniques are subject to variability and can present some risk for injury to athletes. Leggett *et al.* [4••] demonstrated a significant increase in cervical spine strength with a cervical spine-strengthening device (MedEx, Ocala, Florida) used with a series of exercises over a single training session once per week. The strength gain was then maintained with two cervical training sessions per month.

The rationale for using neck strengthening to help prevent injuries to the axial cervical spine comes from basic observation of strength training. Not only do the muscles increase in strength, but the bones and ligaments of the loaded structures also increase in strength [5]. Several studies have demonstrated that muscle mass is an important component of force dissipation and absorption with loading [6,7].

Cervical spine injury

The care of acute cervical spine injury can be appropriately divided into five major concerns that are detailed in Table 1.1.

On-field evaluation

Athletic events should be attended by a designated individual who is trained in rapid assessment and immobilization techniques and who is certified in cardiopulmonary resuscitation. Physicians and athletic trainers often fill this role. A spine board and cervical collar should be readily available and an evacuation plan should precede the event.

Any athlete complaining of severe neck pain, particularly with any neurologic symptom, should be

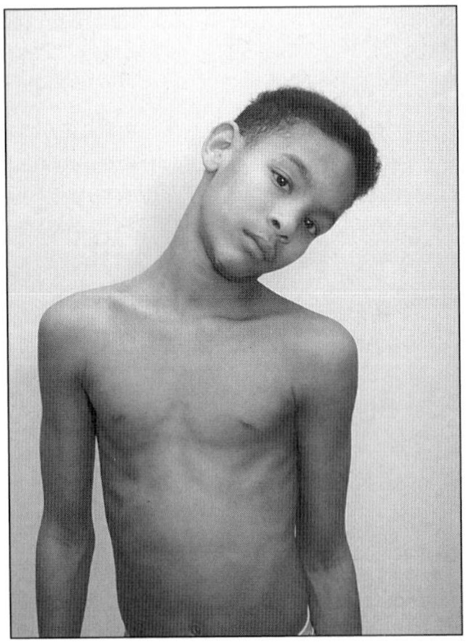

FIGURE 1.1

Asymmetry and decreased cervical range of motion are the most predictable physical findings following significant cervical injury.

Table 1.1	CONCERNS DURING THE CARE OF ACUTE CERVICAL SPINE INJURY

Initial assessment, including transportation and emergency stabilization.
Assessment of the cervical spine, including physical examination and imaging techniques.
Thorough working knowledge of the differential diagnosis related to cervical complaints.
Appropriate treatment for such conditions.
Criteria for return to play following injury.

immobilized immediately. Spinal injuries usually present with pain and spasm. This, however, will not be apparent in the unconscious athlete. Because it is impossible to determine the stability of the injury on the field, the initial tasks for those in charge include simultaneous immobilization of the cervical spine and maintenance of a clear airway (which may simply involve removing a mouth piece or carefully logrolling the face-down athlete with full control of the head and neck). It is critical to address these issues and to avoid any spinal manipulation. The goal is to prevent further injury. Swenson *et al.* [6] demonstrated radiographically that removal of the helmet in football players with shoulder pads increased cervical lordosis. They recommend leaving the helmet in place during transportation. Further evaluation is performed at the hospital [7].

Less dramatic cervical complaints, requiring determination of continued participation, may present during an event. Before allowing an athlete to return to contact competition, four conditions must be met. There should be a normal neurologic examination, a full range of motion, normal strength, and resolved pain. These determinations need to be made away from the coaches, the crowd, and parents who may pressure for the return of the athlete to the event.

Stingers or burners are a common sideline complaint in contact sports, such as gridiron football and rugby. Several mechanisms have been proposed. One involves a brachial plexus traction palsy from ipsilateral shoulder compression and/or contralateral neck flexion. A second mechanism is nerve-root compression from cervical extension with ipsilateral lateral flexion, essentially a Spurling maneuver. Finally, some injuries represent a direct brachial compression at Erb's point in the supraclavicular region. Athletes with these injuries will often present with acute, sharp lancinating pain and tingling in the hand. The upper trunk innervated muscles, biceps, deltoid, and supraspinatus are often transiently involved. The traction neuropraxia mechanism would likely explain the acute transient symptoms, particularly in young athletes.

Conversely, Levitz *et al.* [8] studied 55 athletes at the intercollegiate and professional levels with chronic recurrent symptoms. Eighty-three percent reported a mechanism of cervical extension with ipsilateral lateral deviation. Seventy percent had a positive Spurling sign also consistent with a nerve root compression. Developmental spinal stenosis and cervical disc degeneration were also present.

This chronic burner syndrome likely represents a different pathology than the transient traction palsy incurred by younger school-age athletes. Furthermore, direct peripheral nerve injury must be considered. Perlmutter *et al.* reported on 11 isolated axillary nerve injuries during contact sports. Good function recovery was noted in 10 of these athletes [9]. Suprascapular and long thoracic nerve palsies may also occur.

Consideration for the return to play for the athlete on the field may occur if all symptoms clear within minutes, there is no neurologic deficit or pain, and the range of cervical motion is complete. Conversely, bilateral, prolonged, or lower extremity symptoms, as well as transient quadriplegia, mandates a formal evaluation for spinal stenosis before returning to play. New onset of symptoms should also be considered carefully before allowing continued participation in contact sports [10].

Formal evaluation and treatment

According to a startling report on second-stage cervical spine injury [11], patients with trauma have sustained cervical spine injuries after being transported to a medical care facility. The authors emphasized that in nearly every instance technically acceptable AP, lateral, and open-mouth views of the cervical spine would have detected the cervical spine abnormality and averted further injury. In one case, complete quadriplegia resulted from the obtaining of lateral flexion-extension views before the initial plain-film radiographs were assessed.

Acute macrotrauma to the cervical spine may result in fracture of a vertebrae, facet dislocation, or ligamentous disruption with segmental instability. Acute disc ruptures may result in an anterior cord syndrome or a transient quadriplegia. To assess these problems, the patient is first evaluated under appropriate immobilization with a cross-table lateral view, which includes the superior end plate of T-1. If there is no fracture or displacement and there is no neurologic deficit, the patient proceeds directly to anterior-posterior, lateral, oblique, open-mouth odontoid, and flexion-extension views. Criteria established for instability by White and Panjabi[12] are used. In older adolescents, greater than 3.5 mm displacement or greater than 11 degrees of angulation are considered unstable.

In children and younger adolescents, however, radiographic variations may lead to some confusion in diagnosis. This is due to hypermobility and variation in ossification centers. The child may have a normal atlanto-dens excursion of up to 4.5 mm and an increased excursion at C2-3 and C3-4 [1]. Extension may produce a posterior displacement of C2 on C3 and apparent overriding of the atlas on the odontoid. Loss of normal cervical lordosis in the neutral position and lack of uniform angulation of adjacent vertebrae with cervical flexion may occur up to the age of 16 years (Fig. 1.2). Several physeal variations are of note. The basilar odontoid epiphysis is still visible in 50% of 4- to 5-year-old children, but occasionally is still visible at 11 years of age. These often have an irregular sclerotic border, yet they rarely will appear as a radiolucent line. The apical odontoid epiphysis inconsistently fuses to the odontoid by age 12 and is seen best on the lateral view. Adolescents may also exhibit secondary ossification centers of the spinous processes that may appear as avulsion fractures [11]. Swischuk [14] also demonstrated that anterior wedging of C3 may persist into childhood, possibly due to chronic exaggerated hypermobility and delay in ossification.

In the presence of a neurologic deficit or an unstable fracture on lateral view, computed tomography (CT) is necessary. Unilateral facet dislocations will be present with a 25% displacement, and a bilateral facet dislocation will be present with a 50% displacement on lateral radiography. Intraspinal pathology, such as disc protrusion, may be assessed with myelograph contrast enhanced computed tomography or MRI scanning.

Bailes *et al.* [15] pointed out an important additional aid in the early assessment of cervical spine injury in athletes. They noted that intermediate-weighted MRI scan images are preferable to T_2-weighted

images for detecting minimal spinal cord trauma. They suggested that the brightness of the cerebrospinal fluid on the T2-weighted images may obscure the intraparenchymal high-intensity contusion signal. Other observers [16] have suggested that, in addition to plain-film radiographic assessment of bony spinal stenosis, lateral MRI is particularly useful in determining the relative risk for impingement of the spinal cord on the bony, particularly the distal, elements of the spine. It has also been demonstrated that high-resolution CT myelography with thin contiguous axial section reliably demonstrates nerve-root avulsions in brachial plexus injuries [17].

In this same landmark article, based on the largest review in the literature of cervical spine injuries in the athletically active population, Bailes *et al.* [15] discussed the management of such injuries. The authors divided the patients studied into three types: 1) those with spinal cord injuries that were demonstrable, either clinically or with imaging; 2) those with transient neurologic injuries and structurally intact spines; and 3) those with vertebral column injuries only.

They further noted a subgroup of patients who had definitive spinal cord signs and symptoms initially, but who had complete resolution of neurologic deficit without vertebral column injury or permanent spinal cord sequelae. This latter type of disorder, they observed, may often be underdiagnosed in the initial assessment, unless a careful history, physical evaluation, and new imaging techniques are used.

The authors noted that the first type of injury (permanent damage to the spinal cord) is relatively easy to diagnose. In the second group, however, the careful assessment and differentiation from less seri-

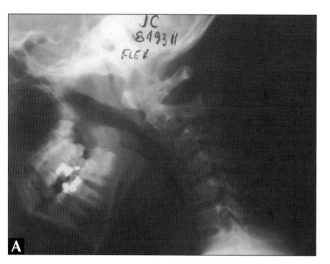

A

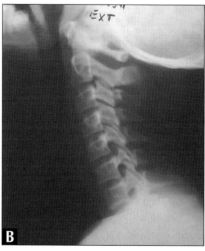

B

FIGURE 1.2

Lateral flexion view (*panel A*) and extension view (*panel B*) reveal pathologic excursion and instability at C2-3 in a young athlete following injury. This is not "physiologic" laxity.

ous injuries, such as brachial plexus neuropathy or neuropraxia (referred to as the burner or stinger injury), must be done. Burner injuries are relatively common. Some studies have found them in as many as 50% of collegiate football players during a single season [18,19]. These injuries usually resolve without significant neurologic sequelae. The radiographic assessments are normal, and there are no findings suggestive of cord involvement, such as bilaterality, lower extremity symptoms, or long-track findings. Electromyographic evidence of neuromuscular injury, however, may be present and persist for a long time after the initial injury, even after apparent full restoration of function has occurred [20]. Bailes *et al.* called attention to "burning hand syndrome," described by Maroon [21]. The syndrome is thought to be a mild variant of central cord syndrome, and it causes burning dysesthesias in both arms and hands with associated weakness. Four patients in this series were classified with burning hand syndrome. All had normal radiographic studies and complete resolution of their symptoms within 48 hours.

Bailes *et al.* believed that the second group of patients, those with transient neurologic findings without residual neurologic deficit, radiologically demonstrable injury, or congenital cervical spine anomaly, could return to full participation in contact sports. The authors state, however, that, if recurrent episodes of spinal cord symptoms occur, these athletes may be at a higher-than-normal risk for catastrophic injury. Limits on participation should therefore be considered.

It is evident that most cases of spinal stenosis fall within this category. In 1986, Torg *et al.* [22] suggested that certain young athletes with transient cord symptoms and with apparent complete resolution were found in retrospect to have a relatively decreased neurocanal size. They further provided criteria for this sizing and noted that the ratio of the neurocanal to the vertebral body width on lateral radiographs was less than 0.8 to 1.0 mm. Bailes *et al.* [15] noted that of their 10 patients with transient spinal cord symptoms, four had a canal diameter less than 14 mm in absolute width.

A certain degree of confusion has been clarified regarding the use of this ratio as a risk factor for injury in contact sports. Herzog *et al.* [16] noted that these criteria would prevent a high percentage of professional football players from participating in this sport. Cantu [10] stressed the importance of functional stenosis secondary to soft tissue impinge-

ment. This is determined using MRI and contrast position CT when indicated. Torg [23] also recently established that this ratio has a poor positive predictive value in determining an athlete's suitability to play. The ratio does not seem to predict catastrophic neurologic injury even with athletes experiencing transient quadriplegia.

Return to play

In type-3 injuries, which show radiographic evidence of abnormality but no neurologic findings, a great deal of individualization is required when return to play is considered. The obvious problem is that a fracture of the cervical spine that appears to have progressed to normal bony union and demonstrates normal physiologic stability on lateral flexion-extension views, may still carry increased risk for injury with the higher loads of sports. This possibility exists even if the cervical spine does not have increased risk for reinjury with normal physiologic ranges of load.

Bailes *et al.* [15] also noted that few experimental or clinical data are available to assess the degree of stability or the strength of a healed fracture or ligament injury of the cervical spine under extreme degrees of stress. Cervical spine posterior ligaments appear to contribute more to stability in flexion, whereas the anterior ligaments are more important in extension. The authors concluded that in the absence of reliable data and objective measure of the degree of stability under dynamic stress, any healed fracture of the spinal column should be considered unsuitable to safely withstand further challenges from impact (with the exception of a healed, isolated, minor vertebral body, lamina, or spinous process fracture).

Injuries with radiographic evidence of abnormality must include those with normal bony architecture that have been demonstrated to have abnormal ranges of motion on flexion-extension views. It is generally accepted that cervical instability exists when there is more than 3.5 mm of horizontal or 11 degrees of angular displacement between adjacent vertebrae. Although a physician may not think it necessary to perform a spinal fusion for normal activities of daily living, it might not be advisable to allow a patient with abnormal range of motion to return to contact sport activities. MRI must be considered an additional risk factor, along with other findings, in the determination of returning the athlete to play. Certainly a relative spinal stenosis with cervical spine anomalies or abnormalities of structure from previous injury may contraindicate heavy-contact sports.

Surgical management

The basis for treatment of cervical spine injury depends on a determination of the potential for stability after the initial injury has healed. In most cases this can be accomplished on the basis of the radiographic architecture from plain-film radiographs, CT, or MRI. In many cervical spine fractures, the application of cervical tong or halo traction, followed by halo vest stabilization, allows satisfactory healing of the bony fracture and a subsequently stable cervical spine. When the cervical spine is judged to be dangerously unstable, with little likelihood of subsequent stability after in situ healing, early cervical spine stabilization and fusion is indicated.

When herniated cervical discs are responsible for persistent symptoms and are anticipated to cause ongoing compromise of the neurocanal anterior discectomy, with or without associated anterior fusion, posterior surgical approach with discectomy may be indicated [22]. In cases in which initial conservative management has been followed by persistent cervical spine instability, such as nonunion at the dens, a second-stage posterior spinal fusion may be indicated [23].

Parenteral methylprednisolone 30 mg/kg bolus, followed by 5.4 mg/kg/hr, over the next 24 hours is recommended in the acute management of most spinal cord injuries.

Prevention

Little information has been available until recently on the prevention of cervical spine injuries in sports.

Schneider's [27] monumental book on head and neck injuries in football, published in 1973, captured the attention of the medical community and the lay public. Attention was directed to the role of the rigid plastic football helmet in decreasing the rate of head injuries but increasing the risk for cervical spine injuries when the head is used as a battering ram. In 1976, the National Collegiate Athletic Association and the National Federation of High School Athletic Associations adopted rules banning "spearing," the use of the top of the helmet as the initial point of contact in striking an opponent during a tackle or a block. Torg [28] noted the dramatic decline in cervical spine injuries between 1976 and 1987, apparently as a result of this rule change (Fig. 1.3). Although football is the only sport to have demonstrated an association between techniques of play, rule interpretations, and changes in implementation, it has been suggested that preventive measures in sports as diverse as rugby, ice hockey, trampoline, and wrestling, in which the mechanisms of injury are now being researched, would similarly help reduce the risk for injury. Torg and other authors have suggested that vertical axial compression is the basic mechanism of cervical spine injury in football, but it also may be implicated as a major mechanism of injury in sports such as diving, rugby, ice hockey [29], and wrestling [30]. Various case reports from other sports, particularly diving, suggest that hyperflexion (or in some cases hyperextension) may also be a mechanism of injury. However, Torg's experimental and clinical observations [31] make a compelling argument that straight axial load in the neutralized neck is a major cause of injury in football.

In rugby, cervical spine injuries have also drawn much attention, and attempts to minimize their frequency have been instituted at the international level

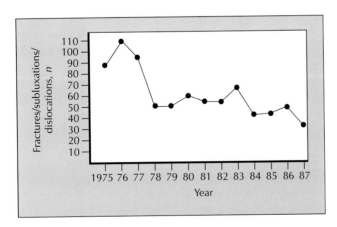

FIGURE 1.3

The yearly incidence of cervical spine fractures, dislocations, and subluxations for all levels of participation (1975–1987) decreased markedly in 1978 and continued to decline during the remaining 9 years as a direct result of the rule changes instituted in the 1976 banning of head-first blocking, tackling, and spearing. (*From Torg et al. [73]; with permission.*)

[32]. One well-recognized mechanism of rugby cervical spine injury occurs during the scrum, another situation in which Torg hypothesizes that the injury is caused by direct axial load rather than hyperflexion, as was once thought [33]. The implementation of the New Zealand rules, in which the force of the impact is minimized by requiring the two opposing sides to touch, pause, bend, and then join, has been shown in one study to decrease the incidence of cervical spine injuries in rugby by 40% [34].

As discussed, the value of careful examination of youth athletes who are at additional risk for cervical spine injury because of previous injury or incomplete rehabilitation has been hypothesized but not proven. Certainly, the more carefully the preparticipation evaluation is performed, the better. Additionally, the role of strengthening and flexibility exercises in helping to prevent cervical spine injury must once again be hypothesized since it has not been clearly proven by studies. Needless to say, it will be extremely difficult to obtain sufficient clinical material to prove that cervical spine strengthening and exercises can significantly decrease the rate of injury in athletes.

THORACIC SPINE AND CHEST WALL

Although they are less common in athletes, injuries to the upper back, chest wall, and thoracic spine can sometimes be problematic. At times they can end athletic careers, especially in throwing sports.

On-field management

Macrotraumatic injuries to the thoracic spine and chest wall occur predictively in such heavy contact sports as football and rugby, but also in light contact sports like soccer and basketball. Acute injuries include contusions, strains, sprains, disc herniations, and visceral injuries. Thoracic vertebral fracture and spinal cord injuries are not common, but are found occasionally in high-velocity sporting activity, such as motor racing. Apophyseal avulsion fractures of the thoracic and lumbar spine are common.

Another potentially serious thoracic injury is a fractured rib. At fieldside it is difficult to determine whether the injury involves muscle or bone. For the team physician, the major challenge in this situation is whether or not to return the athlete to play. In the case of a fractured rib, the obvious concern is the development of a tension pneumothorax because of subsequent trauma and puncturing of the parietal and visceral pleura. Abdominal visceral injury may also occur. One noteworthy case involved a rugby player who had chest pain and did not report the injury immediately to the team official. Midway through the second half of the game he developed respiratory distress and was determined to have a tension pneumothorax. Fortunately, prompt transport to a medical support facility and the installation of a chest tube resulted in a favorable outcome.

Another rib-complex injury that can be very challenging for the team physician in particular is the rib-tip syndrome [35]. These injuries often occur in contact sports, such as gridiron football, lacrosse, or rugby. They are caused by a separation of the anterior margin of the rib from the conjoint anterior costal cartilage. These lesions are slow to heal and subject to reinjury. An athlete with this injury should be advised to expect recurrence of the injury, with symptoms after even minor reinjury for the remainder of the season. Symptoms may take up to 9 to 12 weeks to resolve.

The risk of catastrophic injuries to the thorax has gained increased attention in recent years because of the highly publicized cases of deaths from impact to the anterior chest wall and sternum in young baseball players. These injuries have been assumed to result from either cardiac concussion or cardiac contusion. In the former case, it has been assumed that a direct blow to the mobile sternum of the child may cause impact to the pericardium and cardium, which results in asystole and death. In the latter case (cardiac contusion), direct structural injury to the cardium can be documented.

Most cases of cardiac contusion from blunt trauma are the result of high-impact or motor-vehicle accidents and are rarely seen in sports. There have been several recent reports, however, of cardiac contusions resulting from trauma in boxing [36]. In youth baseball there has been little recognition of the dangers posed by this injury and even less information about mechanisms of prevention, although in 1991, Abrunzo [37•] reported two cases of cardiac asystole. One resulted in death caused by a blow to the chest from a thrown ball. The exact number of such injuries is not known, but the U.S. Consumer Product Safety Commission reported in 1984 that 51 children aged 5 to 14 years died of baseball-related injury between 1973 and 1983. Twenty-three of these deaths resulted from ball impact to the chest [38]. Attempts to prevent this injury have taken two avenues. The more popular appears to be the development by several manufacturers of a reduced-injury-factor baseball. Another proposal is the use of chest protectors, specifically for batters. The softer ball has the obvious advantage of protecting all players from injury. One of the injured players reported by Abrunzo [37•] had been struck by a ball thrown from the outfield.

Baseball-related injuries have received the most attention in regard to catastrophic chest trauma. There have been case reports of similar injuries, however, resulting from impact with a hockey puck or a lacrosse ball [39,40], and Serina and Lieu [41•] reported a relatively high incidence of thoracic injuries in *Taekwon-do*. A demonstration sport in the 1988 Olympics in Seoul, *Taekwon-do* became an official event in the 1992 Barcelona Olympics. *Taekwon-do* is a Korean martial art in which points are scored when contact to the torso or head is sufficient to produce a "trembling shock." Approximately 80% of the competitive strokes are kicks as opposed to hand strikes. In the study cited, it was noted that almost half of all *Taekwon-do* injuries are to the chest wall and thorax, and it was suggested that a high proportion of the *Taekwon-do* kicks carry the risk for serious injury to both skeletal structures and visceral organs when no protective body equipment is used. This study has been thought to highlight the need for adequately designed equipment to protect the thorax against structural injury.

Formal evaluation and treatment

Acute injuries to the thoracic spine usually result in strains of the paravertebral or parascapular musculature. A careful physical examination can generally distinguish the area of maximal tenderness and relate it to the muscular anatomy. With any acute musculotendinous strain, a period of relative rest, icing, medications (including anti-inflammatory agents or muscle relaxants), and physical therapy to restore range of painless motion and muscle strength are indicated. Rehabilitation should be initiated as soon as acute symptoms have been alleviated.

On occasion symptoms may persist beyond the usual 3 to 4 weeks of muscle-tendon strain. In such instances, a differential diagnosis (including injury to the costovertebral joints, intrathoracic injury, and thoracic disc) must be considered.

Some costovertebral joint injuries may persist for several months and be a source of continued pain to the athlete. The diagnosis can often be confirmed by indirect pressure on the appropriate rib, which causes pain centralized to the costovertebral junction.

Careful localization, followed by corticosteroid injection of the affected joint with fluoroscopic assistance, can often be instrumental in relieving symptoms and returning the athlete to play.

Persistent pain associated with particular movements, such as lateral bending or torso rotation, may turn out to be caused by thoracic disc injury. Fortunately, the confirmation of this diagnosis has been greatly aided by the availability of MRI techniques. The problem with thoracic disc injury in the competitive athlete, particularly the contact-sport athlete, is determining a rationale for management and return to play. The thoracic disc has generally been considered the purview of the neurosurgeon. A review of the literature finds wide-ranging opinions regarding its management [42]. Several authorities believe that a thoracic disc prominent enough to cause radicular symptoms, and more particularly cord symptoms, must be addressed quickly with resection. Another body of opinion, however, maintains that, as with the lumbar disc, a period of observation and limited activity may be sufficient to allow long-track and neural symptoms to resolve. Obviously, the decision to allow a competitive athlete with thoracic pain to return to play is difficult because there are no clear guidelines. Ice hockey superstar Wayne Gretzky, who ultimately was allowed to return to play and did not undergo surgical intervention, is a case in point. It is imperative to obtain the opinion of one's neurosurgical colleagues in cases of symptomatic thoracic disc.

Several other athletic injuries to the thoracic spine, although rare, merit attention. Several cases involving vertebral body fractures, caused by direct trauma or falls in athletic competition, have been recorded. In every instance these were stable vertebral compression fractures. Fortunately, it is extremely rare to generate the level of force capable of causing an unstable thoracic spine injury in sports. Nevertheless, one case, involving a young hockey player who struck the boards after an illegal check from behind and sustained an unstable fracture of the high thoracic spine, has been reported. Riding competitions and motor sports have also been implicated.

These fractures are usually sustained with axial loading vertically or in flexion. In the absence of sufficient force to cause a compression fracture, it is prudent to implement a search for a pathologic lesion. The initial evaluation includes AP and lateral radiographs. On lateral radiographs of the thoracic spine, the degree of anterior compression is assessed. When anterior compression is less than 25%, posterior ligamentous injury is unlikely. As the compression reaches 50% posterior disruption is often seen [43]. In this latter circumstance a CT scan is indicated to evaluate the posterior neural arch and foramina. Any neurologic symptom associated with a minimal compression fracture also suggests the need for a CT scan.

Stable thoracic compression fractures may be treated with a thoracolumbar spine orthosis or a Jewett extension brace for 8 to 12 weeks. Physical therapy is started as pain allows. Flexibility and extensor strength are addressed. The athlete is allowed to return to noncontact sports, such as gymnastics, but unless the compression is quite minimal, contact sports remain an area of caution. The risk of reinjury must be understood and accepted by the athlete, parents, and institutions. Severe compression fractures and any thoracic instrumentation are contraindications to contact sports [23].

Unique to the adolescent are the thoracic and lumbar spinous process apophyseal avulsion injuries that occur with rapid torsional, flexion, and extension maneuvers. These are treated with initial rest followed by strength and flexibility rehabilitation. A flak jacket is helpful in facilitating return to contact sports. Another cause of chronic pain complaints in the thoracic spine can be related to postural or structural abnormalities of the spine itself. Classic Scheuermann's kyphosis occurs in the thoracic spine, generally in the mid or upper portions and, by definition, consists of at least three vertebrae with wedging, vertebral endplate changes, and disc space narrowing. This disorder can be a source of pain in the young athlete (Fig. 1.4) [44,45]. Again, the diagnosis can often be confirmed on physical examination. There is an irreversible round-back posture with forward shoulder thrust and associated, rather dramatic tightness of the lower lumbar spine on forward bending. Since Holger Scheuermann first described this condition in 1920 and suggested a traumatic etiology, it has been associated with nonathletic individuals. We now know, however, that water ski jumping has a strong correlation with thoracic Scheuermann's. In competitive skiers, who had 9 years of experience starting before age 15, 100% demonstrated some radiographic changes of Scheuermann's [47]. The pain associated with this deformity generally responds to a program of relative rest and associated periscapular and dorsal extension strengthening exercises. On occasion, bracing is indicated with curves in excess of 50

degrees. The opinion of a specialist in scoliosis and spinal deformity should be sought. Once symptoms have resolved these athletes can always return safely to play.

LUMBAR SPINE INJURIES

Low back pain in the high-performance athlete is a relatively common occurrence. Estimates of the incidence have ranged from 50%–75% [48]. Fortunately, most of these complaints are self-limited, resolve within 3 weeks, and are generally ascribed to minor strains and sprains of the musculoskeletal system. The injuries of major concern to the sports physician are: 1) acute injuries that result in severe pain and limit the athlete's ability to compete or train, and 2) low back pain of insidious onset that increases progressively to the point where training cannot be carried on without significant pain (Table 1.2).

ACUTE LUMBAR SPINE INJURIES
Contusions

Contusions are well-known sports injuries and certainly can occur to the lumbar area of the spine. They are caused by a direct blow. Generally the diagnosis is easily made through a careful history and physical examination. An area of ecchymosis and tenderness is usually apparent posteriorly. Provocative testing of the area, particularly with lateral bending to the opposite side, elicits pain. A careful neurologic assessment should be done to

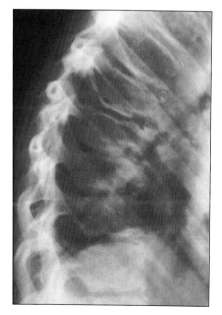

FIGURE 1.4

Classic thoracic Scheuermann's kyphosis with wedging and disc involvement of at least three adjacent vertebrae.

ensure there is no associated neurologic injury. AP and lateral radiographs of the lumbar spine are obtained to ensure that associated injury, such as transverse process fracture, has not occurred. Careful attention should be directed to the possibility of renal injury. Urinalysis should be obtained, and the athlete should be warned to watch for any changes in urinary behavior. The initial treatment consists of rest, ice, compression, and elevation, followed by progressive rehabilitation to the point where the athlete can resume full competition without significant pain. On occasion a simple elastic brace with a plastic insert is employed to provide mechanical protection to the injured area.

Musculotendinous strains

Spasm may be present in the paraspinous muscles, with tenderness at the site of muscle-tendon junction injury. There may be some curvature of the involved area of the spine. Plain-film radiographs show lateral deviation of the lumbar or thoracolumbar vertebrae but no rotation of the vertebrae, as in true idiopathic scoliosis. Again, careful neurologic examination should be done and the results confirmed as negative. The straight-leg raising test may cause pain in the low back, particularly as the leg is brought down during provocative testing. Treatment is expectant, with initial first-aid measures followed by slow, progressive restoration of flexibility and strength to the involved musculature. Return to sport is initiated when the athlete is asymptomatic and fit for competition.

Fractures

Fractures of the lumbar spine are also quite uncommon in the athlete. thoracolumbar compression fractures may be assessed for instability using Denis's 3-column stability method. The anterior longitudinal ligament and anterior half of the vertebral body comprise the anterior column. The middle column goes from the remaining vertebral body to the pedicle origin. The posterior column comprises the bony neural arch and its ligamentous attachments. Stability is determined by stability of the middle column. Involvement of two columns implies instability [49]. In this instance, CT scanning could be indicated to further assess stability. A thoracolumbar orthosis is used to treat stable fractures for 6 weeks. Physical therapy is started as pain allows. Return to sports is usually allowed when the athlete is pain free and has full flexibility.

Unstable fractures that require instrumentation are usually a contraindication to contact sports. A possible exception is a single-level fusion, although in this case, the forces are transferred to the adjacent level and predispose to disc degeneration [25].

Table 1.2		
INJURIES OF MAJOR CONCERN TO THE SPORTS PHYSICIAN		
Repetitive Microtraumatic LBP	Stress reaction	Transitional pseudarthrosis
Contusion	Fracture (spondylolysis)	Facet syndrome
Soft tissue strain, sprain	Displacement (spondylolisthesis)	Adults
Disc herniation	Discogenic LBP	Hyperextension mechanism
Fracture	Hyperflexion mechanism	Degenerative disc disease
Apophyseal avulsion	Discogenic LBP	Spondylolysis
Traumatic spondylolisthesis	Small HNP	Spinal stenosis
Vertebral fracture	Atypical Scheuermann's kyphosis	Chronic soft tissue LBP
Spinal cord injury	Soft tissue LBP	Hyperflexion mechanism
Viscera injury	Single or recurrent strenuous motion	Degeneration disc disease
	Lordotic back pain	Chronic soft tissue strain/sprain
Macrotrauma LBP	Apophyseal avulsion or apophysitis	Arthritic degeneration
Adolescents	HNP	Facet arthrosis
Hyperextension mechanism	Chronic soft tissue strain or sprain	Sacroiliitis
Spondylolytic process	Arthritic degeneration	Transitional pseudarthrosis

Adapted from Gerbino and Micheli [74]; with permission.
HNP—herniated nucleus pulposus; LBP—low-back pain.

Other less common causes of acute-onset back pain in the young athlete include acute traumatic spondylolysis or fracture through the posterior elements, facet fracture, transverse process fracture, or spinous process injury. In the case of spondylolysis, or isthmus fracture, the physician can never be entirely certain whether there were preexistent weaknesses in the pars intraarticularis as a result of repetitive training activities. Some athletes state they had absolutely no pain in their low back before one particular fall or twist. For example, a young gymnast coming down from a vaulting maneuver with acute onset of back pain was subsequently shown to have fractured the isthmus at L-5.

In these instances of acute traumatic injury to the posterior elements of the spine, an exact diagnosis should be made. This can sometimes be extremely difficult. As with overuse injuries, the use of a single-photon emission computed tomography (SPECT) bone scan can sometimes help localize the injury anatomically. It can subsequently be further delineated by high-resolution computed tomographic scanning, with narrower cuts of as little as 2 mm now available.

The treatment is similar to that for the spondylolysis overuse injury. The goal of management should be to obtain bony union. In the case of acute traumatic isthmic fractures we institute rigid antilordotic bracing to maintain a satisfactory apposition of the fragments and to minimize the bending stresses on the posterior elements. Although it might seem logical that apposition of the fragments would be enhanced by inducing lordosis of the lumbar spine and, in effect, bring the fragments closer together, radiographic studies have demonstrated that flattening of the lumbar spine, which renders the posterior elements more vertical and more subject to compression than to bending stress, seems to speed the disappearance of pain and aid in the subsequent bony union (Fig. 1.5).

Disc ruptures

Although less common, acute traumatic injuries to the anterior elements of the spine, vertebral body, and disc can also be encountered in the young athlete. Walters *et al.* [50] described an acute vertebral endplate rupture with the development of a Schmorl's node in a young gymnast, and highlighted the specificity of MRI in assisting the diagnosis. In this instance plain-film radiographs and radionucleotide images were nondiagnostic.

The more common acute anterior element injury is a posterior or posterolateral herniated nucleus pulposus. In the adolescent athlete the presentation of back pain associated with disc herniation is often unlike that in the adult. The adolescent may present with pain in the buttocks only, or extreme tightness in the hamstrings with associated back spasm and/or neurogenic scoliosis (Fig. 1.6) Physical examination shows decreased lumbar motion, positive straight-leg raising and Lesegue's tests, and on

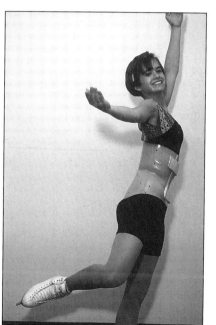

FIGURE 1.5

Lightweight thermoplastic arthrosis used to assist healing of lumbar spondylolysis in a young figure skater.

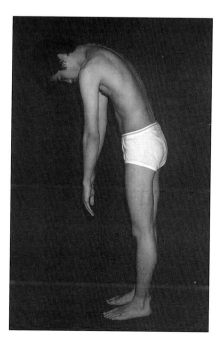

FIGURE 1.6

Dramatic loss of forward flexion in a young tennis player with lumbar disc herniation and little pain.

occasion an acute decrease in strength or change in reflexes.In cases of acute disc herniation, particularly in adolescents or young adults, plain-film radiographs of the lumbar spine are obtained to rule out other associated skeletal injury. An MRI often follows. This approach has generally been sufficient to confirm the diagnosis.

With the exception of herniation with a hinged fibrocartilage piece, the majority of disc herniations respond well to a conservative approach. Following a brief initial period of bed rest to quiet inflammation and spasm, a molded thoracolumbar brace with 15 degrees of lumbar lordosis is often applied. A gradually increasing physical therapy program is started simultaneously. Range of motion (active and passive) is important to enhance the hydrostatic forces for disc nutrition [53]. Obviously, this is begun in a limited pain-free range and increased as tolerated. Aerobic activity, such as walking or water therapy, is initiated early. Progressive resistive exercises (PREs) are implemented when the acute inflammation subsides. The PREs address pelvic tilt, lumbar extensors, abdominals, and all of the muscular attachments to the thoracolumbar fascia, such as latissimus dorsi. Nonsteroidal anti-inflammatory medication and occasionally oral corticosteroids may be used.If the athlete is still symptomatic in 8 to 12 weeks epidural corticosteroids are considered. Jackson has demonstrated a more expeditious return to athletics with this approach [54].

Surgical indications include cauda equina symptoms, worsening motor symptoms, and unresolved pain. The hinged fibrocartilage of an adolescent may also require excision. Decompressive technique should preserve facet joints and interspinous ligaments for segmental stability. The athlete and parents must understand that following complete rehabilitation, return to sports is allowed, although there is a theoretical risk of further degeneration at that level.

Spondylolysis and spondylolisthesis

It has been our experience (and that of several other physicians who treat large numbers of young athletes with complaints of back pain) that a disproportionate number of structural injuries in this age group occur to the posterior elements of the spine. The greatest percentage of these injuries, in turn, occur at the isthmus or the pars intraarticularis of the lumbar spine. Our sports medicine clinic reported a 47% incidence of spondylolysis in adolescents presenting with back pain. The vulnerability of this

anatomic site to repetitive flexion, rotation, or hyperextension injury has been demonstrated in several cadaver and computer-analog models [57]. It is likely that the most common mechanism for this injury is repetitive hyperextension, which is well reported in sports with hyperextension, such as ballet and gymnastics, as well as multiple other sports, including soccer and handball. Seitsalo *et al.* [58] recently reported on the incidence of spondylolysis in the Finnish National Ballet. Nineteen of 60 dancers (32%) had spondylolysis and 15 (25%) had spondylolisthesis.

It is extremely important for the physician dealing with sports injuries to be aware that, although there may be a congenital predisposition to these injuries, they are in great measure acquired in this young athletic population. Therefore, the young athlete who participates in sports that put high demands on the lumbar spine for flexion, extension, or rotation and complains of back pain that is exacerbated by provocative hyperextension testing is suspect for an early stress fracture of the pars intraarticularis. The diagnosis can be extremely accurate if a careful history documents the onset of pain and the movements that particularly increase it. These movements normally include the back walkover or back flip in gymnasts, the arabesque in young dancers, and the down position of interior football linemen. As with stress fractures in general, and particularly stress fractures occurring in a distraction environment, such as the pars intraarticularis of the lumbar spine, the bony changes observable by plain-film radiograph occur late, if at all. SPECT imaging has proven useful in detecting spondylolytic lesions [59]. Plain-film radiographs may sometimes show spina bifida occulta, which has a higher than normal incidence in this group of symptomatic athletes.

If the pars intraarticularis defect is already present on the oblique views of the lumbar spine, to the point where frank breakthrough has occurred, the lesion has been present for considerable time. On occasion, a plain-film (oblique view) radiographic fracture appears on one side of the lumbar spine, whereas bony and nucleotide bone scans show increased uptake on the opposite side. This apparent paradox has been referred to as Wilkinson's sign. Computed tomographic scans are sometimes used in this situation to clarify the lesion. In our experience this lesion generally represents a unilateral nonunion of one pars and a reactive hypertrophy of the opposite pars in response. One recent case demonstrated a positive SPECT scan on one side with a dysplastic facet on the opposite side.

We have encountered rare cases of slow onset of back pain with sciatica in young athletes. The lesion in these cases can by a spondylolysis at L-5, with involvement of the L-5 nerve roots by the overgrown pseudoarthritic tissue at the site of nonunion of the pars. In other instances combined lesions of spondylolysis and disc herniation at the level above the spondylolysis have occurred. In these cases of back pain with associated sciatica that is exacerbated by hyperextension testing, we recommend plain-film radiographs and SPECT bone scan for diagnosis and also MRI of the lumbar spine.

We make every effort to attain bony union in the spondylolytic lesion. The potential for attaining bony union and preventing the complete breakthrough and development of a nonunion at this site is good if detected early, particularly in young individuals. We use a 0-degree orthosis combined with physical therapy addressing peripelvic stretching and abdominal strengthening. Once the athlete is free of pain and flexible, usually within 6 weeks, they may return to any sports that allows the brace to be worn.

We have never documented a case of significant progression of this athletically induced spondylolysis into a spondylolisthesis. We therefore believe that this lesion is stable and can safely withstand the stresses of athletic competition, including contact sports. Several authors, most recently Muschik *et al.* [61], have reported on the low risk of slip progression in the athlete with spondylolisthesis. They reported on 86 athletes between the ages of 6 and 20. Thirty-six subjects showed no progression. Thirty-three showed only an average of 10.5% increase in slippage. Seven subjects showed a decrease in slippage. Furthermore, these athletes had no associated symptoms during an average 4.8 year period of training. Similarly, Seitsalo [58] reported no association of pain in his group of Finnish ballet dancers. It may be that the athletic training helps to stabilize the involved segment.

Overuse injuries to the disc

Certain cases of gradual-onset low back pain in young athletes may be caused by insidious disc herniations, often in combination with relatively narrowed neuroforamina and short pedicles. The disc herniations and bulges are often present at multiple levels, rendering them less than ideal for surgical

intervention. Fortunately, a high proportion of these injuries respond to conservative management, with relative rest of the back followed by careful physical therapy to restore normal range of motion and flexibility. Attention to lumbar extension strengthening combined with trunk stabilization has been demonstrated by Risch [63]. In some instances, however, normal range of motion and flexibility, as well as pain-free return to activities, have not been possible despite all efforts.

Several studies have greatly increased our understanding of repetitive microtrauma or overuse injuries to the lumbar spine in athletes. Needless to say, repetitive training that involves the use of the lumbar spine is intrinsic to numerous sports activities. Three studies of lumbar spine injury in competitive gymnasts all used MRI to determine evidence of lumbar spine deterioration or disruption in athletes versus control subjects [60,61,62]. Although at first the conclusions of these studies seem quite different, further review of their data suggests that their findings are remarkably similar.

A Finnish study [64] reviewed a group of 35 girl and boy gymnasts whose mean age was 12.0 ± 2.6 years and compared them with control subjects. Of these gymnasts, 11 had complained of low back pain during the previous training period and three had MRI evidence of degenerative disc.

Another study of young gymnasts by Goldstein *et al.* [65] divided their participants into three groups based on level of participation and age. The first group, preelite female gymnasts, had a mean age of 11.8 years, very similar to that of the Finnish group. The second group, elite gymnasts, had a mean age of 16.6 years. The third group, former national or Olympic-level gymnasts, had a mean age of 20.7 years. Using MRI criteria for spinal abnormalities, the authors found a 9% incidence of abnormalities in the young pre-elite gymnasts, a 43% incidence in the elite gymnasts, and a 63% incidence in the Olympic-level gymnasts. This latter figure was contrasted with 15.8% incidence in a control group of swimmers in the appropriate age range. The authors concluded that gymnasts who train more than 15 hours per week show a significant increase in degenerative changes of their lumbar spines.

A third study from Sweden [66] observed 24 male elite gymnasts who were former members of the Swedish national team and compared them with 16 male nonathletes of similar age (18 to 29 years). Evidence of spinal deterioration was found in 75% of the gymnasts versus 31% of the control subjects.

The authors also noted a significant correlation between complaints of clinical back pain and abnormalities on MRI.

Taken together these three studies are very important for their scientific exploration of the relationship between athletic training and overuse injuries. They show a dramatically increased incidence of degenerative spinal changes in gymnasts and suggest that gymnastics training that exceeds 15 hours per week appears to pass the threshold of increased risk for lumbar spine injury. It is additionally important to note that these incidence rates may actually underestimate the problem. Studies from our own clinic have found that a large proportion of lumbar spine injuries in gymnasts are actually overuse injuries of the bony posterior elements of the spine that are not readily detectable by MRI. We have also encountered cases with both posterior and anterior element involvement.

The combination of vertebral endplate and vertebral body wedging that occurs over 2 or 3 levels in the thoracolumbar junction or upper lumbar area has been characterized as atypical Scheuermann's disease (Fig. 1.7). The pain from these entities is generally insidious in onset, and it has been presumed that this condition represents repetitive microinjuries with resultant pain and reactive muscle spasm. The pain is increased with flexion testing. Our observation is that in every instance of this condition there has been a remarkable straightness of the thoracic and lumbar spines, with hypokyphosis of the thoracic spine and hypolordosis of the lumbar spine (flat back). In these cases the biomechanical concentration of force appears to occur at the thoracolumbar junction (Fig. 1.8).

We have instituted a program of hyperextension strengthening, stretching, and hyperextension bracing for atypical Scheuermann's disease. A 15-degree thoracolumbar orthosis is initiated and advanced as tolerated. Our young patients usually become asymptomatic in 4 to 6 weeks. They are then allowed to gradually resume activities, including sports, over a period of 3 to 6 months. Despite the resolution of symptoms and restoration of more normal back mechanics, anterior body remodeling and reformation may be relatively modest in these cases as opposed to the more typical Scheuermann's disease of the thoracic spine.

Mechanical low-back pain

There is another group of young athletes with insidious onset of low back pain. We have chosen to classify them as subject to mechanical back pain [67]. These young people have a history of back pain, usually following practice of their sports activities. They often have back pain after prolonged sitting, standing, or walking and may have just experienced a significant adolescent growth spurt [64]. On physical examination, they tend to show tight hamstrings, hip flexion contractures, tight lumbodorsal fascia, weak abdominal muscles, and a limited ability to bend forward and touch their toes. Further assessment, including neurologic examination, imaging,

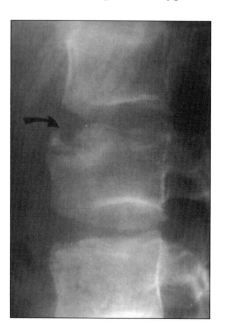

FIGURE 1.7

Atypical Scheuermann's kyphosis at thoracolumbar junction (*arrow*). Note "flat back."

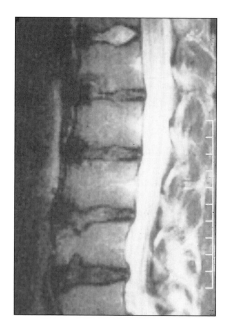

FIGURE 1.8

Multiple levels of disc deterioration with Schmorl's nodes in a young athlete initially diagnosed with back strain.

and bone scans, is unremarkable. These individuals may have apophyseal injuries to the spinous processes and iliac crest that might be picked up on a bone scan that is looking for spondylolysis. If careful assessment is followed by a specific physical therapy regimen that emphasizes range of motion, flexibility, and strengthening exercises of the lumbar and peripelvic musculature, pain-free resumption of sports is possible in almost every instance.

Arthritic Degeneration

Transitional vertebrae such as hemisacralization of L-5 will often have an enlarged lateral mass or bar. A pseudarthrosis may develop from the lateral mass to the sacral ala or iliac wing. Repetitive extension motion, as seen for example in gymnasts, is thought to produce degenerative changes and inflammation in the pseudarthrosis as described by Bertolotti [69]. Confounding the issue is an occasional coexisting disc herniation at the level above the pseudarthrosis. Treatment entails relative rest and corticosteroid injections into the pseudarthrosis. The disc above, however, may be the cause of pain. A molded TLSO can be quite helpful to relieve the inflammation. A bone scan with SPECT may localize the sight of inflammation (Fig. 1.9). Resection of the bar has been described. Gymnasts and other athletes involved in hyperextension sports are cautioned about returning to such provoking activity [66].

Facet arthropathy is difficult to diagnose. There are no unique radiographic, historical, or physical findings [71]. In some athletes, however, who have refractory point tenderness over a unilateral zygapophyseal joint with reproducible pain on extension, a negative evaluation for other disease states, and some radiographic support, a facet corticosteroid block has been helpful.

SCOLIOSIS

Scoliosis has been associated with ballet, possibly as a result of the hormonal effects of the female triad. Athletes with asymmetric loading to the trunk, such as javelin throwers, have been reported to have up to 80% incidence of scoliosis, though with small curves [72].

Adolescent-onset idiopathic scoliosis does not normally cause pain and is not a contraindication to sports. Plain-film radiographs are recommended to ensure there are no congenital elements, such as a lack of formation or segmentation in the spinal curvature. Even in advanced cases of idiopathic scoliosis that require part-time bracing for a maximum of 18 hours per day, full athletic participation and training (up to and including the elite levels) is possible. Where fusion is required, most surgeons advise against participation in full-contact sports. In certain cases involving single-level fusion, such as basal fusions for symptomatic or advanced spondylolysis or spondylolisthesis, return to sports should be individualized. In general, these athletes can reasonably expect to return to full sports participation, including contact sports.

NEOPLASMS AND INFECTIONS

The physician dealing with sports injuries must be well aware that back pain associated with neoplasms or infections may present initially as part of sports training. Unfortunately, this tendency can delay timely diagnosis because the physician a assumes that the pain is caused by acute or repetitive injury from sports. In the young athlete back pain that does not respond as expected to conservative management techniques within 3 to 6 weeks, particularly continued painful scoliosis or spinal deviation, should be assessed for unusual causes, such as infection or tumor. Osteoblastoma, osteoid osteoma, intraspinal tumor, giant cell tumor, and even osteogenic sarcoma and Ewing's sarcoma have been reported in these instances.

Infection, both osteomyelitis and discitis, can present as back pain in the young athlete. Complete blood count with erythrocyte sedimentation rate and imaging techniques, including bone scans or MRI, may be necessary to make an exact diagnosis

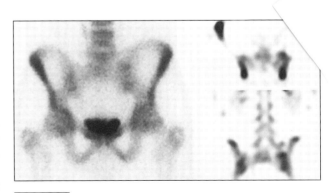

FIGURE 1.9

Bone scan (frontal and axial views) with increased activity at the left L5-S1 pseudarthrosis of a transitional vertebrae.

REFERENCES AND RECOMMENDED READING

Recently published papers of particular interest have been highlighted as:

- • Of special interest
- •• Of outstanding interest

1.•• Pizzutillo PD: Spinal consideration in the young athlete. *Instr Course Lect* 1993, 42:463–472.

Excellent review of the current concepts of assessing and managing spinal problems in young athletes.

2.• American Academy of Pediatrics Committee on Sports Medicine and Fitness: Atlantoaxial instability in downs syndrome (Subject Review). *Pediatrics* 1995, 96:151–154.

This committee report reviews the available data regarding the screening of atlantoaxial instability in youth with Down syndrome including radiographs and clinical observations.

3.• Tan JC, Nordin M: Role of physical therapy in the treatment of cervical disk disease. *Orthop Clin North Am* 1992, 23:435–449.

Review of current physical therapy management for cervical dysfunction.

4.•• Leggett SH, Graves JE, Pollock ML, *et al.*: Quantitative assessment and training of isometric cervical extension strength. *Am J Sports Med* 1991, 19:653–659.

Validation of the cervical spine strength measuring devices (*eg*, MedEx, Ocala, Florida) and significant measured strength gains with training once per week.

5. Tipton CM, Matthes RD, Maynard JA, *et al.*: The influence of physical activity on ligaments and tendons. *Med Sci Sports* 1975, 7:165–175.

6. Swenson TM, Lauerman WC, Blanc RO, *et al.*: Cervical spine alignment in the immobilized football player: radiographic analysis before and after helmet removal. *Amer J Sports Med* 1997, 25:226–230.

7.• Torg JS, Glasgow SG: Criteria for return to contact activities following spine injury. *Clin J Sport Med* 1991, 1:12–26.

Excellent clinical criteria for team physicians regarding patient counseling for spinal stenosis.

8. Levitz CL, Reilly PJ, Torg JS: The pathomechanics of chronic, recurrent cervical nerve root neuropraxia: the chronic burner syndrome. *Am J Sport Med* 1997, 25: 73–76.

9. Perlmutter GS, Leffert RD, Zarins B: Direct injury to the axillary nerve in athletes playing contact sports. *Am J Sports Med* 1997, 25: 65–68.

10. Cantu RC: Head and spine injuries in youth sports. *Clin Sports Med* 1995, 14:517–532.

11. Davis JW, Phreaner DL, Hoyt DB, *et al.*: The etiology of missed cervical spine injuries. *J Trauma* 1993, 34:342–346.

12. White AA, Panjabi MM: *Clinical Biomechanics of the Spine.* Philadelphia: JB Lippincott; 1978.

13. Bohlman HH, Rekate HL, Thompson GH: Problem fractures of the cervical spine in children. In *Problematic Musculoskeletal Injuries in Children.* Edited by Houghton GR, Thompson GH. London: Butterworths; 1981:101–120.

14. Swischuk LE, Swischuk PN, John SD: Wedging of C-3 in infants and children: usually a normal finding and not a fracture. *Radiology* 1993, 188:523–526.

15.•• Bailes JE, Hadley MN, Quigley MR, *et al.*: Management of athletic injuries of the cervical spine and spinal cord. *Neurosurgery* 1991, 29:491–497.

In-depth review of the largest survey of sports-related cervical spine injuries yet reported.

16.• Herzog RJ, Wiens JJ, Dillingham MF, *et al.*: Normal cervical spine morphology and cervical spine stenosis in asymptomatic professional football players: plain film radiography, multiplanar computed tomography, and magnetic resonance imaging. *Spine* 1991, 16:S178–S186.

Notes that Torg criteria for spinal stenosis may be an oversensitive measure for professional football.

17. Walker AT, Chaloupka JC, de Lotbiniere AC, *et al.*: Detection of nerve rootlet avulsion on ct myelography in patients with birth palsy and brachial plexus injury after trauma. *Amer J Roentgenol* 1996, 167:1283–1287.

18. Clancy WG Jr, Brand RL, Bergfeld JA: Upper trunk brachial plexus injuries in contact sports. *Am J Sports Med* 1977, 5:209–216.

19. Robertson WC, Eichman PL, Clancy WG: Upper trunk brachial plexopathy in football players. *JAMA* 1979, 241:1480–1482.

20.• Bergfeld JA, Hershman EB, Wilbourn AJ: Brachial plexus injuries in sports: a five year follow-up. *Orthop Trans* 1988, 12:743–744.

Five-year follow-up of "burner" injuries that found persistent electromyographic abnormalities in most injured players.

21. Maroon JC: "Burning hands" in football spinal cord injuries. *JAMA* 1977, 238:2049–2051.

22.• Torg JS, Pavlov H. Genuario SE, *et al.*: Neurapraxia of the cervical spinal cord with transient quadriplegia. *J Bone Joint Surg* 1986, 68A:1354–1370.

Hypothesizes developmental spinal stenosis as an explanation for transient cervical quadriplegia.

23. Torg JS, Naranja RJ, Palov H, *et al.*: The relationship of developmental narrowing of the cervical spinal canal to reversible and irreversible injury of the cervical spinal cord in football players. *J Bone Joint Surg* 1996, 78A:1308–1314.

24. Meyer PR, Heim S: Surgical Stabilization of the Cervical Spine. In *Surgery of the Spine Trauma.* Edited by Meyer PR. New York: Churchill Livingstone; 1989:397–523.

25. Micheli LJ: Sports following spinal surgery in the young athlete. *Clin Orthop* 1985, 198:152–157.

26. Swischuk LE: Anterior displacement of C2 in children: physiologic or pathologic? *Radiology* 1977, 122:759–763.

27. Schneider RC: *Head and Neck Injuries in Football.* Baltimore: Williams & Wilkins; 1973.

28.•• Torg JS: Epidemiology, pathomechanics, and prevention of football-induced cervical spinal cord trauma. *Exerc Sport Sci Rev* 1992, 20:321–338.

This reviews the cervical spinal cord injuries in football with emphasis on tackling technique, evaluation and prevention.

29. Tator CH: Neck injuries in ice hockey: a recent, unsolved problem with many contributing factors. *Clin Sports Med* 1987, 6:101–114.

30. Torg JS: Mechanisms and pathomechanics of athletic injuries to the cervical spine. In *Athletic Injuries to the Head, Neck and Face*, ed. 3. Edited by Torg JS. Philadelphia: Lea & Febiger; 1993:139–154.

31. Torg JS: Injuries to the cervical spine and cord resulting from water sports. In *Athletic Injures to the Head, Neck and*

Face, ed. 2. Edited by Torg JS. Philadelphia: Lea & Febiger, 1991:157–173.

32.• Scher AT: Rugby injuries of the spine and spinal cord. *Clin Sport Med* 1987, 6:87–99.
Good review of the mechanisms of cervical spine injury in rugby.

33. Taylor TKF, Coolican MRJ: Spinal cord injuries in australian footballers: 1960–1985. *Med J Aust* 1987, 147:109–110.

34.• Burry HC, Calcinai CJ: The need to make rugby safer. *Brit Med J Clin Res Ed* 1988, 296:149–150.
Classic article on injury prevention in rugby football.

35. McBeath AA, Keene JS: The rib-tip syndrome. *J Bone Joint Surg* 1975, 57A:795–797.

36. Bellotti P, Chiarella F, Domenicucci S, *et al.*: Myocardial contusion after a professional boxing match. *Am J Cardiol* 1992, 69:709–710.

37.• Abrunzo TJ: Commotio Cordis: The single, most common cause of traumatic death in youth baseball. *Am J Dis Child* 1991, 145:1279–1282.
First in-depth report of this worrisome, catastrophic childhood sports injury.

38. Rutherford GW, Kennedy J, McGhee L: *Hazard Analysis: Baseball and Softball–Related Injuries to Children 5-14 Years of Age.* Washington, DC: United States Consumer Product Safety Commission; 1984.

39. Karofsky PS: Death of a high school hockey player. *Phys Sportsmed* 1990, 18:99–103.

40. Edlich RF, Mayer NE, Fariss BL, *et al.*: Commotio cordis in a lacrosse goalie. *J Emerg Med* 1987, 5:181–184.

41.• Serina ER, Lieu DK: Thoracic injury potential of basic competition *Taekwon-do* kicks. *J Biomech* 1991, 24:951–960.
Good example of biomechanics applied to a clinically relevant problem.

42. Albrand OW, Corkill G: Thoracic disc herniation: treatment and prognosis. *Spine* 1979, 4:41–46.

43. Keene JJ, Thoracolumbar fractures in winter sports. *Am J Sports Med* 1987, 216:39.

44. Blumenthal SL, Roach J, Herring JA: Lumbar Scheuermann's: a clinical series and classification. *Spine* 1987, 12:929–932.

45.• Sward L, Hellstrom M, Jacobsson B, *et al.*: Back pain and radiologic changes in the thoraco-lumbar spine of athletes. *Spine* 1990, 15:124–129.
Careful review of disc and apophyseal injuries of the thoracolumbar spine in sports.

46. Sward L, Hellstrom M, Jacobsson B, *et al.*: Vertebral ring apophysis injury in athletes: is the etiology different in the thoracic and lumbar spine? *Am J Sports Med* 1993, 21:841–845.

47. Horne J, Cockshott WP, Shannon HS: Spinal column damage from water ski jumping. *Skeletal Radiol* 1987, 16:612–616.

48.• Ferguson RJ, McMaster JG, Stanitski CL: Low back pain in college football linemen. *J Sports Med* 1974, 2:63–69.
Classic article noting higher incidence of spondylolysis in these athletes.

49. Denis F: Spinal instability so defined by the three column spine concept in acute spinal trauma. *Clin Orthop* 1984; 189:65–76.

50. Walters G, Coumas JM, Akins CM, *et al.*: Magnetic resonance imaging of acute symptomatic Schmorl's node formation. *Pediatr Emerg Care* 1991, 7:294–296.

51. Mundt DJ, Kelsey JL, Golden AL, *et al.*: An epidemiologic study of sports and weight lifting as possible risk factors for herniated lumbar and cervical discs: the northeast collaborative group on low back pain. *Am J Sports Med* 1993, 21:854–860.

52. Keller, RH: Traumatic displacement of the cartilaginous vertebral rim: a sign of intervertebral disc prolapse. *Radiology* 1974, 110:21–24.

53. Mooney V: Where is back pain coming from? *Annals Med* 1989, 21:373–379.

54. Jackson DW, Rettig A, Wiltse LL: Epidural cortisone injections in the young athletic adult. *Am J Sports Med* 1980, 8:239–243.

55. Takahashi H, Suguro T, Okazima Y, *et al.*: Inflammatory cytokines in the herniated disc of the lumbar spine. *Spine* 1996, 21:218–224.

56. Komori H, Shinomiya K, Nakai O, *et al.*: The natural history of herniated nucleus pulposus with radiculopathy. *Spine* 1996, 21:225–229.

57. Kraus H: Effect of lordosis on the stress in the lumbar spine. *Clin Orthop* 1976, 117:56–58.

58. Seitsalo S, Antila H, Karrinaho T, *et al.*: Spondylolysis in ballet dancers. *J Dance Med Sci* 1997, 1:51–54.

59. Bellah RD, Summerville DA, Treves ST, *et al.*: Low back pain in adolescent athletes: detection of stress injury to the pars intraarticularis with SPECT. *Radiology* 1991, 180:509–512.

60. Merbs CF. Incomplete spondylolysis and healing. *Spine* 1995, 20:2328–2334.

61. Muschik M, Hahnel H, Robinson PN, *et al.*: Competitive sports and progression of spondylolisthesis. *J Ped Orthop* 1996, 16:364–369.

62. Marchetti PG, Bartolozzi P: Classification of spondylolisthesis as a guideline for treatment. In *The Textbook of Spinal Surgery*. Edited by Bridwell KH, Dewald RL. Philadelphia: Lippincott-Raven; 1997:1211–1254.

63. Risch SV, Norvell NK, Pollock ML, *et al.*: Lumbar strengthening in chronic low back pain patients: physiologic and psychological benefits. *Spine* 1993, 18:232–238.

64.• Tertti M, Paajanen H, Kujala UM, *et al.*: Disc degeneration in young gymnasts: a magnetic resonance imaging study. *Am J Sports Med* 1990, 18:206–208.
Of 35 young Finnish gymnasts, only three showed disc disease by MRI criteria. These children trained 12.0 + 5.5 h/wk, low hours by North American criteria.

65.•• Goldstein JD, Berger PE, Windler GE, *et al.*: spine injuries in gymnasts and swimmers: an epidemiologic investigation. *Am J Sports Med* 1991, 19:463–468.
Study showed a progressively increasing percentage of disc disease by age in young gymnasts, significantly higher than in age-matched swimmer control subjects.

66.• Sward L, Hellstrom M, Jacobsson B, *et al.*: Disc degeneration and associated abnormalities of the spine in elite gymnasts: a magnetic resonance imaging study. *Spine* 1991, 16:437–443.
This study underlines the disc and thoracolumbar changes associated with sports involving repetitive flexion and extension.

67. Micheli LJ: Low back pain in the adolescent: differential diagnosis. *Am J Sports Med* 1979, 7:362–364.

68. Marshall JL, Tischler HM: Screening for sports guidelines. *NY J Med* 1978, 78:243–249.

69. Bertolotti M: Contributo alla conoscenza dei vizi di differenzazione regionale dei rachide con speciale riguardoallo assimiliazone sacrale della v lombare. *Radial Med (Toriono)* 1917, 4:113–144.

70. Santavirta S, Tallroth K, Ylinen P, *et al*.: Surgical treatment of bertolotti's syndrome: follow-up of 16 patients. *Arch Orthop Trauma Surg* 1993, 112:82–87.

71. Dreyer SJ, Dreyfus PH: Low back pain and zygapophyseal (facet) joints. *Arch Phys Med Rehab* 1996, 77:290–300.

72. Sward L: The thoracolumbar spine in young elite athletes: current concepts on the effects of physical training. *Sports Med* 1992, 13:357–364.

73. Torg JS, Vegso JJ, O'Neil MJ, *et al*.: The Epidemiologic, pathologic, biomechanical, and cinematographic analysis of football-induced cervical spine trauma. *Am J Sports Med* 1990, 18:50–57.

74. Gerbino PG, Micheli LJ: Low back injuries in the young athlete. *Sports Med Arthroscopy Rev* 1996, 4:122–131.

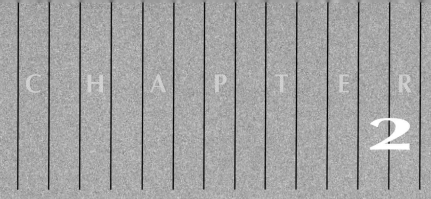

SURGICAL MANAGEMENT OF SHOULDER AND UPPER ARM INJURIES

Claude E. Nichols III

The problems facing orthopedic surgeons addressing sports-related shoulder injuries are becoming more complex as the relationship between the various components of the glenohumeral and scapulothoracic articulations becomes clearer. A major problem facing the surgeon managing these injuries is apparent when selecting the optimal intervention for a particular pathologic entity. As with most issues, the more information that is available, the more difficult it becomes to proceed. Fortunately, the recent literature confronts many of these issues.

Currently, the results of arthroscopic stabilization procedures still do not approach those of the open techniques. The development of new types of suture anchors and absorbable materials has made it easier to reattach the disrupted glenolabral complex. New techniques to decrease the volume of the capsule have been described as well. The issue of when to intervene has also been addressed to optimize the results of these procedures. Early intervention may also decrease the recurrence rate in a young, active population.

Understanding the underlying pathology surrounding anterior instability is fundamental to developing an optimal treatment plan. Taylor and Arciero [1] prospectively evaluated intra-articular pathology in first-time dislocators within 10 days of injury. Ninety-seven percent of the shoulders arthroscopically examined demonstrated disruption of the capsuloligamentous complex from the glenoid. There was no gross evidence of intracapsular injury. The control group declined surgery. The recurrence rate in the control group was 90%. This suggests that at the time of the first dislocation, the primary injury is an avulsion of the labrum from the glenoid with very little capsular injury, implying that surgical repair of the glenocapsular attachment in first-time dislocators may have a favorable effect on the recurrence rate in a high-risk population.

The results of arthroscopic procedures in a high-demand population have been addressed by Bacilla *et al.* [2]. To date, the failure rate of arthroscopic repairs for anterior instability has dampened enthusiasm to their widespread use. The intermediate follow-up of arthroscopic anterior capsulolabral reconstructions using suture anchors, performed by Bacilla *et al.* (Fig. 2.1), led to a 7.5% recurrence rate at an average of 30 months after surgery. This finding was a marked improvement over a previous report by the same authors, in which a 15% recurrence rate was noted after stabilization with a suture punch technique. In comparison, Montgomery and Jobe [3] reported a 97% good-to-excellent result for the open modified anterior cap-

sulolabral reconstruction, with an average 27-month follow-up.

Guanche *et al.* [4•] reviewed their experience with arthroscopic versus open stabilizations of patients with Bankart lesions. They documented inferior results of the arthroscopic procedure in satisfaction, stability, apprehension, and loss of forward flexion. The authors believe that capsular laxity is an issue to be addressed in the arthroscopic procedures. The inability to purposefully decrease capsular laxity is also a point in the authors' [5] review of their clinical experience with arthroscopic stabilization using the Suretac device. Second-look arthroscopies were used to evaluate postoperative instability in seven patients. The Bankart lesion was completely healed in 43%, partially healed in 14%, and had recurred in 43%. Warner *et al.* concluded that complete healing of the Bankart lesion is not a requisite for shoulder stability.

Closure of the rotator interval has been demonstrated to decrease pathologic laxity about the shoulder in specific patients and has been proposed as an

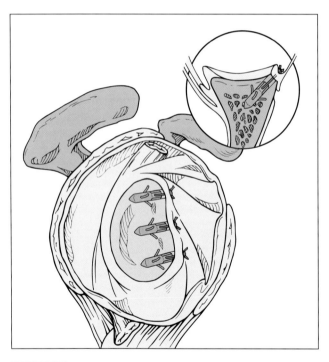

FIGURE 2.1

Arthroscopic Bankart reconstruction. In most cases three anchors are inserted into the glenoid neck, shifting the capsule superiorly and repairing the avulsed capsulolabral structures to the glenoid.

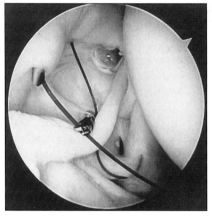

FIGURE 2.2

Initiation of intra-articular rotator interval repair. Note the suture transport device through the subscapularis tendon and middle glenohumeral ligament and the spinal needle through the anterior margin of the supraspinatus tendon and adjacent capsule. A nonabsorbable monofilament suture is being advanced through the spinal needle. A lateral plication stitch (*bottom*) is in place. A second, more medial stitch is being completed as the transporter device retrieves the suture out the anterior portal.

integral step in open stabilization procedures. Treacy *et al.* [6] recently described their experience with arthroscopic closure of the rotator interval capsule closure (Fig. 2.2). Anecdotal preliminary evidence suggests that this may be a helpful adjunct to improve the results of arthroscopic stabilization. This strategy fits very well with present ideas of decreasing the size of the glenohumeral joint capsule to add to the stability of the joint. In the future, laser or thermal energy may provide a way to decrease capsular volume in a reliable fashion. However, data from clinical trials using these technologies are pending.

At this time, I continue to approach recurrent anterior instability with an open anterior capsulorrhaphy with a horizontal capsulotomy, repair of the Bankart lesion, and decreasing the volume of the joint capsule by closing the rotator interval and capsulotomy— very similar to the anterior capsulolabral reconstruction described by Jobe (Fig. 2.3). First-time dislocators are rarely encountered in my practice, so in light of the unfavorable recurrence rates following arthroscopic stabilization in chronic cases, I only perform open procedures.

SUBSCAPULARIS RUPTURE

Traumatic rupture of the subscapularis tendon, previously thought to be rare, was first brought to general attention by Gerber and Krushell [7] in 1991. They reported on 16 cases and and described the clinical and radiographic manifestations of the injury. They described the "lift-off test," a maneuver that demonstrates subscapularis injury in the physical evaluation (Fig. 2.4). Deutsch *et al.* [8••] recently reported their technique for physical diagnosis, imaging, and treatment of this injury. A positive lift-off test was reported in only two of 14 patients. Interpretation of the results of this maneuver was made more difficult due to pain experienced during the testing. Magnetic resonance imaging (MRI) studies (Fig. 2.5) were believed to be

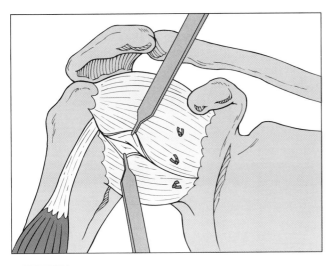

FIGURE 2.3
Closure of the horizontal capsulotomy after reattachment of labrum in the anterior caspsolabral reconstruction.

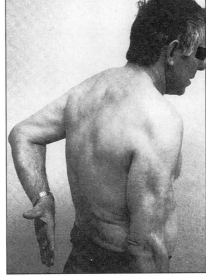

FIGURE 2.4
The "lift off" test. Normal test on the left.

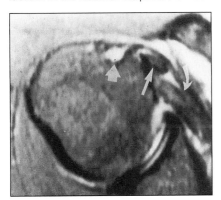

FIGURE 2.5
T_2-weighted axial–gradient recalled image demonstrating medial dislocation of the biceps tendon (*straight arrow*), with an empty sheath noted laterally (*arrowhead*). The subscapularis tendon is thinned and irregular (*curved arrow*).

diagnostic; however, studies performed and evaluated at other facilities were not correctly diagnosed. Biceps tendon injuries were commonly found at the time of surgery. Surgical treatment is recommended in view of the persistent pain and dysfunction associated with the untreated subscapularis injury.

In my experience, a high index of suspicion is necessary to identify this lesion. As in Deutsch *et al*.'s [8••] study, the lesion is often overlooked by radiologists interpreting the MRI studies. Although a positive lift-off test is not diagnostic, it should alert the examiner to the possibility of subscapularis injury. Anterior shoulder pain after a traumatic episode that does not respond to conservative treatment is suggestive of a subscapularis injury. The intraoperative pathology is often difficult to identify, even with obvious MRI abnormalities.

LABRAL INJURIES

With the widespread use of arthroscopy as a diagnostic tool to identify shoulder pathology, the presence of labral lesions has generated interest.

Unfortunately, diagnosing this problem in the clinical setting presents a problem. The history can be suggestive, but findings on physical examination can be nonspecific. Kibler [9] described the anterior slide test as clinical test to aid in the diagnosis of labral pathology. This test is performed with the patient either standing or sitting with their hands on their hips. The examiner stands behind the patient with one hand on top of the shoulder to be tested and the index finger applying pressure to the anterior aspect of the glenohumeral joint. The examiner's other hand is placed behind the elbow to be tested and a slight superior and anterior force applied (Fig. 2.6). The patient is asked to resist this force. Pain under the examiner's finger, a pop or click, or recreation of symptoms is considered a positive test. In his experience, the test is 78% sensitive and 91% specific compared with arthroscopic findings.

Liu *et al*. [10] reported on the crank test as another clinical test to evaluate labral pathology. This test is performed with the patient in the upright and supine positions. The arm is elevated to 160° in the scapular plane. One hand applies an axial load

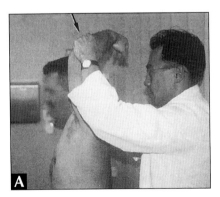

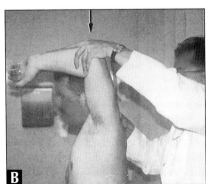

FIGURE 2.6

Application of force for anterior slide test.

FIGURE 2.7

In the upright position, the examiner performs the crank test by elevating the patient's arm to 160° in the scapular plane, applying joint load along the axis of the humerus with one hand (*arrow*) while externally (**A**) and internally (**B**) rotating the humerus with the other hand.

along the axis of the humerus while the humerus is rotated (Fig. 2.7). A positive test elicits pain or reproduction of symptoms. The sensitivity of this test is 91% and the specificity is 93%, with a positive predictive value of 94% and negative predictive value of 90% when compared with arthroscopic findings.

I use these clinical tests, as well as the O'Brien test, as part of the physical examination. When positive, these maneuvers can be a helpful adjunct in the diagnosis of labral pathology, but at our institution, MR arthrography provides information not only on the labrum, but also on the associated lesions commonly seen with this type of injury.

ROTATOR CUFF REPAIR

Methods to address full-thickness rotator cuff injuries are evolving. Mini-open and arthroscopic techniques are gaining popularity in an effort to reduce morbidity and enhance cosmesis. Some of the difficulties in performing arthroscopic rotator cuff surgery, including the ability to determine the size of the tear, the tendon quality, ability to mobilize the torn tendon, and suture placement, have been investigated by Gartsman [11]. In 50 patients, he determined that

arthroscopic means of determining the aforementioned parameters compared favorably with open assessment. The technical difficulties encountered with mobilization of the cuff is emphasized.

Blevins *et al.* [12] evaluated their experience with a mini-open deltoid splitting technique. This procedure entailed arthroscopically controlled acromioplasty and acromioclavicular joint surgery followed by a deltoid splitting approach to the greater tuberosity and fixation of the cuff using suture anchors (Fig. 2.8). The results compared favorably to those reported with open techniques; however, the authors emphasize the demanding nature of the surgery and echo Gartsman's [11] observation regarding mobilization of the cuff tissue.

Results of rotator cuff repair in contact athletes was reviewed by Blevins *et al.* [13], involving both full-thickness and partial-thickness injuries. In their series of 10 athletes, nine were able to return to active participation in football. Partial thickness tears involving more than 50% of the thickness of the tendon were debrided and repaired.

The issue of partial rotator cuff tears has been addressed in a preliminary report by Payne *et al* . [14•]), who identified two patient groups. One group experienced a traumatic episode with result-

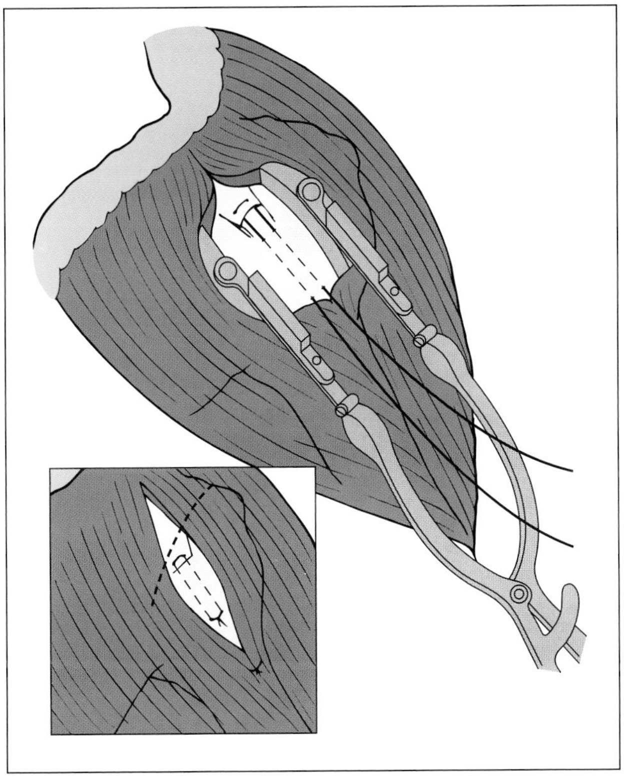

FIGURE 2.8

Mini-open exposure. **A,** Horizontal skin incision in Langer's lines (*dotted line*). Rotator cuff tear has been repaired through deltoid splitting exposure. **B,)** A self-retaining Cloward-type retractor is used to retract the deltoid to acromion to prevent progression of split and possible axillary nerve injury.

ing cuff injury. The other group experienced symptoms that were insidious in onset, with increased translation noted on the examination under anesthesia. All groups underwent debridement of the cuff injury, repair of labral lesions if present, and appropriate subacromial surgery (debridement, acromioplasty, or both). The group with insidious onset of symptoms demonstrated good pain relief following debridement, but often failed to return to their preinjury level of sports participation. Those patients with traumatic causes achieved pain relief and were frequently able to return to sports. These findings highlight the conundrum of rotator cuff injury in the face of subtle instability: does the increased laxity predispose to these cuff injuries? If so, what diagnostic tests can help us improve our results of treatment?

LAXITY

The issue of shoulder joint laxity versus instability has recently been the focus of two papers. McFarland *et al.* [15] evaluated posterior laxity of the shoulder in 356 athletes undergoing routine physical examination. Over 55% of the shoulders could be subluxated posteriorly. These athletes were asymptomatic and the laxity was considered to be normal. Female patients demonstrated more posterior and inferior translations than male patients. Lintner *et al.* [16] examined 76 Division 1 collegiate athletes and noted laxity up to 2+ and asymmetry in laxities in many of these asymptomatic subjects. These studies show that instability is a clinical phenomenon and that the laxity present in varying degrees in many shoulders should not necessarily be considered pathologic.

REFERENCES AND RECOMMENDED READING

Recently published papers of particular interest have been highlighted as:

- • Of special interest
- •• Of outstanding interest

1. Taylor DC, Arciero RA: Pathologic changes associated with shoulder dislocations: arthroscopic and physical examination findings in first-time, traumatic anterior dislocations. *Am J Sports Med* 1997, 25:306–311.

2. Bacilla P, Field LD, Savoie FH III: Arthroscopic Bankart repair in a high demand patient population. *Arthroscopy* 1997, 13:51–60.

3. Montgomery WH, Jobe FW: Functional outcomes in athletes after modified anterior capsulolabral reconstruction. *Am J Sports Med* 1994, 22:352–358.

4.• Guanche CA, Quick DC, Sodergren KM, Buss DD: Arthroscopic versus open reconstruction of the shoulder in patients with isolated Bankart lesions. *Am J Sports Med* 1996, 24:144–148.

A retrospective comparison of two techniques with subjective and objective outcome measures.

5. Warner JJP, Miller MD, Marks P, Fu FH: Arthroscopic Bankart repair with the Suretac device. Part I: Clinical Observations. *Arthroscopy* 1995, 11:2–13.

6. Treacy SH, Fields LD, Savoie FH: Rotator interval capsule closure: an arthroscopic technique. *Arthroscopy* 1997, 13:103–106.

7. Gerber C, Krushell RJ: Isolated rupture of the tendon of the subscapularis muscle: clinical features in 16 cases. *J Bone Joint Surg Br* 1991, 73:389–394.

8.•• Deutsch A, Altchek DW, Veltri DM, Potter HG, Warren RF: Traumatic tears of the subscapularis tendon: clinical diagnosis, magnetic resonance imaging findings, and operative treatment. *Am J Sports Med* 1997, 25: 13–22.

A complete review of the clinical evaluation, diagnostic work-up, and treatment of this previously obscure entity.

9. Kibler WB: Specificity and sensitivity of the anterior slide test in throwing athletes with superior glenoid labral tears. *Arthroscopy* 1995, 11:296–300.

10. Liu SH, Henry MH, Nuccion SL: A prospective evaluation of a new physical examination in predicting glenoid labral tears. *Am J Sports Med* 1996, 24:721–725.

11. Gartsman GM: Arthroscopic assessment of rotator cuff tear reparability. *Arthroscopy* 1996, 12:546–549.

12. Blevins FT, Warren RF, Cavo C, Altchek DW, Dines D, Palletta G, Wickiewicz TL: Arthroscopic assisted rotator cuff repair: results using a mini-open deltoid splitting approach. *Arthroscopy* 1996, 12:50–59.

13. Blevins FT, Hayes WM, Warren RF: Rotator cuff injury in contact athletes. *Am J Sports Med* 1996, 24:263–267.

14.• Payne LZ, Altchek DW, Craig EV, Warren RF: Arthroscopic treatment of partial rotator cuff tears in young athletes: a preliminary report. *Am J Sports Med* 1997, 25:299–305.

This study identifies two groups of patients with partial-thickness rotator cuff tears with different responses to surgical treatment.

15. McFarland EG, Campbell G, McDowell J: Posterior shoulder laxity in asymptomatic athletes. *Am J Sports Med* 1996, 24:468–471.

16. Lintner SA, Levy A, Kenter K, Speer KP: Glenohumeral translation in the asymptomatic athlete's shoulder and its relationship to other clinically measurable anthropometric variables. *Am J Sports Med* 1996, 24:716–720.

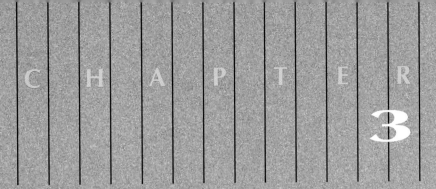

CHAPTER 3

ELBOW AND FOREARM TRAUMA

James R. Andrews and
Yvonne E. Satterwhite

Findings and developments from cadaveric and biome-chanic research have contributed a vast amount of new knowledge of elbow physiology and function in both static and, more importantly, dynamic states. These developments have improved techniques for evaluating and managing upper-extremity injury in athletes. The elbow in particular has been of significant interest because of the many bony and soft-tissue injuries that may be incurred from direct and indirect trauma.

As in the evaluation of any injury, acute or chronic, great attention must be paid to the athlete's history. The physical examination is systematic and must include a thorough neck and shoulder assessment because pathology in these areas can refer symptoms to the distal upper extremity (*ie*, the elbow and forearm). The elbow examination should include an evaluation of the asymptomatic contralateral elbow for comparison. Radiographic assessment begins with a standard series (antero-posterior, internal, and external oblique views and an axial projection). In addition, radiographic stress testing can be used when a ligament injury is suspected. Gadolinium-enhanced magnetic resonance imaging (MRI), computed tomographic (CT) arthrography, electromyography/nerve conduction studies, and diagnostic arthroscopy are also in the physician's armamentarium to aid in establishing a definitive diagnosis. Treatment regimens follow a specific algorithm, but they are individualized to each athlete's personality and degree of injury.

This chapter highlights several of the current, frequently diagnosed entities of elbow and forearm trauma in sports medicine. We emphasize the philosophy of our institution for management of these disorders.

ELBOW FLEXION CONTRACTURE

Previous clinical studies have estimated that up to 50% of baseball pitchers insidiously develop a flexion contracture. A mild flexion contracture (less than ≈20°) does not appear to interfere with the athlete's throwing ability. However, a significant posttraumatic flexion contracture as a sequelae of acute trauma (*eg*, dislocation or fracture) can be debilitating for any athlete who requires a sport-specific range of motion to function adequately. Conservative treatment is attempted first with stretching exercises and serial casting or splinting. Previous surgical options have included an open anterior release or an extensile release followed by aggressive rehabilitation [1]. Currently, we perform a capsular release arthroscopically with our previously described anterolateral, straight-lateral, medial, and posterior portals [2]. A closed manipulation is also performed if necessary. A Dynasplint (Dynasplint Systems, Baltimore, MD) type of orthosis may be added to the postoperative protocol. Normal preinjury range of motion is difficult to restore, but significant improvements can be obtained and maintained.

DISTAL BICEPS TENDON RUPTURES

Rupture of the distal biceps tendon is caused by tensile overload in the presence of an eccentric biceps contraction. This injury is more commonly seen in competitive weightlifters and bodybuilders than in any other type of athlete. The presenting symptom is subjective weakness with minimal cosmetic deformity. In the surgical repair of these lesions, a two-incision approach is advocated to allow improved protection of the posterior interosseous nerve. D'Alessandro *et al.* [3] recently reported their results with distal biceps tendon repairs, noting that 10 athletes treated surgically returned to full unlimited activity, had a return of strength to within 25% of normal, and regained muscle contour.

REFRACTORY LATERAL EPICONDYLITIS

"Tennis elbow" is a frequently diagnosed condition resulting from a chronic inflammatory reaction to microtearing and focal degeneration that originates in the extensor carpi radialis brevis tendon. As a differential diagnosis, posterior interosseous nerve entrapment should be ruled out (but is known to coexist with lateral epicondylitis in 10% of cases). Once the diagnosis of epicondylitis has been established clinically, an extensive period of conservative treatment is initiated, including an aggressive rehabilitation program to restore strength and flexibility, a tennis elbow strap, oral nonsteroidal anti-inflammatory medication, and, in certain cases, local steroid injection. This treatment is successful in 90% to 95% of cases, although the time to recovery can be prolonged. In patients who do not respond to conservative measures, the surgical option of a lateral release with debridement is offered. A postoperative rehabilitation program is always instituted. The success rate for this procedure is approximately 90% satisfactory results.

Morrey [4] studied 13 patients who had an unsatisfactory outcome after lateral release and required reoperation. The reasons for failure were defined as inadequate initial release, incorrect initial diagnosis (posterior interosseous syndrome instead of epicondylitis, intra-articular abnormalities, or ligamentously unstable elbow), or postoperative complications (capsular fistula, incidental release of the lateral collateral ligament with ensuing instability, or formation of an adventitial bursa). Of 13 patients, 11 underwent further surgery to address the appropriately delineated pathology, 85% of whom had a satisfactory outcome. Recently, Baker (Paper presented at the 1997 Arthroscopy Associates of North America Specialty Day meeting at the American Academy of Orthopaedic Surgeons [AAOS] annual meeting, San Francisco, 1997) has advocated an arthroscopic technique for the treatment of lateral epicondylitis. Using a 4.0-mm, 30° arthroscopic resector, the capsule at the lateral epicondyle is removed to expose the underlying diseased portion (≈2 cm) of the extensor carpi radialis brevis tendinous origin, which is then debrided. The adjacent lateral epicondyle and lateral epicondylar ridge are decorticated with an arthroscopic burr to complete the procedure. Long-term clinical results are pending.

POSTERIOR ROTATORY INSTABILITY OF THE ELBOW

In 1991, O'Driscoll *et al.* [5] described an unusual instability pattern of the elbow. Posterolateral rotatory instability has been diagnosed with increasing frequency as our clinical skills and recognition of this entity have improved. Presenting symptoms may include recurrent catching, locking, and episodes of frank instability, particularly if there has been a traumatic dislocation in the past [6]. The definitive clinical test to demonstrate this instability is the posterolateral rotatory instability test (Fig.

3.1). In this maneuver, the patient is supine and the arm is forward and flexed overhead. With external humeral rotation prevented, the patient's forearm is supinated with the elbow extended; then, as a valgus force and axial compression load are applied, the elbow is flexed. At approximately 40° of flexion, this maneuver produces a posterolateral subluxation of the ulnohumeral joint and dislocation of the radiohumeral joint, which spontaneously reduce as the elbow is flexed further (*see* Fig. 3.1). The cause of the instability appears to be loss of integrity of the ulnar part of the ulnar collateral ligament (UCL). Treatment requires surgical repair or reconstruction of this ligament followed by a period of bracing and rehabilitation. Results with surgical repair have been very good in the small population of patients diagnosed with this disorder.

OSTEOCHONDROSES AND OSTEOCHONDRITIS DISSECANS OF THE LATERAL ELBOW

Panner's disease is an osteochondrosis (avascular necrosis) of the capitellar epiphyses occurring in skeletally immature patients during initial ossifica-tion of the capitellum or radial head when the vascular supply to this area is limited. It has been previously described in young baseball pitchers, and the reason for its prevalence in gymnasts becomes apparent. The cause appears to be related to repetitive valgus compression and shear forces to the lateral side of the elbow. The young athlete, typically age 9 to 12 years of age, presents with complaints of elbow pain during sports activities. Physical examination demonstrates tenderness to palpation of the radiocapitellar joint and, occasionally, loss of motion, local swelling, crepitation, and pain with valgus loading across the elbow [7]. Radiographic findings include sclerosis, fissuring, and irregular margins of the capitellum (Fig. 3.2). In the early stages, MRI is helpful if plain-film radiographs are negative. Treatment includes cessation of the inciting activity and restoration and maintenance of motion. Once the symptoms have abated and there is radiographic resolution of the disease, the athlete is placed on a specific conditioning program for the elbow, including instruction in proper biomechanics if needed.

When diagnosed early and treated appropriately, Panner's disease usually heals without residual sequelae. However, if the patient presents to the

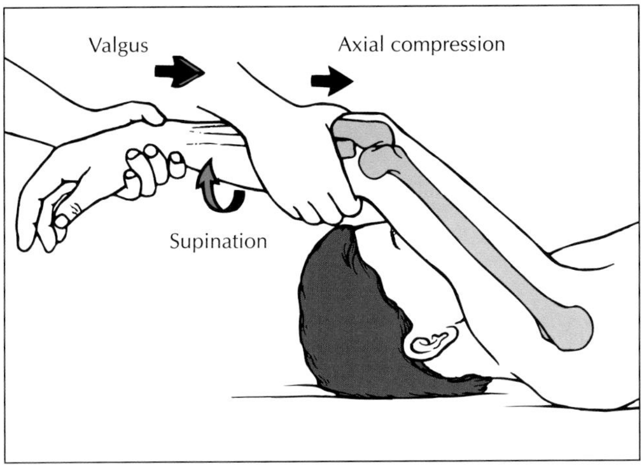

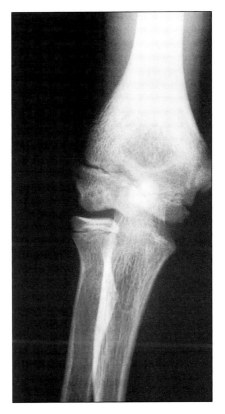

FIGURE 3.2

Anteroposterior radiograph of Panner's disease.

FIGURE 3.1

Posterolateral rotatory instability maneuver. (*Adapted from O'Driscoll et al.* [5]; with permission of the *Journal of Bone and Joint Surgery.*)

physician late, after continued overuse of the symptomatic elbow, there may be signs of capitellar growth arrest and collapse. Radial head overgrowth may be seen, resulting from the hyperemic response occurring during the repair phase. In the most severe cases, loss of joint congruity may result and can lead to secondary osteoarthritis. Rehabilitation of these elbows is difficult. Arthroscopic intervention with radiocapitellar debridement may be indicated to alleviate symptoms and improve function [8,9].

Osteochondritis dissecans of the capitellum, or radial head, is a subchondral focal area of avascular necrosis occurring in skeletally immature athletes around the time of the adolescent growth spurt. Like Panner's disease, it results from chronic, repetitive, lateral compression stress. Some authors believe that osteochondritis dissecans is on a continuum with Panner's disease as a progressive endochondral ossification disorder in which the presenting signs and prognosis depend on the patient's age at presentation. In osteochondritis dissecans, the athlete's symptoms may include lateral elbow pain, locking, catching, swelling, and loss of motion. Clinical examination results are consistent with radiocapitellar disease and possibly a loose body. Radiographic findings are subarticular rarefaction, cyst formation, cortical fragmentation or flattening, loose bodies, and, in the later stages, isolated loss of the radiocapitellar joint space (Fig. 3.3). Early diagnosis and treatment is critical. Results are improved if the disease occurs and is appropriately managed before physeal closure. As in Panner's disease, treatment includes cessation of the aggravating sports activity and the use of physical therapy to attempt to restore motion and alleviate discomfort.

If the patient's symptoms do not improve, we proceed with an arthroscopic debridement of articular surface defects. We rarely perform pure drilling of these areas. If a loose body is thought to be present clinically, but is not seen on plain radiographs, it may be demonstrated with CT arthrography. In all cases, the loose body should be removed; this may be performed arthroscopically. If left indwelling, a loose body will accelerate degenerative changes in these elbows.

Postoperatively, these patients are placed in a rehabilitation program and then slowly returned to sport. Not all baseball players return to throwing, and not all gymnasts return to their previous level of competition. Symptoms do improve, however, and we have noted good overall results in this difficult patient group [10,11].

Many physicians and baseball coaches are concerned that the risk of developing osteochondroses is increased in very young pitchers who attempt to incorporate the curve ball into their routine selection of pitches before achieving skeletal maturity. In the American Sports Medicine Institute's biomechanics laboratory, critical evaluation of the force differences created at the elbow between the fast ball and curve ball has provided objective data that suggest increased forces during the curve ball pitch. Thus, our present recommendation is for this pitch to be avoided in the young throwing athlete.

ELBOW DISLOCATIONS

Elbow dislocations are seen in athletes who fall onto an outstretched hand with the elbow extended and the forearm pronated, subjecting the elbow to an axial load. The resulting posterior or posterolateral dislocation can usually be treated with a closed reduction maneuver. The elbow is checked for varus-valgus stability and then immobilized for 3 to 5 days. Range-of-motion exercises are then begun, with emphasis on obtaining extension. A removable protective brace may be used for the first few weeks

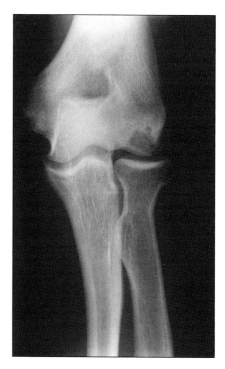

FIGURE 3.3

Anteroposterior radiograph of capitellar osteochondritis dissecans lesion.

after injury. Clinical results have not been shown to be significantly improved with immediate surgical repair of the injured medial or lateral ligamentous complex in these posterior dislocations. If neurovascular compromise is present or there are associated fractures (*eg*, an entrapped medial epicondyle fragment), surgical intervention is necessary.

CORONOID FRACTURES

Coronoid fractures occur most commonly in association with a posterior elbow dislocation. Regan and Morrey [12] have classified coronoid process fractures of the ulna into four types based on the percentage of articular involvement. Treatment depends on the type of fracture and the presence or absence of associated elbow instability. Coronoid tip fractures (type 1) result from avulsion of the anterior capsular or brachialis tendon. Early protected range-of-motion exercise is instituted but modified as necessary when elbow stability is questionable. Type 2 coronoid fractures involve greater than 50% of the articular surface. Open reduction and internal fixation (ORIF) and early range-of-motion exercise yield the best results. When significant soft-tissue ligamentous injury has also occurred, an external fixator is used concomitantly to augment initial stability. Comminuted coronoid fractures (type 3) are frequently associated with an elbow dislocation. Type 4 injuries, by definition, include a radial head fracture and an elbow dislocation. Type 3 and 4 injuries are managed as a type 2 injury regarding the coronoid. Additional injuries are treated traditionally.

RADIAL HEAD FRACTURES

Fractures of the radial head can be isolated or associated with an elbow dislocation. They are caused by axial compression or a valgus lateral load to the elbow. The radial head contributes to elbow stability and, therefore, should be salvaged whenever possible—particularly if there is concomitant medial UCL compromise. In Mason type 1 nondisplaced fractures, sling immobilization with early range-of-motion exercise is the preferred treatment. More emphasis has been placed recently on attempting ORIF of the Mason type 2 fractures, especially when they are associated with elbow dislocation or Essex–Lopresti injury (distal radioulnar joint disruption). In the treatment of severely comminuted Mason type 3 fractures, radial head excision is advocated, preferably immediately.

In the presence of an Essex–Lopresti injury or medial elbow instability, implantation of a radial head silicone prosthesis is warranted for 6 months to 1 year or until soft tissues are completely healed [13].

CAPITELLAR FRACTURES

Capitellar fractures are rarely seen. The mechanism of injury may be either a fall directly onto a fully-flexed elbow or an outstretched hand with the elbow partially flexed, creating a shear force from the radial head across the capitellum. The resulting fracture can be classified as one of three types. The type 1 (Hahn–Steinthal) fracture involves a large portion of the anterior capitellum and may include the immediately adjacent trochlea. If displaced, this fracture is best treated with ORIF. The type 2 (Kocher–Lorenz) fracture occurs in the area of the subchondral plate of the capitellum; the fragment is small and, if significantly displaced, should be excised. The type 3 capitellar fracture is an extensively comminuted pattern requiring excision of the fragments. Early protected range-of-motion exercise is instituted in all cases [14].

OLECRANON PHYSEAL FRACTURE NONUNION

First described by Torg and Moyer [15] in 1977, this injury is thought to be secondary to the repetitive traction forces exerted by the triceps across the olecranon physes as the elbow is rapidly extended (*eg*, in the throwing motion of a baseball pitcher) [15,16]. Our cases have involved the late-adolescent or college-age throwing athlete who presents with complaints of posterior elbow pain exacerbated by the acceleration and follow-through phases of throwing. Clinical examination demonstrates tenderness of the proximal posterior olecranon and pain with forced passive extension of the elbow. Radiographically, the olecranon physeal line is widened with sclerotic margins that may obliterate the medullary canal. Technetium bone scan may be used to confirm the diagnosis. Histologically, these lesions show fibrous metaplasia with poorly organized connective tissue and no physeal zones. This presentation is consistent with a nonunion of a physeal stress fracture, rather than with delayed physeal union. Treatment usually requires surgical debridement of the nonunion (with care not to violate the olecranon articular surface) and internal fixation. We use a single cannulated screw and, as needed, a tension-band wiring technique (Fig. 3.4). Bone grafting is recommended but not always necessary. The athlete may return to throwing once signs of clinical and radiographic healing are present.

OLECRANON FRACTURES

Olecranon fractures may be categorized into three types: 1) Mayo classification, based on the amount of fragment; 2) comminution and displacement; and 3) the degree, if any, of elbow instability [17]. Type 1 fractures demonstrate no elbow instability, and the olecranon fragment is minimally comminuted, dis-

placed less than 2 mm, and amenable to splinting or, in the athletic population, ORIF and tension-band wiring. If displacement exceeds 2 mm (type 2 fracture) in a stable elbow, tension-band wiring is performed. However, if comminution is present, an ORIF with a neutralization plate is preferred. If comminution is significant and plate fixation cannot guarantee elbow joint stability, the olecranon fragments are excised and the triceps tendon insertion reattached. The elbow is unstable in a type 3 fracture, independent of fracture appearance, and is best treated by ORIF. Postoperatively, a hinged brace is used with flexion limited to less than 90° initially to decrease triceps stress.

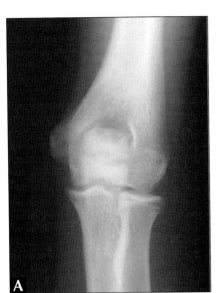
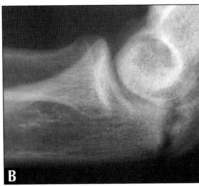
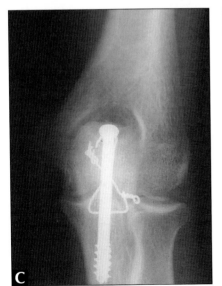
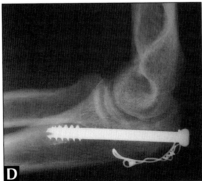

FIGURE 3.4

Preoperative (*panels A* and *B*) and postoperative (*panels C* and *D*) radiographs of olecranon physeal fracture nonunion.

TRICEPS TENDON AND OLECRANON TIP INJURY

Repetitive, forceful triceps contractions can result in several symptomatic posterior elbow lesions. These occur most frequently in those athletes who must actively force the elbow into full extension over their heads. Triceps tendonitis is an inflammatory reaction to tensile microtearing and focal degeneration of the triceps tendon insertion, and it can lead to a reactive synovitis causing diffuse posterior elbow pain. Olecranon tip fractures are caused by partial avulsion of the triceps insertion. Olecranon tip osteophytic formation may occur as a response to the chronic traction forces exerted across the olecranon tip by the triceps. These lesions are usually treated symptomatically with rest, ice, nonsteroidal medication, and technique modifications. In the case of an olecranon tip osteophyte that is large enough to limit full extension and interfere with function (or, less likely, that has fragmented and left a loose body in the posterior compartment), arthroscopy is performed to debride the osteophyte and olecranon tip and to remove any loose bodies (Fig. 3.5) [18]. Postoperatively, attention is paid to achieving full range of motion.

FATIGUE FRACTURE OF THE ULNA

In both skeletally mature and immature athletes, fatigue fractures of the ulna have been reported to occur while bodybuilding, fencing, and playing tennis. Most recently, Tanabe *et al.* [19] discussed their findings in fast-pitch softball pitchers. These athletes presented with complaints of pain in the forearm that worsened with their specific sports activity. Clinically, there was localized tenderness, swelling, and pain with manual force applied across the ulnar shaft. Radiographs often demonstrated a transverse fracture, with periosteal new bone formation. The fracture occurred most commonly in the middle third of the ulna, followed in frequency by the distal third and then proximal third, including the olecranon (the latter is a nonphyseal injury). The forearm is subjected to strong pronation forces during the windmill type of delivery seen in both fast-pitch softball and the tennis serve. The middle third of the ulna is biomechanically inferior to the proximal and distal ulna in resisting torsional stress because of its triangular shape, thinner cortex, and smaller cross-sectional area. These differences may explain why fatigue injuries occur most frequently in the midulna. Treatment is usually symptomatic and includes avoidance of upper-extremity loading and stress until clinical and radiographic signs of complete healing are present.

WHEELS AND FOREARM FRACTURES

In-line skating and skateboarding have gained in popularity, especially in male adolescents. Injuries are common, and over one third occur within the first week of initial exposure to these sports. Upper extremity fractures predominate, with an incidence as high as 80% of all injuries. During in-line skating, in which speeds can exceed 30 mph, radial head fractures account for approximately 10% of all fractures. Distal radius fractures are most common [20]. Skateboarding injuries often consist of a midthird forearm fracture, followed in frequency by distal one-third forearm and wrist fractures. "Skateboard elbow" refers to a shattered olecranon process that results when the skateboarder falls forcibly onto the posterior tip of the elbow [21]. Injury rates or the severity of injury may be decreased by the use of protective gear (pads and splints) and appropriate instruction in performance and falling techniques.

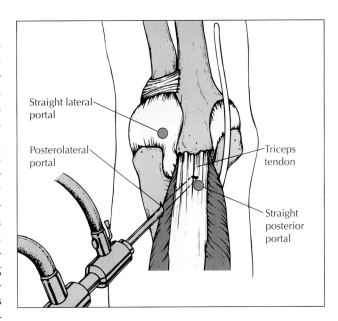

FIGURE 3.5

Arthroscope placement in the posterior compartment. (*Adapted from* Andrews and Craven [18]; with permission.)

VALGUS EXTENSION OVERLOAD SYNDROME

Valgus extension overload is a complex of lesions originating from chronic, repetitive compressive forces to the posteromedial elbow in the pitching arm [11]. The cocking phase of throwing creates significant tensile forces across the medial elbow ligamentous structures as the elbow is placed in extreme valgus extension. This position forces the posteromedial olecranon to impinge on the olecranon fossa. In addition, an extension is rapidly initiated and further compression forces occur in this posterior area. These repetitive forces cause the formation of an osteophyte along the posteromedial olecranon tip (Fig. 3.6). A corresponding area of chondromalacia can form on the posterior trochlea in the olecranon fossa; this area of articular surface degeneration is referred to as the "kissing lesion."

There appears to be a correlation between UCL injury and development of valgus extension overload. There is a possibility that the formation of a posteromedial osteophyte may in some cases be a compensatory response to stabilize the medial elbow in the face of UCL injury. The athlete with valgus extension overload presents with complaints of posterior elbow pain during the pitching motion and a sense of loss of control over the pitch during the pitching motion. On physical examination, the posteromedial elbow may be tender to palpation. Pain is evoked on forced passive elbow extension combined with valgus stress. Radiographs frequently demonstrate a posterior osteophyte at the tip of the olecranon; the posteromedial extent of the osteophyte can be seen on an axial projection with the elbow flexed to 100°. We also obtain internal and external oblique projections to further delineate the osteophyte. (In the general population, a small posterolateral olecranon spur may be present, but this is a normal variant and of no clinical significance).

Our treatment protocol begins with a period of active rest during which flexibility, strengthening, and conditioning of the athlete are emphasized. The athlete is also placed on a program of shoulder conditioning to avoid the development of any shoulder complaints once throwing is reinstituted. If these conservative measures are unsuccessful or symptoms recur on return to throwing, surgical intervention is offered. Although previously we used an open approach to address the posteromedial lesions, we now routinely perform the procedure entirely arthroscopically [22]. A complete diagnostic arthroscopy of the entire elbow is performed first. Then, through our previously described posterior and posterolateral portals, a small osteotome, synovial resector, and motorized burr can be introduced to effectively accomplish resection of the posterior-posteromedial osteophyte and debridement of the kissing lesion, if needed (Fig. 3.7). Postoperatively, immediate range-of-motion exercises are begun. The pitcher may return to throwing within an average of 3 months. Recovery may be accelerated in professional pitchers; however, we have seen a higher recurrence rate in pitchers who return too quickly.

FLEXOR–PRONATOR SPRAIN

A flexor–pronator sprain is a fairly common overuse syndrome seen in the throwing athlete, particularly in spring training or the early season. The flexor–pronator muscle group stabilizes the medial elbow dynamically, assisting the UCL dur-

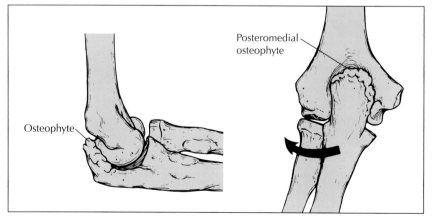

Posteromedial osteophyte

Osteophyte

FIGURE 3.6

Valgus extension overload lesion. (*Adapted from* Wilson *et al.* [22]; with permission.)

ing resisting the extreme valgus forces exerted across the elbow during the cocking phase of throwing. Appropriate conditioning and strengthening, as well as correct biomechanics, can decrease the occurrence rate of these types of injuries. On initial presentation, the athlete complains of pain with throwing and nonthrowing activities. Clinically, there is tenderness to palpation of the flexor–pronator origin from the medial epicondyle, often continuing distally for several centimeters. Pain is elicited with active resisted wrist flexion and forearm pronation; there may be a loss of elbow extension as well. Treatment is directed toward the resolution of inflammatory symptoms with ice, rest, anti-inflammatory medication, and local modalities (such as phonopheresis), followed by a flexibility and strengthening program.

ACUTE MEDIAL ELBOW RUPTURES

An acute traumatic disruption of the entire medial elbow soft-tissue complex can occur when an athlete sustains a severe, direct blow to the lateral elbow or falls onto the upper extremity, sustaining a marked valgus force across the elbow [23]. On clinical examination, the elbow hinges open medially, with valgus stress testing at 30° (Fig. 3.8). Symptoms and signs of a concomitant ulnar nerve traction injury may be present as well. Radiography may show an avulsion fracture of the medial epicondyle, particularly in skeletally immature athletes, and displacement greater than 5 mm indicates significant medial injury. Unlike the treatment of posterior elbow dislocations, we advocate immediate surgical repair of an isolated medial elbow disruption, especially if it has occurred in the dominant extremity. If unrepaired, residual medial instability may result. This condition leads to chronic ulnar nerve irritation and difficulty in throwing, pushing, or pulling.

The surgical technique consists of a medial approach, with immediate identification and protection of the ulnar nerve. If a medial epicondyle fracture is present, the fragment is reduced and secured with a screw and, if necessary, a soft-tissue spiked washer (Fig. 3.9). In the absence of a frac-

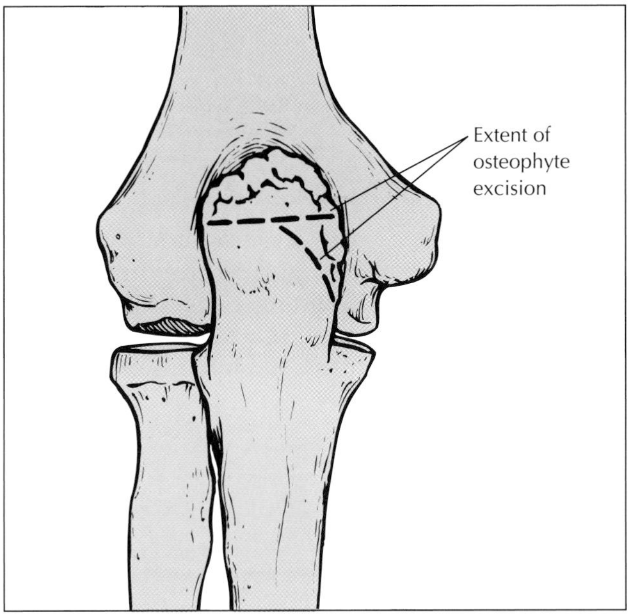

FIGURE 3.7

Excision of valgus extension overload lesion. (*Adapted from* Wilson *et al.* [22]; with permission.)

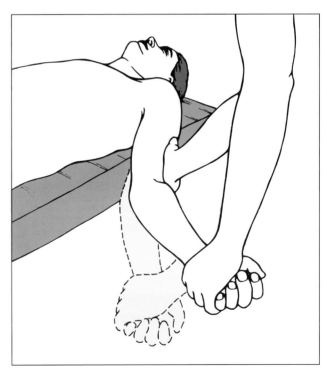

FIGURE 3.8

Valgus stress test for medial instability. (*Adapted from* Norwood *et al.* [23]; with permission.)

ture, the UCL is treated in any of several ways, depending on the site of injury. If the ligament has been avulsed proximally, it is repaired to bone through two drill holes at its site of origin beneath the medial epicondyle. Midsubstance ruptures are repaired directly with care to advance the stretched ligament ends. The flexor–pronator muscle mass is usually avulsed in the more severe injuries and repaired as well. We no longer repair the anterior capsule to avoid contributing to the posttraumatic loss of extension that often accompanies these injuries, and the ulnar nerve is not routinely transposed. Postoperatively, a splint is used for the first several days, followed by a single-axis elbow orthosis blocking the terminal 30° of extension for 6 weeks.

Protected motion is allowed, and full range of motion is obtained at 4 to 6 weeks. A full elbow rehabilitation program emphasizing muscle strengthening is begun once medial elbow healing is complete (≈ 6 weeks).

ULNAR COLLATERAL LIGAMENT INJURIES FROM REPETITIVE OVERLOAD

The anterior bundle of the UCL is analogous to the anterior cruciate ligament of the knee in its importance in providing stability to the elbow. Recent research has focused on defining the exact origin and insertion of the anterior, posterior, and transverse

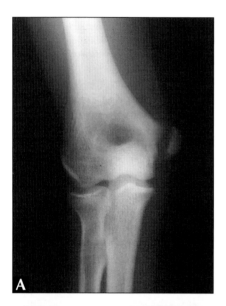

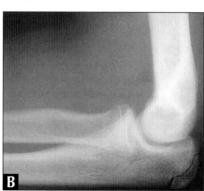

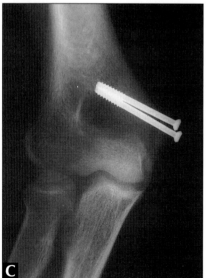

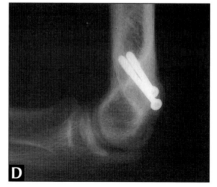

FIGURE 3.9

Preoperative (*panels A* and *B*) and postoperative (*panels C* and *D*) radiographs of medial epicondyle avulsion fracture and anteroposterior radiograph of normal contralateral elbow.

bundles of the UCL; its histology, biomechanical function, and response to stress; and the appropriate techniques for the diagnosis and management of UCL injury. UCL injury in the throwing athlete may occur acutely, with a single off-balance or hard throw; more commonly, the etiology is chronic. In the throwing motion, extreme valgus forces are generated during the cocking phase, creating a significant tensile load across the medial elbow joint. The anterior oblique bundle of the UCL is the primary static restraint for the medial elbow and must be able to withstand and resist these valgus forces on a recurrent basis. With repetitive stress and overuse, the throwing athlete may develop microtearing in the UCL. This microtearing can progress to a partial or complete tear or even an avulsion injury with compromise of the functional integrity of the ligament.

The symptomatic athlete complains of medial elbow pain with throwing, a loss of accuracy or velocity in the throw, a sense of instability, local swelling, and, occasionally, tingling in the small and ring fingers (ulnar neuritis symptoms). An initial diagnosis may have been a flexor–pronator strain that did not resolve with standard treatment. Clinical examination may show a valgus deformity or flexion contracture of the elbow, as well as tenderness at the proximal, mid-, or distal portions of the anterior bundle of the UCL. Also, pain may be evoked with forced valgus stress testing of the elbow at 30°, or frank medial joint line opening may

be detected. All tests should be performed on the contralateral elbow for comparison. A positive Tinel's sign may be present if there is chronic irritation of the ulnar nerve. Sensory and motor examinations of ulnar nerve function should be performed, and a standard series of radiographs (anteroposterior, lateral, axial, internal, and external obliques) should be obtained. Associated pathology, such as signs of a loose body or a posteromedial osteophyte from valgus extension overload (VEO), is assessed in addition to any findings consistent with an UCL injury. These findings may include a large medial epicondyle avulsion, a small avulsion fleck of bone distal to the medial epicondyle, heterotopic ossification along the proximal or distal end of the ligament, and medial joint–space widening. If the question of a UCL injury remains, we obtain stress radiographs in which the elbow is secured in partial (30°) flexion in a Telos machine (Austin and Associates, Fallston, MD), and graded valgus stresses are applied as an anteroposterior radiograph is obtained. Contralateral elbow stress radiographs are used for comparison and the amount of medial joint–space widening is measured. The elbows should be within 1 mm of each other for each stress radiograph. A difference of more than 1 mm implicates UCL injury; however, a negative stress test does not rule out a partial tear (Fig. 3.10).

Other ancillary tests that may be performed to further evaluate the medial elbow include CT arthrogra-

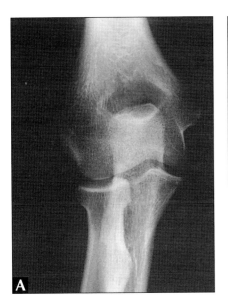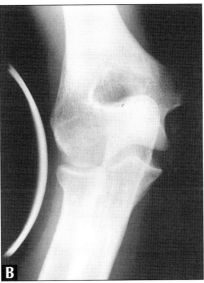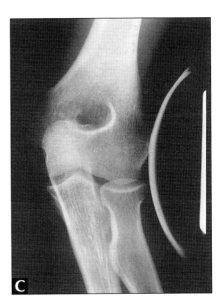

FIGURE 3.10

Telos stress radiographs of 0-kPa–stress injured elbow (*panel A*), 15-kPa–stress injured elbow (*panel B*), and 15-kPa–stress normal elbow (*panel C*).

phy. More recently, fat-depressed, spin-echo, T_1-weighted, intra-articular, gadolinium-enhanced MRIs have been performed. Our studies indicate that MRI arthrography has a capability similar to that of CT arthrography in demonstrating complete UCL tears and surpasses CT in detecting partial or incomplete tears. One type of partial tear that can be demonstrated with either technique is the partial undersurface tear. This tear is classified by the deep ligamentous fibers that detach from their bony insertion, but the superficial fibers and adjacent capsule are intact. In these instances, there is no gross leakage of contrast dye; however, there may be a diagnostic "T-sign" (as we refer to it). The T-sign is a T-shaped accumulation of contrast material between the undersurface of the UCL and its bony sites of deep ligamentous attachment that, when intact, allow no contrast to accumulate (Fig. 3.11). Partial intersubstance tears appear on gadolinium MRI as areas of increased signal within the ligament itself.

Once the diagnosis of chronic UCL injury has been established, the athlete begins a conservative "active rest" program that includes a rehabilitation protocol and nonsteroidal anti-inflammatory medication. For partial tears, this regimen is used for approximately 6 to 8 weeks with mild injury and up to 3 or 4 months with moderate injury. We administer no corticosteroid injections in the management of UCL injuries secondary to the deleterious effects of local steroid on collagen tissue. With an acute complete UCL rupture (such as from a single pitch), the athlete's elbow is placed in a functional brace with range of motion limited to between 15° and 100° for the first 6 weeks. Swelling and pain are treated with ice and oral nonsteroidal medication; wrist and elbow isometrics are instituted. From 6 to 10 weeks, range of motion is progressively increased by 5° of extension and 10° of flexion per week. Isotonic exercises for the wrist and elbow and a rotator-cuff maintenance program are added as well. At 10 to 14 weeks, the rehabilitation program is advanced, with emphasis on eccentric and plyometric motion for strengthening. The athlete is also instructed in neuromuscular control exercises. After 14 weeks, an interval throwing program is initiated, and at approximately 18 weeks, the athlete may return to full activity if asymptomatic and all rehabilitation criteria have been met.

In chronic UCL injuries, the conservative protocol described is followed; splinting may be used initially for comfort. In our experience, the success rate for the conservative treatment of partial tears, although fair at best, is more favorable than that of complete tears, particularly chronic complete tears. If the conservative program is unsuccessful, surgery is recommended. In complete UCL tears, surgery is advocated more quickly in acute than in chronic injuries.

The surgery begins with an examination under anesthesia. Valgus stress testing and range of motion are assessed bilaterally, and arthroscopy is then performed. The patient is placed in the supine position with the arm suspended overhead by sterile fingertraps and the elbow flexed to 90°. After elbow distension with saline, the anterolateral portal is made and a 30° arthroscope introduced. The UCL is visualized and pathology noted. A valgus stress test is performed, and the medial ulnohumeral joint space is observed for any signs of opening. A gap under stress of more than 1 mm is thought to be consistent with loss of UCL integrity. (It is important to note that our cadaveric studies showed that only the anterior 20% to 30% of the anterior oblique bundle can be seen arthroscopically with an anterolateral portal). The remainder of the elbow articular surfaces are examined, and any loose bodies are removed. If a VEO lesion is known to be present, it is best addressed during the open part of the procedure. The hand is then removed from the fingertrap suspension and the upper extremity placed on a hand table. A medially based curvilinear incision is made. The medial antebrachial cutaneous nerve is identified and protected, and the ulnar nerve is identified and, if warranted, mobilized.

In the classic approach described by Jobe *et al.* [24,25], the origin of the common flexor bundle is incised and elevated, leaving a small tendinous stump for later reapproximation. This allows adequate expo-

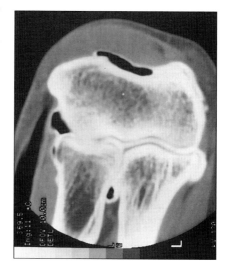

FIGURE 3.11

Computed tomographic arthrogram demonstrating "T-sign."

sure of the ulnar nerve and the bone insertion sites for the UCL. The integrity of the UCL can also be assessed through a separate small-flexor mass-muscle split. Recent cadaveric dissections explored the feasibility of performing an entire UCL reconstruction through a new extensile-muscle splitting approach. The split is created through the raphe between the flexor carpi ulnaris and the common flexor mass from the medial humeral epicondyle to a point approximately 1 cm distal to the UCL attachment to the sublime tubercle of the ulna. Overall, this is an internervous plane between the motor distributions of the ulnar and median nerves. Within this "safe zone" or "watershed," the UCL may be repaired or reconstructed with minimal disruption of the flexor pronator mass (Fig. 3.12). The ulnar nerve is not routinely mobilized unless an anterior transposition of the nerve is planned; thus the risk of postoperative paresthesias or neuropathy is decreased (Jobe and Thompson, Paper presented at the 1997 American Shoulder and Elbow Society Specialty Day meeting at the AAOS annual meeting, San Francisco, 1997) [26].

Altchek (Personal communication) has accumulated data on 40 patients who underwent ulnar collateral reconstruction through this extensile muscle split approach. No postoperative complications relative to the approach developed in any of the patients. If a VEO posteromedial osteophyte is present, a capsulotomy is made posterior to the trochlea. As valgus stress is applied, visualization of the posterior olecranon is excellent. A small osteotome and rongeur are used to debride the posterior and posteromedial olecranon, and attention is then directed toward exploration of the UCL. If the ligament has an acute midsubstance

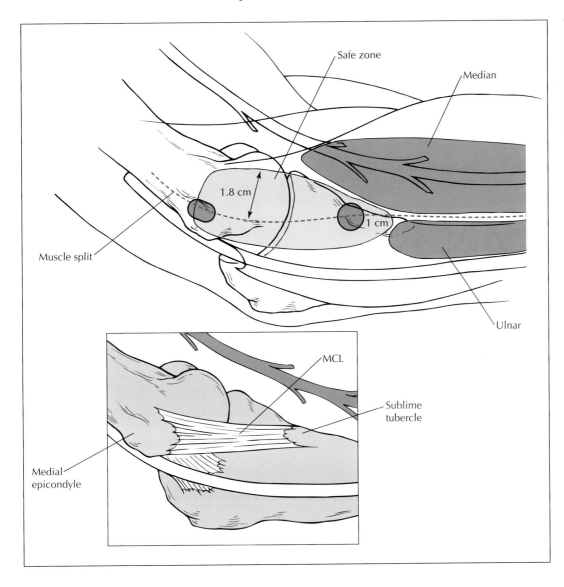

FIGURE 3.12

Medial extensile-muscle splitting approach safe zone. (*Adapted from* Smith *et al.* [26]; with permission.)

rupture, a repair is performed. If the tissue appears unhealthy, serious consideration is given toward augmenting the repair with an autogenous palmaris longus, plantaris, or toe extensor tendon graft. Additional graft sources include autogenous quadriceps, patella, Achilles tendon, or similar allograft tissues. If there is an acute proximal or distal rupture, the ligament may be reattached to its site of avulsion through bony drill holes. If the repair appears inadequate, an augmentation procedure should be performed. In chronic ruptures, a completely torn UCL is debrided, the ends are repaired as possible, and a reconstruction is performed as described by Jobe *et al.* [25] using autogenous tissue (Fig. 3.13). In a chronic partial tear, the injured anterior oblique bundle may need to be incised longitudinally. This technique allows inspection of the fibers in their midsubstance and undersurface to delineate the extent and site of microtearing and degeneration or partial avulsion. The area of injury is debrided, and surgery proceeds with a standard ligament reconstruction. The iatrogenic split in the original UCL is repaired once the bone tunnels have been made and the graft has been passed. The ends of the graft are sutured with the elbow flexed to 30° and slight varus stress is applied. In addition, we suture the graft to the remaining underlying UCL ligament fibers. Next, when indicated, a subcutaneous subfascial transposition of the ulnar nerve is performed. The wound is closed over a drain, and a well-padded posterior splint is applied.

Postoperatively, the rehabilitation protocols for the acute UCL repair and the autogenous reconstruction of chronic UCL injuries are identical for the first 3 months. For the first 10 days to 2 weeks, the posterior splint is worn. Wrist range-of-motion, grip strengthening, and shoulder isometric exercises are performed as frequently as tolerated. The posterior splint is then exchanged for a functional brace set at 30° to 100°. At the third week, the brace is advanced to 15° to 110°, and, by the fourth week, 15° to 120°. At the sixth week, full range of motion is allowed, the brace is discontinued, and elbow concentric exercises are initiated. Eccentric exercises are added at 8 weeks. Isokinetic testing and an interval throwing program begin at 3 months in patients with acute repair and 4 months in those with chronic autogenous reconstruction. The predicted time for return to activity depends on the athlete, injury, type of surgery, and rate of rehabilitation. In an acute repair, return may be as soon as 4 to 6 months, whereas chronic reconstruction cases may require 6 months to 1 year before the athlete returns to competitive throwing. After ulnar col-

lateral reconstruction for a chronic injury, the success rate for returning baseball athletes to their previous level of function or higher is 65% to 80% (Azar *et al.*, Paper presented at the 1997 American Orthopaedic Society for Sports Medicine Specialty Day meeting at the AAOS annual meeting, San Francisco, 1997) [27].

SPORTS-INDUCED NEUROPATHIES

Sports-induced neuropathies may be either acute or chronic and tensile or compressive. Acute nerve injury can result from a direct blow or contusion to the nerve, a laceration or stretch injury associated with a fracture or dislocation, or compression and ischemia (as occurs with a compartment syndrome). Chronic injuries are secondary to repetitive tensile overload, compression from muscular hypertrophy, aberrant anatomy leading to entrapment, nerve hypermobility, or irritation from repetitive exertion in the surrounding muscle compartment [28,29].

Median nerve

In the athlete, median nerve compression is more likely to occur proximally in the forearm than distally at the wrist. Sites of compression may be at the lacertus fibrosis, between the two heads of the pronator teres, at a fibrous arch in the flexor digitorum sublimis, or, rarely, by the ligament of Struthers. Subtle differences in the clinical examination may

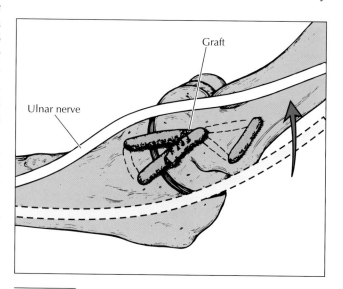

FIGURE 3.13

Jobe's reconstruction of the ulnar collateral ligament. (*Adapted from* Jobe *et al.* [25]; with permission of the *Journal of Bone and Joint Surgery*.)

help differentiate between these possible sites. Localized tenderness is always a helpful finding, and pain with repetitive or resistive forearm pronation and wrist flexion may indicate pronator teres compression. Painful resisted elbow flexion at 120° with forearm supination correlates with lacertus fibrosis compression, and exacerbation or reproduction of symptoms with resisted long finger flexion may be consistent with flexor digitorum sublimis arch compression. Sensory symptoms may be intermittently present in the distribution of the median nerve. Routine radiographs should be obtained to rule out a medial supracondylar bony process of the humerus. Electromyography is not usually helpful. Treatment is conservative initially (as with most entrapment neuropathies) and includes rest, nonsteroidal anti-inflammatory medication, and physical therapy for flexibility exercises and local modalities. Modification in the athlete's biomechanics may ameliorate symptoms as well. When conservative management is unsuccessful, surgical exploration and decompression of the median nerve is recommended. The surgical success rate may approach 100% if either the flexor digitorum sublimis or the pronator teres alone is the cause of the compression syndrome. However, if both the flexor digitorum sublimis and the pronator teres are involved, then successful results decrease to less than 80% (Glowocki *et al.*, Paper presented at the 1997 AAOS Annual Meeting Scientific Program, San Francisco, 1997).

Anterior Interosseous Nerve

The anterior interosseous nerve (a pure motor branch from the median nerve) innervates the flexor pollicis longus, the pronator quadratus, and the flexor digitorum profundus muscles of the index and (occasionally) the long finger. Injury leads to the inability of the athlete to form an "OK" sign, with weakness in pinching. The nerve may be injured during internal fixation of a proximal radius fracture, by entrapment by fibrous bands from the flexor digitorum sublimis or the deep head of the pronator teres, or by an accessory slip of the flexor pollicis longus. Surgical exploration is warranted if symptoms do not resolve with conservative management.

Radial Nerve

The radial nerve may be subject to compression at four different sites along the radial tunnel that lies between the radial head and the supinator muscle.

These sites include a fibrous band tethering the posterior interosseous nerve to the radial head, a fan-shaped arcade of the recurrent radial artery and vein anterior to the lateral humeral epicondyle, a sharp tendinous edge of the extensor carpi radialis brevis tendon, and (more commonly) the fibrous arcade of Frohse along the proximal edge of the supinator. Clinical signs include tenderness over the supinator and pain with elbow extension and resisted forearm supination (supinator muscle compression) or forearm pronation and wrist flexion (arcade of Frohse compression), unless the entrapment is at the radial head, in which case pain will be present with extreme supination with the elbow in a flexed position. The lateral epicondyle is rarely tender except with compression of the nearby radial recurrent nerve or a concomitant lateral epicondylitis. Motor loss, if any, is incomplete. There may be a tendency toward radial deviation with active wrist dorsiflexion because of weakness of the extensor carpi ulnaris. Sensory deficits indicate that the compression site is proximal to the division of the radial nerve into the superficial radial and posterior interosseous nerves. Elimination of pain with injection of a local anesthetic into the radial tunnel is believed by some authors to be diagnostic of a radial tunnel syndrome [29]. Electromyography may be helpful. If motor deficits are present and do not show signs of resolution after 2 to 3 months of conservative treatment, a surgical exploration with decompression should be performed. In the absence of motor loss, conservative measures may be used for 6 to 12 months before surgery is elected.

Lateral Antebrachial Cutaneous Nerve

Compression neuropathy of the lateral antebrachial cutaneous nerve is rare, but it should be included in the differential diagnosis for causes of lateral elbow pain. This nerve is the terminal branch of the musculocutaneous nerve and has a pure sensory function. In baseball pitchers, during the follow-through phase of pitching (as the elbow extends and the arm pronates), this lateral sensory nerve may become entrapped between the lateral margin of the bicipital aponeurosis and the brachial fascia. Described in 1982 by Bassett and Nunley [30], this syndrome produces anterolateral elbow pain with paresthesias or dysesthesias radiating into the proximal forearm. Physical examination may demonstrate local tenderness, a positive Tinel's sign, and subjective sensory loss along the distribution of the nerve. A selective steroid-anesthetic injection may be diagnostic and therapeutic. Other treatment modalities include periodic splinting with the terminal 20° to 40° of elbow extension blocked, anti-inflammatory medication, and, in recalcitrant cases, surgical decompression with possible partial wedge resection of the impinging biceps tendon and aponeurosis.

Ulnar Nerve

The ulnar nerve is the most injury-prone nerve in the elbow and forearm. It occupies a superficial position in the cubital tunnel with adjacent bony and soft-tissue constraints that can contribute to its impingement and compression when certain external forces are applied. Direct trauma to the ulnar nerve is an acute cause of neuropathy, usually secondary to a fall or a blow to the area. Indirect trauma may be seen in baseball, racquet sports, and weightlifting. In the cocking phase of baseball pitching, tensile forces are generated across the elbow as it assumes an extreme valgus position. In the presence of an incompetent UCL, unresisted valgus forces further increase medial elbow stress. In turn, the ulnar nerve develops chronic irritation from repetitive traction. Cubital tunnel spurring, UCL hypertrophy, arcuate ligament fibrosis, and a congenitally hypermobile ulnar nerve are additional aggravating etiologic factors. Other sites of compression include the flexor carpi ulnaris or an anomalous anconeus epitrochlears (reported in weightlifters). Symptoms of ulnar neuritis are tingling and sensory changes in the small finger and ulnar half of the ring finger as well as posteromedial pain, particularly when the elbow is flexed and the shoulder abducted. When present, motor complaints may be described by the athlete as a feeling of clumsiness in the hand and fingers. Physical examination includes a complete neurologic assessment of the upper extremity. The elbow examination should include bilateral measurement of elbow range of motion, degree of flexion contracture, amount of valgus deformity, lack of UCL integrity, tenderness in the cubital tunnel, palpable medial epicondyle osteophytes or soft-tissue hypertrophy, medial snapping sensation with elbow range of motion, nerve subluxation from the groove with the shoulder abducted and the elbow flexed, a positive Tinel's sign, and reproduction of symptoms with the elbow held in a flexed position for 5 minutes. Routine radiographs are obtained to demonstrate any bony abnormalities at the cubital tunnel, including signs of ulnar collateral ligament injury. Ancillary tests (*eg*, electromyographic and nerve conduction studies) may be performed, but a normal study does not rule out a symptomatic neuropathy.

Initial treatment is nonoperative and includes splinting, anti-inflammatory medication, physical therapy, and alteration of throwing mechanics, if necessary. Surgery is recommended if symptoms do not resolve after an appropriate time. Results are better for athletes whose electromyographic studies, prior to surgery, are normal rather than positive for a motor defect (Brach and Sotereanos, Paper presented at the 1997 AAOS annual meeting scientific program, San Francisco, 1997). Ulnar nerve decompression with anterior transposition is the surgical technique most frequently selected, especially in the athlete. The transposition may be submuscular, subcutaneous subfascial, or subdermal [31,32]. In the submuscular transfer, the flexor–pronator origin may be divided or elevated by detachment with a portion of the medial epicondyle. However, osteotomy of the medial epicondyle may not be desirable in the competitive overhead athlete. We prefer a subcutaneous subfascial transposition either in patients undergoing UCL reconstruction who have concomitant ulnar neuritis or in the athlete with symptomatic ulnar nerve subluxation.

In the subcutaneous subfascial technique, two fascial slings are constructed from the flexor–pronator muscle group fascia. These slings are proximally based flaps originating anterior and just distal to the medial epicondyle and measure approximately 2.5 cm in length and 1 cm in width. A small amount of muscle is left on the undersurface of each flap. The ulnar nerve is decompressed and freed from soft-tissue constraints proximally and distally so that it may be placed without tension anteriorly onto the flexor-pronator mass. The two fascial slings are loosely laid over the ulnar nerve and sutured to fascia, thus maintaining the nerve in its new anterior position. The elbow is gently placed through a full range of motion to ensure that no kinking of the nerve occurs and no residual areas of compression exist. Postoperatively, a well-padded posterior splint is applied with the elbow flexed to 90°. Wrist range-of-motion and grip-strengthening exercises are begun immediately. After 1 week, elbow range of motion is allowed to within 15° of full extension; at 3 weeks, the splint is discontinued, and full range of motion is encouraged. Flexibility and progressive resistance exercises are also begun at this time. The throwing athlete will begin an interval throwing program at 8 to 12 weeks.

CONCLUSIONS

Techniques for evaluating elbow and forearm injuries in sports medicine continue to improve. However, growth in this area cannot replace the critical importance of a detailed history and physical examination, but will serve to enhance the ability to manage athletes more effectively and return them to their preinjury level of competition. Coaches, trainers, and physicians dealing with young athletes should take care not to accelerate them beyond the skeletal limitations imposed by their ages. Conditioning and flexibility programs for the competitive athlete will receive more emphasis in the future as further knowledge of injury prevention is gained.

REFERENCES AND RECOMMENDED READING

1. Morrey BF: Post-traumatic contracture of the elbow. *J Bone Joint Surg Am* 1990, 72:601–617.

2. Tedder JL, Andrews JR: Elbow arthroscopy. *Orthop Rev* 1992, 21:1047–1053.

3. D'Alessandro DF, Shields CL Jr, Tibone JE, Chandler RW: Repair of distal biceps tendon ruptures in athletes. *Am J Sports Med* 1993, 21:114–119.

4. Morrey BF: Reoperation for failed surgical treatment of refractory lateral epicondylitis. *J Shoulder Elbow Surg* 1992, 1:47–55.

5. O'Driscoll SW, Bell DF, Morrey BF: Posterolateral rotatory instability of the elbow. *J Bone Joint Surg Am* 1991, 73:440–446.

6. Imatani J, Hashizume H, Ogura T: Acute posterolateral rotatory subluxation of the elbow joint: a case study. *Am J Sports Med* 1997, 25:77–80.

7. Gill TJ, Micheli LJ: The immature athlete: common injuries in overuse syndromes in the elbow and wrist. *Clin Sports Med* 1996, 15:401–423.

8. Chan D, Aldridge MJ, Maffulli N, Davies AM: Chronic stress injuries of the elbow in young gymnasts. *Br J Radiol* 1991, 64:1113–1118.

9. Ruch DS, Poehling GG: Arthroscopic treatment of Panner's disease. *Clin Sports Med* 1991, 10:629–636.

10. Bauer M, Jonsson K, Josefsson O, Linden B: Osteochondritis dissecans of the elbow. *Clin Orthop* 1992, 284:156–160.

11. Jackson DW, Silvino N, Reiman P: Osteochondritis in the female gymnast's elbow. *Arthroscopy* 1989, 5:129–136.

12. Regan W, Morrey BF: Fractures of the coronoid process of the ulna. *J Bone Joint Surg Am* 1989, 71:1348–1354.

13. Geel CW, Palmer AK, Reudi T, Leutenegger AF: Internal fixation of proximal radial head fractures. *J Orthop Trauma* 1990, 4:270–274.

14. Jupiter JB, Morrey BF: Fracture of the distal humerus. In *The Elbow and its Disorders*. Edited by Morrey BF. Philadelphia: WB Saunders; 1993:328–366.

15. Torg JS, Moyer RA: Non-union of a stress fracture through the olecranon epiphyseal plate observed in an adolescent baseball pitcher. *J Bone Joint Surg Am* 1977, 59:264–265.

16. Pavlov H, Torg JS, Jacobs B, Vigorita V: Nonunion of olecranon epiphysis: two cases in adolescent baseball pitchers. *Am J Radiol* 1981, 136:819–820.

17. Cabanela ME, Morrey BF: Fractures of the proximal ulna and olecranon. In *The Elbow and its Disorders*, ed 2. Edited by Morrey BF. Philadelphia: WB Saunders; 1993:405–428.

18. Andrews JR, Craven WM: Lesions of the posterior compartment of the elbow. *Clin Sports Med* 1991, 10:637–652.

19. Tanabe S, Nakahira J, Bando E, *et al.*: Fatigue fracture of the ulna occurring in pitchers of fast-pitch softball. *Am J Sports Med* 1991, 19:317–321.

20. Calle SC, Eaton RG: Wheels in-line roller skating injuries. *J Trauma* 1993, 35:946–951.

21. Fountain JL, Meyers MC: Skateboarding injuries. *Sports Med* 1996, 22:360–366.

22. Wilson FD, Andrews JR, Blackburn TA, McCluskey G: Valgus extension overload in the pitching elbow. *Am J Sports Med* 1983, 11:83–87.

23. Norwood LA, Shook JA, Andrews JR: Acute medial elbow ruptures. *Am J Sports Med* 1981, 9:16–19.

24. Jobe FW, EL Attrache NS: Treatment of ulnar collateral ligament injuries. In *Master Techniques in Orthopedic Surgery: The Elbow*. New York: Raven Press Limited; 1994:149–168.

25. Jobe FW, Stark H, Lombardo SJ: Reconstruction of the ulnar collateral ligament in athletes. *J Bone Joint Surg Am* 1986, 68:1158–1163.

26. Smith GR, Altchek DW, Pagnani MJ, Keeley JR: A muscle splitting approach to the UCL of the elbow: neuroanatomy and operative technique. *Am J Sports Med* 1996, 5:575–580.

27. Conway JE, Jobe FW, Glousman RE: Medial instability of the elbow in throwing athletes. *J Bone Joint Surg Am* 1992, 74:67–83.

28. Cabrera JM, McCue FC III: Nonosseous athletic injuries of the elbow, forearm, and hand. *Clin Sports Med* 1986, 5:681–700.

29. Weinstein SM, Herring SA: Nerve problems and compartment syndromes in the hand, wrist, and forearm. *Clin Sports Med* 1992, 11:161–186.

30. Bassett FH, Nunley JA: Compression of the musculocutaneous nerve at the elbow. *J Bone Joint Surg Am* 1982, 64:1050–1052.

31. Rettig AC, Ebben JR: Anterior subcutaneous transfer of the ulnar nerve in the athlete. *Am J Sports Med* 1993, 21:836–840.

32. Eaton RG, Crowe JF, Parkes JC: Anterior transposition of the ulnar nerve using a non-compression fasciodermal sling. *J Bone Joint Surg Am* 1980, 62:820–825.

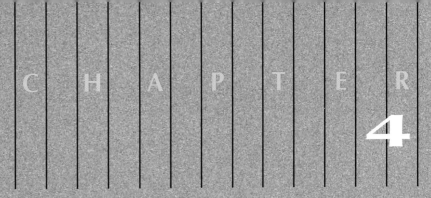

4

ATHLETIC INJURIES TO THE HAND AND WRIST

Frank C. McCue III,
Harry H. Dinsmore,
and David L. Kowalk

Injuries to the hand and wrist are common during athletic competition, accounting for up to 14% of all athletic injuries [1]. Characteristically, the hand is in front of the athlete and frequently absorbs the initial contact or repetitive stresses. Because of this, injuries may range from dislocations and fractures to overuse tendinitis. Appropriate diagnosis and treatment of these injuries is imperative for speedy recovery and optimal final functional result. Whereas most injuries can be treated nonoperatively with proper protection and a good rehabilitation program, there is a small percentage of injuries for which primary surgical management provides the most optimal outcome.

THE WRIST

The complex anatomy of the wrist understandably leads to a complex array of possible injuries. Thus, an athlete with "wrist pain" is often a challenging diagnostic problem. A standard approach of evaluation, however, can help to avoid missing some of the more subtle injuries.

In addition to a thorough history and physical examination, a standard radiographic profile should be obtained. The profile should include a neutral posteroanterior view, anteroposterior and posteroanterior views in radial and ulnar deviation, a true lateral view in the neutral position, a carpal tunnel view, and a closed fist view with the forearm in supination. If obtaining a carpal tunnel view is difficult after an acute injury, much of the same information can be obtained with an oblique view with the forearm in midsupination or pronation. Secondary diagnostic studies can include wrist arthrography under fluoroscopic control, bone scan, plain or computed tomography scan, cineradiography, magnetic resonance imaging, and arthroscopy.

CARPAL INSTABILITIES

Carpal instabilities are generally classified as dissociative or nondissociative. Dissociative instabilities are the result of disruption of intrinsic carpal ligaments between the carpal bones, which causes the proximal carpal row to dissociate from each other and no longer function as a unit. Nondissociative instability is caused by the disruption of extrinsic carpal ligaments with resulting instability at the radiocarpal or the midcarpal joints. This concept of classifying carpal instabilities as dissociative and nondissociative is based on the understanding that the proximal carpal row is an intercalated segment between the forearm and the distal carpal row. The proximal carpal bones have no muscular attachments and move in response to forces applied to them through adjacent articular surfaces and liga-

mentous restraints. The two most common instability patterns are dorsal intercalary segment instability (DISI) and volar intercalary segment instability (VISI). Both of these are dissociative instabilities. Ulnar translation and midcarpal instabilities are nondissociative instabilities. These are less common and will be discussed only briefly.

Carpal instabilities are often the result of a fall on an outstretched hand with the wrist in extension, ulnar deviation, and forced carpal supination. This pattern produces a progression of ligamentous disruption around the lunate beginning on the radial side with either a scaphoid fracture or scapholunate ligament disruption. Further disruption may occur, resulting in lunotriquetral ligament disruption or complete lunate dislocation (Fig. 4.1).

Dorsal intercalary segment instability

Dorsal intercalary segment instability may be the result of either a scaphoid fracture or a tear of the scapholunate ligament. Scaphoid fractures are discussed later, but, in brief, displaced fractures should be reduced and fixed anatomically or, if they are completely nondisplaced, immobilized until union. Disruption of the scapholunate ligament allows the

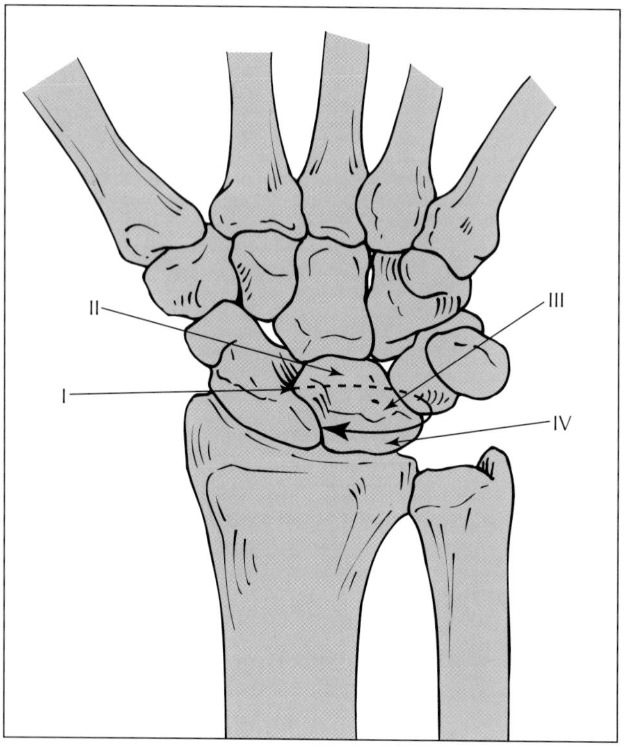

FIGURE 4.1

Mayfield's classification of progressive perilunate instability. I—scapholunate instability; II—capitate dislocation; III—lunotriquetral instability; IV—anterior dislocation lunate. (*Adapted from* Bednar *et al.* [3]; with permission.)

scaphoid and lunate to dissociate from each other. With this, the scaphoid tends to flex, and the lunate tends to extend. This produces the DISI pattern that is seen on the lateral radiograph with an increased scapholunate angle greater than 70° (normal 30° to 60°). On the anteroposterior film, the scapholunate interval is widened, the scaphoid is shortened with a cortical ring sign, and the lunate appears trapezoidal in shape (Fig. 4.2). On physical examination, hypermobility of the proximal pole of the scaphoid can be demonstrated by applying dorsally directed pressure on the volar aspect of the distal scaphoid as the wrist is brought from ulnar to radial deviation (Watson's maneuver). If scapholunate instability is present, an uncomfortable "clunk" will be noted as the proximal pole of the scaphoid is subluxed dorsally in the radioscaphoid fossa.

Acute scapholunate ligament disruptions should be treated with either open ligament repair and K-wire fixation, or closed anatomic reduction and percutaneous K-wire fixation. These should be immobilized in a cast for 8 weeks followed by 4 weeks in a removable splint. Partial ligament disruptions may be treated by a period of immobilization. Chronic scapholunate ligament tears may be treated with ligament reconstruction using a strip of the flexor carpi radialis or a dorsal capsulodesis if the deformity is reducible (Fig. 4.3) [2]. If the deformity is irreducible, but without advanced degenerative changes, the position of the scaphoid may be maintained with a limited intercarpal fusion such as a scaphotrapeziotrapezoid fusion [3]. Chronic scapholunate instability will eventually result in a scapholunate-advanced-collapse (SLAC) wrist

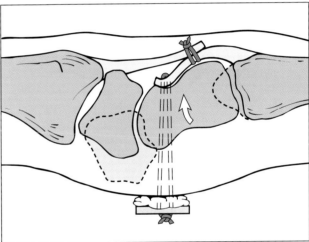

FIGURE 4.3

Blatt capsulodesis. (*Adapted from* Garcia-Elias [9]; with permission.)

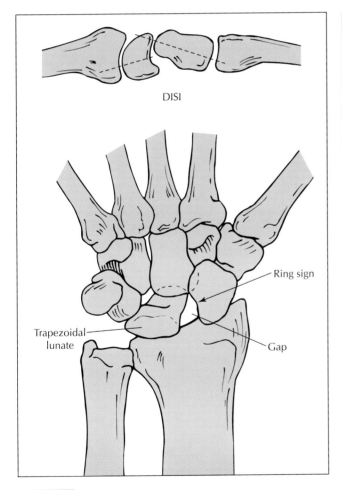

FIGURE 4.2

Dorsal intercalary segment instability (DISI). (*Adapted from* Bednar *et al.* [3]; with permission.)

deformity. This pattern of degenerative arthritis spares the radioulnate articulation due to its spherical configuration, as opposed to the radioscaphoid joint which is elliptical and is eroded with malrotation of the scaphoid. SLAC wrist deformities are best treated with either a wrist fusion or a proximal row carpectomy with the capitate articulating in the intact radiolunate fossa.

Volar intercalary segment instability

This deformity is the result of disruption of the lunotriquetral ligament. In this pattern, the lunate flexes with the scaphoid and the triquetrum extends. This VISI pattern can be seen on the lateral radiograph. The anteroposterior film shows shortening of the flexed scaphoid (a triangular-shaped

lunate), the disruption of the smooth arc of the proximal row between the lunate and triquetrum, and the overlap of these two bones (Fig. 4.4). Acute injuries may be treated by open ligament repair or by closed reduction and percutaneous K-wire fixation with protective immobilization. Partial ligament injuries may be treated with a period of immobilization. Chronic injuries may be treated with reconstruction using tendon autograft (Fig. 4.5) or limited intercarpal (lunotriquetrohamate or lunotriquetral) fusions.

Nondissociative instabilities

Acute traumatic midcarpal instabilities, with disruption between the proximal and distal carpal rows, may be treated by a trial of immobilization. Chronic cases, however, are best treated by triquetrohamate fusion, because immobilization and ligamentous reconstruction have been less successful in maintaining stability in chronic cases.

Ulnar translation of the entire carpus is usually the result of high-energy motor vehicle accidents and is rarely seen in sporting injuries. These injuries are the result of severe disruption of the radiocarpal ligaments with resulting translation of the carpus down the slope of the radius. Soft tissue reconstructions often result in either recurrence or excessive stiffness. Radioulnate arthrodesis will control ulnar translation and give a satisfactory result more often.

TRIANGULAR FIBROCARTILAGE COMPLEX TEARS

Lesions of the triangular fibrocartilage complex (TFCC) are common causes of ulnar-sided wrist pain. Activities that load the wrist, such as weight-

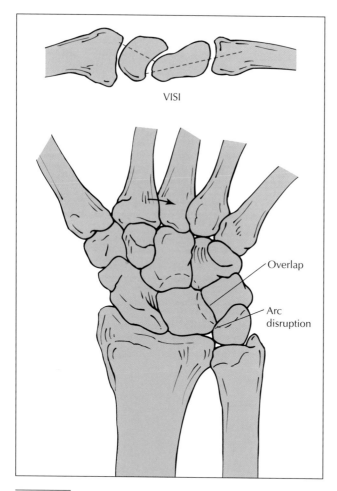

FIGURE 4.4

Volar intercalary segment instability (VISI). (*Adapted from* Bednar *et al.* [3]; with permission.)

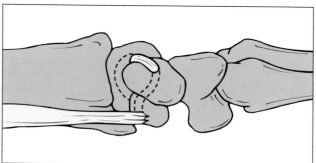

FIGURE 4.5

Lunotriquetral ligament reconstruction using a section of flexor carpi ulnaris. (*Adapted from* Bednar *et al.* [3]; with permission.)

bearing activities, especially during supination and pronation, are common mechanisms of injury. Clinical presentation includes local tenderness at the ulnocarpal joint, and stress maneuvers may elicit a painful click or catch. Arthrography and magnetic resonance imaging are helpful in establishing the diagnosis. Arthroscopy is often more helpful for diagnostic and therapeutic purposes.

The central and radial attachment of the TFCC is avascular, whereas the peripheral attachment is more vascular and, thus, has the ability to heal. Injuries to the TFCC as well as concomitant partial ligamentous injuries of the ulnar side of the wrist may respond well to a short course of protective casting.

Those injuries refractory to conservative management may benefit from further evaluation and treatment. At arthroscopy, tears classified by Palmer as ulnar avulsions may be repairable; all others should be debrided.

More chronic situations with a positive ulnar variant recalcitrant to conservative measures may be candidates for ulnar shortening. Gymnasts with positive ulnar variance also present with chronic disruption of the TFCC. Those with posttraumatic degenerative change of the distal radioulnar joint, particularly in young patients with loss of pronation and supination, may be candidates for further reconstruction. We have successfully used the Suave–Kapandji procedure, which incorporates a fusion of the distal radioulnar joint and pseudoarthrosis just proximal to the ulnar head.

WRIST TENDINITIS

Overuse of the wrist and hand in athletics can result in a wide spectrum of tendinitis occurring near the wrist. deQuervain's tenosynovitis of the first extensor compartment is commonly seen in golf, racquet sports, and fly fishing. Production of pain over the first dorsal compartment with the thumb flexed and ulnar deviation of the wrist (Finkelstein's test) confirms the diagnosis. Intersection syndrome is an inflammatory condition at the intersection of the first dorsal compartment muscles (the abductor pollicus longus and the extensor pollicus brevis) and the radial wrist extensors. This is most commonly seen in oarsmen and weightlifters. Flexor carpi ulnaris tendinitis can also occur; this should be differentiated from a synovitis around the pisiform or arthritis of the pisiform triquetral articulation. Lastly, tendinitis can occur within the tunnel of the flexor carpi radialis.

Treatment consists of splinting, nonsteroidal anti-inflammatory medications, and, occasionally, cortisone injection. Surgical decompression with release of the respective compartments is the final option in refractory cases. For chronic flexor carpi ulnaris tendinitis, pisiform excision is often curative.

ULNOCARPAL IMPACTION SYNDROME

Patients typically present with ulnar-sided wrist pain and crepitus, especially with ulnar deviation and loading. Plain films reveal ulnar positive variance and sclerotic or cystic changes of the lunate, ulnar head, or both.

Physeal stress injuries of the distal radius have been described in young gymnasts [4]. Repetitive compressive and tensile injuries to the epiphysis may be responsible for premature closure (acquired Madelung's deformity).

Treatment is individualized and usually starts with supportive therapy. This includes epiphyseal rest in children. Surgical options include ulnar shortening and wafer osteotomy. Ulnar head resection, Suave–Kapandji procedure, or matched resection may be appropriate treatments in patients with more severe degenerative changes

DORSAL IMPACTION SYNDROME

Dorsal impaction syndrome is the result of repetitive loading of the wrist in extension with impaction of the distal radius and the carpus. This syndrome is seen in gymnasts and may result in the formation of a bony hypertrophic ridge and synovitis [5]. Conservative treatment consists of restriction of wrist extension activities, strengthening of wrist flexors, steroid injection, and immobilization. Surgical treatment consists of synovectomy and cheilectomy.

SCAPHOID FRACTURES

Fracture of the scaphoid accounts for 70% of all carpal bone injuries. The mechanism of injury is often a fall on the outstretched hand, which is apt to occur in almost any sport. Pain on power grip and tenderness over the "anatomic" snuffbox, even in a wrist with negative radiographs, should be treated cautiously. A 2-week period of casting with reevaluation by radiograph, physical examination, and possibly bone scan should be employed. Missed fractures resulting in mal- or nonunions have been shown to lead to DISI with resulting SLAC wrist and degenerative arthritis.

Nondisplaced fractures may be treated with a thumb spica cast. Fractures that are unstable and displaced need primary open reduction and internal fixation with either K-wires or a Herbert screw, and, sometimes, primary grafting. Delayed unions, which occur most frequently in fractures of the proximal pole, may necessitate bone grafting with or without fixation. Healing can take up to 3 or 4 months. Evaluation of the union may be confirmed by either plain or computed tomography scans. An alternative is excision of the proximal pole and replacement with a carved silicone spacer. There are reports of silicone-induced synovitis and poor outcomes with this treatment, but we have experienced good results even in throwing-sport athletes.

Fracture of the scaphoid does not necessarily preclude one from athletic participation. A protective silicone rubber splint has been developed that conforms to the rules of collegiate football (Fig. 4.6). This splint may be worn during games and practices and then replaced with a bivalved fiberglass cast at other times. However, acutely unstable injuries, as well as those in the immediate postoperative course, may not be amenable to such an early form of less-protected care. Such a decision should be left up to the operating surgeon. Open reduction and internal fixation of acute stable fracture is a viable option. Some authors reported returning a patient to sports 6 weeks after open reduction and internal fixation with healing rates similar to other treatment modalities [6].

HAMATE HOOK FRACTURES

Because of its anatomic location (projecting toward the palmar surface of the hand), the hook of the hamate bone is susceptible to injury. Both the transverse carpal and the pisohamate ligaments attach to this bone, and both the flexor digiti minimi brevis and opponens digiti minimi muscles arise from it. The hook is surrounded by the flexor digitorum profundus to the small finger on the radial side and the motor branch of the ulnar nerve on the ulnar side.

The hook of the hamate may be fractured due to direct trauma in a fall, but breaks most commonly occur during a tennis, baseball, or golf swing. These may represent stress fractures from repetitive impaction, the butt of the equipment handle may strike the hook, or a violent contraction of the flexor

carpi ulnaris (which pulls through the pisohamate ligament) may cause the hook to fracture.

The athlete with a hamate fracture will present with wrist pain, poor grip strength, and tenderness over the base of the hypothenar eminence. Due to the proximity of the ulnar nerve, the patient may also exhibit symptoms of nerve compression. The most effective radiographic view is the carpal tunnel view. An oblique view with the wrist maximally radially deviated and partially supinated may also show the fracture. If the diagnosis remains uncertain, a computed tomography scan of both wrists will often provide conclusive information.

The treatment of acute undisplaced fractures is applied using a short gauntlet cast with extension to the little finger. The incidence of nonunion, however, is significant due to the muscular and tendinous attachments. In a symptomatic nonunion, the displaced hook should be surgically excised. Such treatment may be used in the acute setting, as healing time for operative care may be less than that required for conservative management.

NERVE COMPRESSION

Compression of the median nerve in the carpal tunnel or the ulnar nerve in Guyon's canal can both manifest as problems in the athlete's wrist. Symptoms are usually referable to the distribution of the particular nerve involved. Fortunately, in the young, healthy athlete, a conservative program of

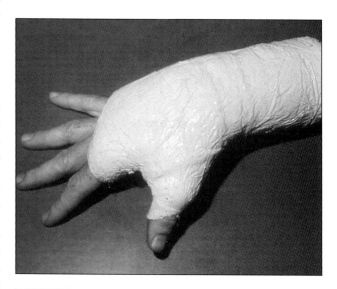

FIGURE 4.6

Protective splint for scaphoid fractures.

rest and anti-inflammatory medication will resolve most problems. Surgical decompression of either nerve should be a rare occurrence.

A particularly unique situation occurs in touring cyclists, who develop ulnar nerve compression at Guyon's canal as a result of continued pressure of the ulnar nerve on the handlebars. This condition may be relieved by wearing gloves and thickly padding the handlebars. Additionally, one must be wary of fractures of the pisiform or hamate, which can also lead to secondary compression of the canal with symptoms.

CARPOMETACARPAL JOINT DISLOCATIONS OF THE THUMB

Complete traumatic dislocations of the carpometacarpal joint of the thumb are rarely seen. Much more common are sprains or partial tears of the volar carpometacarpal ligament complex. The injury occurs most commonly as a result of hyperextension, hyperabduction, or both forces across the volar aspect of the thumb metacarpal. Clinically, the patient presents with a diffusely swollen basilar area with pain and inability to pinch. Often times, the dislocation cannot be appreciated secondary to spontaneous reduction of the injury. Evaluation should include standard anteroposterior and lateral radiography with occasional stress views for those injuries that appear to have reduced spontaneously.

For those injuries judged to be stable following closed reduction, 6 weeks of immobilization in a short-arm thumb spica followed by an active exercise program is appropriate. For those cases where reduction is difficult to maintain, the reduced position can be held with a transarticular K-wire. Ligamentous reconstruction is occasionally required in those cases exhibiting residual laxity.

METACARPAL FRACTURES OF THE THUMB

The usual mechanism of injury for metacarpal fractures of the thumb in athletes is axial compression. The four basic fracture patterns include the two intra-articular types (Bennett's and Rolando's) and the two extra-articular types (oblique and transverse). The intra-articular types are seen more frequently.

The Bennett's fracture dislocation is hallmarked by a small medial fragment anchored to the strong volar ligament. The remaining shaft is subject to the deforming force of the abductor pollicis longus.

Closed reduction and percutaneous pin fixation is the treatment of choice. Rolando's fracture (a proximal, intra-articular, T-shaped fracture) more often requires open reduction to restore joint congruity. Fractures of the metacarpal shaft are often angulated, but a well-molded gauntlet cast can usually hold an acceptable reduction. Continued athletic participation can be allowed in many sports with proper protection. Predictably, bony union occurs in 6 weeks. Union should be followed by a period of protected splinting until normal function of the digit has been restored.

METACARPOPHALANGEAL JOINT DISLOCATIONS OF THE THUMB

This injury occurs secondary to forceful hyperextension of the metacarpophalangeal joint with disruption of the membranous portion of the volar plate. In a simple dislocation, the proximal phalanx lies dorsal to the metacarpal head paralleling the shaft of the metacarpal. Longitudinal traction should be avoided, as this may lead to volar plate incarceration. This reduction maneuver is a push against the dorsal surface of the proximal phalanx with counterpressure of the metacarpal head dorsally.

The complex dislocation involves interposition of the volar plate between the metacarpal and proximal phalanx. Radiography may show a sesamoid bone within the widened joint space. A dimple may be seen on the palmar skin on physical examination. Closed reduction is usually unsuccessful but involves adduction of the thumb metacarpal and flexion of the metaphalangeal joint to relax the intrinsics. This maneuver is followed by hyperextension of the proximal phalanx and a dorsal push to its base. Open reduction is often required for this complex dislocation. This is carried out through a radial midlateral approach; release of the volar plate and accessory collateral ligament may be necessary. The volar plate may be reduced through either a dorsal or volar approach. Postreduction care consists of immobilization for 2 weeks followed by protection in a removable splint for an additional 3 weeks.

COLLATERAL LIGAMENT INJURIES OF THE THUMB

Ulnar collateral ligament injuries (game keeper's thumb) are often associated with skiers; however, these injuries are seen in many sports today, and result from any forceful abduction of the thumb.

New designs in ski poles have helped decrease the incidence of this injury. Clinical examination reveals swelling about the ulnar border of the thumb proximal phalanx and metacarpal as well as tenderness over the ligament. If clinical determination of stability is in question, stress radiography can be used. Side-to-side differences of greater than 10° to 15° or an opening of greater than 35° is consistent with a complete tear (Fig. 4.7). The test should be performed in extension and 30° of flexion. In partial tears, adequate treatment can be provided by a thumb spica cast worn for 3 weeks. Following this, mobilization with part-time protection during sports is encouraged for an additional 3 weeks. In complete tears, the ligament is usually torn from its attachment to the proximal phalanx. Occasionally, this is accompanied by a small bone fragment. Small nondisplaced fractures can be treated in a thumb spica. However, acute complete ligamentous injuries should be treated with open repair and reconstruction. Greater than 50% of these injuries will have the so-called Stener's lesion, which is characterized by the interposition of the adductor pollicis aponeurosis between the torn ends of the tendon. On examination, it is often palpable as a mass. Closed treatment is usually unsuccessful, and the results of long-term reconstruction are not as favorable. Long-term laxity, however, should be addressed in instances to relieve pain, improve stability and improve thumb-index pinch strength. Repaired ligaments, overall, achieve good long-term stability and strength with only slight loss of metacarpophalangeal joint motion [7]. Pull-out sutures over a button and small suture anchors both provide adequate means of ligament repair [8].

Radial collateral injuries are much less common than those that occur on the ulnar side of the digit. The mechanism of injury involves forceful adduction and tortion of the flexed metaphalangeal joint. This is most commonly seen in volleyball players. The ligament is more frequently avulsed from the base of the proximal phalanx. Volar subluxation of the joint can be commonly seen on lateral radiographs. Immobilization for 3 weeks in a thumb spica is adequate treatment for partial tears. Although complete tears may heal more readily on the radial side without the problem of interposing soft tissues, a surgical repair gives a much more predictable result. This is particularly true in those injuries resulting in a volar subluxation pattern.

METACARPAL FRACTURES

The metacarpals are among the most frequently injured bones in athletes. Most commonly, fractures occur through the shafts or the metacarpal neck; however, intra-articular fractures at either end of the bone also occur.

Fractures of the proximal bones are controlled by the transverse intermetacarpal ligament and are generally stable. Those fractures that are only minimally displaced may be treated and protected in a well-molded short-arm cast for 4 to 6 weeks. Long, oblique, and spiral fractures can result in rotatory deformities; therefore, care should be taken to control rotation of the digit by buddy-taping in addition to cast immobilization. Failure to maintain adequate reduction may require percutaneous pinning or open reduction and internal fixation. Multiple, displaced metacarpal-shaft fractures are also an indication for open reduction. Stable internal fixation allows for early range of motion and may provide more rapid return to play.

Boxer's fracture is a metacarpal neck fracture of either the fourth or fifth metacarpal. Both of these bones are more slender and less supported than the shafts of the second and third metacarpal. Because of the increased mobility at the base of the fourth and fifth metacarpals, up to 40° to 50° of angularity deformity is acceptable. Rotation is easily corrected by closed reduction using the 90/90 technique. Four to 6 weeks of immobilization is usually adequate

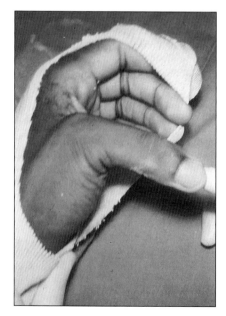

FIGURE 4.7

Ulnar collateral ligament tear.

treatment. In the rare instance in which a fracture is extremely unstable and an acceptable alignment cannot be maintained by splint or cast alone, viable alternatives include either closed reduction and percutaneous pinning or, occasionally, open reduction with internal fixation.

In those fractures involving the articular surface of the metacarpal head, the fracture must be anatomically reduced. More than a 1-mm step-off in the articular surface should be treated with open reduction and internal fixation.

Fractures occurring at the base of the fifth metacarpal are analogous to the intra-articular fractures occurring at the base of the first. However, the deforming force here is the extensor carpi ulnaris. A 30° pronation view may assist in determining whether nondisplaced fractures may be treated with cast immobilization. If the fracture is displaced, closed or open reduction with pinning is needed.

PHALANGEAL FRACTURES

Extra-articular fractures of either the proximal or middle phalanges can occur secondary to either direct or indirect mechanisms. They may appear as spiral, transverse, or oblique. Both bones are subject to the deforming forces of the intrinsic and extrinsic muscles of the hand. Nevertheless, most of these injuries can be treated by closed methods. Attempts should be made to obtain as near anatomic alignment as possible. Usually, longitudinal traction alone with some degree of flexion or extension of the fragments (depending on the deforming forces acting on them) can obtain adequate alignment. The nondisplaced and stable reduced fractures should be treated with immobilization of the joint proximal and distal for 3 weeks. Early mobilization (2 to 3 weeks) should then be the goal. Fractures that are either too unstable or too comminuted should be addressed by either closed reduction and percutaneous K-wire fixation or open reduction and internal fixation techniques. In cases where stable fixation has been achieved, almost immediate range of motion should be permitted.

PROXIMAL INTERPHALANGEAL JOINT INJURIES

Nondisplaced, intra-articular fractures of the proximal interphalangeal (PIP) joint, occurring on either side of the joint, should be treated with 3 weeks of immobilization followed by an additional 4 to 6

weeks of protection for sports. Indications for open reduction and internal fixation include displaced articular surfaces constituting greater than one fourth of the articular surface, displaced volar-lip fractures leading to joint instability, and dorsal-avulsion fractures.

A proper treatment plan for fracture dislocations of the PIP joint should be determined following an attempt at closed reduction. Most commonly, dorsal dislocations lead to fractures of the volar lip. If the joint is stable following reduction, the digit should be splinted in flexion with a dorsal splint with the PIP joint at 30°. If unstable, operative reduction and pinning are needed. Early flexion exercises should begin at 3 weeks and protection for sports is needed for an additional 4 to 6 weeks. On rare occasions, an avulsion of the central slip of the extensor mechanism with a bone fragment can result in a volar subluxation of the middle phalanx. These injuries more commonly require open reduction.

On occasion, the volar subluxation of the joint is secondary to significant comminution resulting from a longitudinal compression force. These acute fractures and those healed in a chronically subluxed position are managed best with excision of the comminution or volar lip and advancement and interposition of the volar plate.

Dislocations of the PIP joint most commonly occur in a dorsal direction but can also occur laterally or volarly. Reduction of the dorsal dislocation is usually easily achieved, and the joint is generally stable because the collateral ligament system has remained intact. Once reduced, the joint should be immobilized in 20° to 30° of flexion for 3 weeks. Extension of the joint can advance weekly, as pain allows, until full extension is obtained in about 3 weeks. Mobilization should then begin with buddy-taping for protection for at least an additional 2 weeks or until the digit is pain-free with a restored range of motion.

Lateral dislocations are slightly more complex, requiring tearing of both the collateral ligament and the volar plate. Most of these injuries may also be treated with 3 weeks of immobilization. However, open dislocations and those dislocations with a rotatory component may require open reduction and repair. Rotation of the distal portion of the digit may result in button-holing of the head of the proximal phalanx between the central slip and the lateral band, making closed reduction unobtainable.

Volar dislocations of the PIP joint usually result in disruption of the central slip of the extensor tendon over the PIP joint, producing the Boutonniere deformity. Following reduction, the digit should be maintained in full extension for 6 to 8 weeks. Protective splinting should be continued during competition for an additional 6 to 8 weeks or until full flexion and maximum extension of the finger have returned. The Boutonniere deformity can occur even without dislocation of the joint and should be suspected with any injury associated with a lag of more than 30° in PIP extension and tenderness directly over the base of the middle phalanx. These injuries should be treated as a dislocation. Any residual, restricted, passive extension at the PIP joint can often be corrected with dynamic splinting techniques.

Open dislocation requires adequate irrigation and debridement in addition to the aforementioned treatment regimens. The wound may be loosely closed as needed.

An acute injury to the volar plate can occur as a result of hyperextension with or without a dislocation of the joint. These injuries should be treated with splinting of the PIP joint in 20° to 30° of flexion for 2 to 3 weeks. Buddy-taping and protected motion may be begun as pain allows.

Chronically, a volar-plate injury can result in either a hyperextension or flexion deformity of the PIP joint. Distal disruption of the volar plate can produce a "swan neck" deformity. Symptomatic swan neck can be treated with distal advancement of the volar plate with sublimis tenodesis. Damage to the proximal membranous portion of the plate produces the "pseudo–Boutonniere deformity." In this case, the central slip is intact, but contracture of the volar plate prevents extension at the PIP joint leading to slight hyperextension of the distal interphalangeal (DIP) joint.

Radiographic evidence of calcification under the distal end of the proximal phalanx is not uncommon. Those deformities resistant to stretching and maintained beyond 40° of flexion may be treated surgically.

DISTAL INTERPHALANGEAL JOINT INJURIES

Dislocations of the DIP joint can occur dorsally and, much less commonly, volarly. Dislocations should be reduced and splinted during athletic activity for at least 3 weeks or until tenderness subsides and a good range of motion is regained.

MALLET FINGER

Extensor mechanism injuries at the DIP joint are common, particularly in football players, baseball catchers and fielders, and basketball players. There are several distinct anatomic types of extensor mechanism injuries. The extensor tendon can be attenuated, ruptured, or avulsed from the base of the distal phalanx with or without a piece of bone (Fig. 4.8). Forced flexion of the DIP joint or an acute hyperextension injury account for this spectrum of injury. Those injuries seen within 12 weeks following initial injury can usually be treated with the DIP joint splinted continuously in extension or slight hyperextension for 8 weeks. An additional 6 to 8 weeks of splinting should be employed during athletics. Mallet fingers involving fractures of greater than 30% of the articular surface and those resulting in volar subluxation of the distal phalanx should be treated with open reduction and internal fixation.

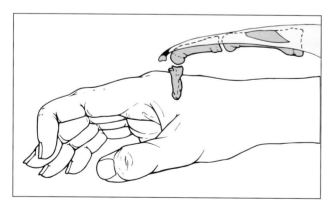

FIGURE 4.8
Mallet finger.

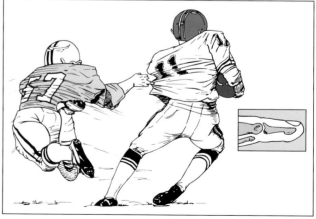

FIGURE 4.9
Jersey finger.

FLEXOR DIGITORUM PROFUNDUS AVULSION

Avulsion of the flexor digitorum profundus is more often called "The Jersey Finger." The injury most commonly occurs to the ring finger in football while grabbing an opponent's jersey. While the ring finger gets caught, the little finger often slips away, resulting in a forced extension of the digit while it is attempting to actively flex. Often, the diagnosis is difficult and the injury is missed. However, typically, there is pain and swelling in the affected finger with loss of active flexion of the DIP joint. Radiographs may or may not reveal bony avulsion from the base of the distal phalanx (Fig. 4.9).

There are three common levels of retraction of the profundus, hence leading to the classification of the injury into three types. In type I injuries, the tendon retracts into the palm, losing its blood supply from both the bone and vincular system. These injuries require reattachment within 7 to 10 days to avoid necrosis of the tendon, resulting in the need for secondary reconstruction. This may also present as a painful mass in the palm. In type II injuries, the tendon retracts to the level of the PIP joint and is held there by the still intact vincula. With the tendon's blood supply intact, a reattachment can be successful up to 6 weeks post-injury. Beyond this point, contractures of the joints often develop, leading to a need for secondary reconstructive procedures. In Type III injuries, there is an avulsion of a large fragment of bone by the tendon from the base of the distal phalanx. Retraction of the tendon is halted at the A-4 pulley. Delayed repair can also be successful in these injuries.

In chronic cases, the digit may be left alone without further sequelae. However, in the young individual requiring the additional dexterity of the digit, a secondary reconstruction can be performed. In delayed repair, efforts should be made to prevent joint contractures prior to surgery. If the only complaint is instability of the distal joint, then fusion of the DIP is an additional alternative form of surgical care. Repair of the tendon to the distal phalanx can be accomplished with either a pull-out suture over a button or with small suture anchors [8].

CONCLUSIONS

Injuries to the hand and wrist are the most common injuries incurred by the athlete. Neglect of such injuries may result in irreparable damage to the hand or wrist. We have summarized the more common injuries to these areas seen in the athlete with a description of the recognition and treatment, giving insight into the multiple considerations the athlete and coach must have. Even seemingly minor injuries must be carefully evaluated and treated by a physician. Early diagnosis, accurate and precise treatment, and proper rehabilitation are extremely important to regain optimal function after these injuries. These injuries may have a significant impact, not only in athletic competition, but also in the athlete's selection of an occupation and function later in life. It is psychologically important, also, that the participant be returned to his particular sport as soon as possible. Most of the injuries can be controlled by conservative means. However, when surgical repair is indicated, it is important for the surgeon to be trained and familiar with the anatomy and techniques of surgery of the hand and wrist.

REFERENCES AND RECOMMENDED READING

1. Rettig AC, Patel DV: Epidemiology of elbow, forearm, and wrist injuries in the athlete. *Clin Sports Med* 1995, 14:289–297.

2. Cooney WP, Linscheid RL, Dobyns JH: Carpal instability: treatment of ligamentous injuries of the wrist. *Instr Course Lect* 1992, 41:33–44.

3. Bednar, JM, Osterman, AL: Carpal instability: evaluation and treatment. *J Am Acad Orthop Surg* 1993, 1:10–17.

4. Plancher KD, Minnich JM: Sports-specific injuries. *Clin in Sports Med* 1996, 15:207–218.

5. Halikis MN, Taleisnik J: Soft-tissue injuries of the wrist. *Clin in Sports Med* 1996, 15:235–260.

6. Rettig, AC, Kollias, SC: Internal fixation of acute stable scaphoid fractures in the athlete. *Am J Sports Med* 1996, 24(2):182–186.

7. Downey DJ, Moneim MS, Omer GE: Acute gamekeeper's thumb: quantitative outcome of surgical repair. *Am J Sports Med* 1995, 23:222–226.

8. Skoff HD, Hecker AT, Hayes WC, *et al.*: Bone suture anchors in hand surgery. *J Hand Surgery* 1995, 20:245–248.

9. Garcia-Elias M: Rotary subluxation of the scaphoid. In *Techniques in Hand Surgery*. Edited by Blair WF. Baltimore: Williams and Wilkins; 1996:550.

HIP AND THIGH INJURIES

Joseph A. Abate III
and Jack T. Andrish

Evaluation of injuries to the hip, pelvis, and thigh may often be complex because there are a variety of structures that may be involved with injury in this region. Furthermore, the injuries may be acute or chronic, and this may influence treatment options. A thorough history and physical examination is required for an accurate diagnosis of the athlete's problem in order to effectively treat injuries in this region (Table 5.1).

ACUTE TRAUMATIC SKELETAL INJURIES

Hip dislocation and subluxation

Although hip dislocations usually involve major traumatic events, they have been reported to occur in athletics [1–3]. Most dislocations are posterior, whereas anterior dislocations account for only 10% to 15% percent of the total number. In a posterior hip dislocation, the leg will normally be held in a flexed, adducted, and internally rotated position. In anterior dislocations, the leg will be extended, abducted, and externally rotated. It is critical to document the neurovascular status of the involved extremity prior to any attempts at reduction. The sciatic nerve is particularly vulnerable to injury and must be carefully assessed. In general, reductions should never be performed on the field of play and as this is a true orthopedic emergency, the patient should be immobilized and sent to an emergency department for definitive treatment as soon as possible [4••].

Radiographic evaluation is critical before reduction of a dislocated hip because it can document the direction of dislocation, the presence of femoral neck or head fractures and associated acetabular fractures. Radiographs should also be obtained after reduction to confirm concentric reduction and to exclude fractures. The hip can also be brought gently through a range of motion to assess the stability after reduction. Computed tomography (CT) scan is not routinely used prior to reduction, but it can be extremely useful to document eccentric reduction of the hip and the presence of fracture fragments within the hip joint after reduction (Fig. 5.1) [5•].

In contrast to hip dislocations, the diagnosis of hip subluxation may be quite difficult because the athlete may have only mild hip discomfort after this injury. The true incidence of hip subluxation is difficult to quantify. Hip subluxation implies abnormal motion of the femoral head out of the acetabulum but not complete dislocation. Injuries to the articular cartilage or soft tissues, such as the labrum, may still occur [6]. In contrast to hip dislocation, athletes who have sustained a hip subluxation are usually able to walk, although they may have hip discomfort and an antalgic gait.

Treatment

A dislocated hip is an orthopedic emergency. Early reduction is required because the risk of avascular necrosis (AVN) of the femoral head increases the longer the hip remains unreduced. This risk becomes significant when the hip stays dislocated longer than 6 hours. Normally the hip can be reduced by gentle closed reduction. This can be accomplished either in the emergency room under analgesia and sedation or may also be performed under general anesthesia if there are difficulties performing the procedure in the emergency room. Usually one or two gentle attempts that fail to produce a satisfactory closed reduction will require an open reduction because there may be some type of anatomic block [7]. The key is to perform the reduction in a gentle manner to minimize further damage

to the articular surface or to prevent fracture of the femoral neck, which is a serious injury in a young patient. After reduction, it is again advisable for the patient to undergo a CT scan or tomograms of the hip to ensure that the patient has a concentric reduction, that there are no bone or cartilage fragments interposed between the femoral head and acetabulum, and that there are not significant fractures of the acetabular wall that may require surgical stabilization. A recent report even describes a Bankart-type repair of the capsule and labrum and the use of allograft to reinforce the posterior rim of the acetabulum for recurrent dislocation of the hip [8].

Following reduction, the athlete should be maintained at bed rest for a short period of time with skin traction until pain and muscle spasm have subsided. Range-of-motion exercises are allowed, and the patient should be instructed in non–weight-bearing crutch ambulation. Protected weight bearing may begin as early as 3 to 4 weeks after the injury. This can be progressed to full weight bearing in 6 to 8 weeks, which should allow adequate healing of soft tissue [5•]. If there are significant fractures of the acetabular wall, this period of protected weight bearing may need to be lengthened to allow adequate bony healing. Progressive resistance exercises may also begin. The patient will continue to work on improving range of motion of the hip. Return to activity is permitted only when full strength, motion, and soft tissue healing have been achieved. Three to 6 months are generally required for this to occur. Serial radiographs should be obtained for the next 2 to 3 years to monitor for the onset of avascular necrosis, chondrolysis of the articular surface, the onset of post-traumatic osteoarthritis, and to document the healing of any fractures. [7].

Table 5.1	HIP AND THIGH INJURIES IN THE ATHLETE	
Acute traumatic skeletal injuries	**Soft tissue injuries**	**Chronic overuse injuries**
Hip dislocation and subluxation	Hip pointer	Stress fractures
Avulsion fractures	Anterior thigh injuries	Femoral neck
Anterior superior iliac spine	Quadriceps contusion	Femoral shaft
Anterior inferior iliac spine	Heterotopic ossification	Snapping hip syndrome
Ischial tuberosity	Compartment syndrome	Osteitis pubis
Lesser trochanter	Medial thigh injury	Iliotibial-band syndrome
Greater trochanter	Posterior thigh injury	
Hip fracture		

For hip subluxations, the treatment program is markedly different than for true dislocations. As the hip is usually stable after this injury, the patient can normally begin strengthening and range-of-motion exercises very early. A period of protected weight bearing with crutches may be needed if the athlete has significant pain with ambulation after the injury. The patient may return to sports when hip range of motion and lower extremity strength have returned to normal.

Complications

Acute complications of hip dislocations can include injury to the sciatic nerve, femoral neck fractures, osteochondral injuries to the femoral head, and acetabular wall fractures. Vascular injuries, which occur more often with anterior dislocations, are rarely seen [9]. The major, long-term complication of hip dislocation is avascular necrosis, which has a reported incidence of approximately 10% [10]. Avascular necrosis and resulting premature post-traumatic arthritis of the hip joint is a devastating injury to any young athlete. The factors reported as important in relation to the development of avascular necrosis include delay in reduction greater than 6 hours, severity of injury to the hip joint, and age of the patient who is over 5 years old [11].

Hip subluxations and their subsequent complications are much more infrequent than hip dislocations. However, avascular necrosis and chondrolysis after hip subluxation in a professional football player have been reported in the literature [6].

Avulsion fractures

Avulsion injuries occur most commonly in children and young adults participating in strenuous sporting activities, but these injuries can also be seen in adult athletes [12]. In young athletes, the injury normally occurs at an open apophysis as a result of a sudden violent muscular contraction or a sudden excessive passive lengthening of a muscle, as can happen to cheerleaders or gymnasts who perform splits. The most common sites for avulsion fractures are the anterior–superior iliac spine (ASIS), the anterior–inferior iliac spine (AIIS), the lesser and greater trochanter, and ischial tuberosity.

In general, athletes with avulsion fractures complain of pain at the site, which can be severe. They may have noticed a "popping" sensation associated with the extreme effort that caused the injury. The injury can often be confirmed with plain radiographs that show an avulsed piece of bone. In patients who have older or chronic injuries, there may be a significant amount of callus at the injury site, and this must not be confused with a malignant process [13,14].

Characteristic muscle involvement associated with avulsion fractures about the hip and pelvis include the sartorii at the ASIS, the superior head of the rectus femoris at the AIIS, the insertion of the hamstrings at the ischial tuberosities, the iliopsoas muscle at the lesser trochanter and the gluteus medius and minimus, and the external rotators of the hip at the greater trochanter.

Anterior–superior iliac spine treatment

For avulsion of the anterior superior iliac spine, nonsurgical treatment is usually recommended. An initial period of relative rest with ice, analgesics, and crutch ambulation can be followed by a gradual return to activity. Most athletes will return to activity approximately 6 to 8 weeks after the injury [14,15]. One recent report supports open reduction and internal fixation to shorten the period of disability and allow a quicker return to full activity in highly competitive athletes [16].

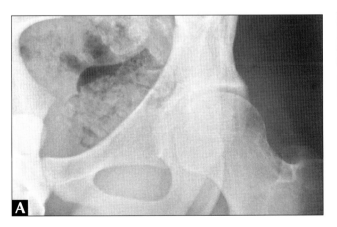

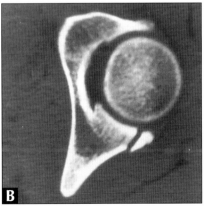

FIGURE 5.1

A, Plain radiograph of a dislocated hip with associated acetabular wall fracture. **B,** Computed tomography scan of a dislocated hip with nonconcentric reduction from interposed bony fragment.

Anterior–inferior iliac spine treatment

For avulsion of the anterior inferior iliac spine, which is much less common than the superior spine or ischial tuberosity, the treatment is again usually nonsurgical. The majority of athletes can usually return to full participation in 6 to 8 weeks after their injury [14,15].

Ischial tuberosity treatment

Controversy exists with regard to treatment for ischial tuberosity avulsion fractures. For minimally displaced ischial tuberosity avulsion fractures, most authors report good results with nonoperative management [14,15]. Operative intervention has been advocated for fractures that are displaced 2 cm or more. If the avulsed bony fragment is large enough, it is usually repaired by open reduction and screw fixation (Fig. 5.2) [17,18].

Lesser trochanter treatment

For lesser trochanter avulsion fractures, the treatment is again nonsurgical in virtually all cases. The athlete will normally resume full activities in 10 to 12 weeks [19].

Greater trochanter treatment

There is debate in the literature regarding the recommended treatment for avulsion fractures of the greater trochanter. If the fragment is displaced more than 1 cm, several authors have recommended open reduction and internal fixation [5•]. For fractures with minimal or no displacement, the treatment can usually be nonsurgical. Progression to full weight-bearing activities should occur as the patient's symptoms resolve. It may take 8 to 10 weeks before the patient is able to return to full competitive activities.

Hip fractures

Fractures of the hip in young athletes are infrequent events because they usually require significant high-speed trauma. In contrast, senior athletes may have increasingly osteoporotic bone and therefore may sustain hip fractures during moderate level activities. This is more commonly seen in alpine or cross-country skiing in the senior populations [20]. Not only are the young and elderly athletes different in the amount of trauma needed to sustain a hip fracture, but the treatment of subsequent hip fractures is different in each group.

As with hip dislocations, the most serious complication of a femoral neck fracture is the loss of vascularity to the femoral head from the injury. Therefore, in young athletes there is an extremely high incidence of avascular necrosis after this injury that can be particularly disabling [21]. The other problem encountered in young athletes who have an interruption of the vascular supply to the femoral head may be injury to the growth plate of the proximal femur and premature closure of the physes. Whether this closure is partial or complete, the result may be a varus deformity of the femoral head and neck and subsequent problems later in life [22].

For young athletes and adults less than 55 years of age, hip fractures require emergent reduction and operative stabilization to avoid the problems of avascular necrosis, chondrolysis, and posttraumatic arthrosis. In the more senior athletic population, the patient's bone quality, symptoms of preexisting hip arthritis, current medical problems, and normal activity level will determine the timing and type of operative intervention. This is too broad a topic to be covered further in this chapter.

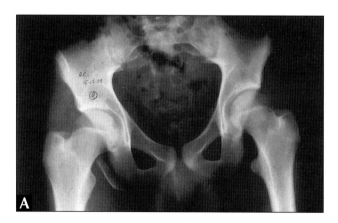
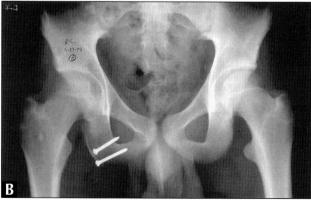

FIGURE 5.2

A, Radiograph of a displaced ischial tuberosity avulsion fracture. **B,** Ischial tuberosity fragment repaired with two screws.

SOFT TISSUE INJURIES
Hip pointer

The term "hip pointer" is often confusing in the literature as it has been used to describe contusions, avulsions, and fractures of the iliac crest. In the literature, "hip pointer" has referred to avulsion injuries in the area of the iliac crest [1,4••]. More commonly, however, the term refers to a contusion of the iliac crest with resulting subperiosteal hematoma formation and disability [5•].

In this condition, athletes normally present with pain and tenderness over the iliac crest, and resisted abduction of the hip causes pain. Plain radiographs may require oblique and comparison views of the opposite side to rule out fractures and avulsion injuries of the iliac crest.

Treatment

Regardless of the underlying etiology, a hip pointer can normally be treated with conservative measures. Treatment should be directed to control bleeding from the injury site with ice, compression, and rest [23•]. Modalities that can cause increased bleeding (*eg*, heat, massage, aspirin and other nonsteroidal anti-inflammatory medications, or aggressive physical therapy) should be avoided in the first 48 hours. If a hematoma does occur, aspiration or open drainage should be avoided because this can lead to infection and is rarely necessary. Protected weight bearing with crutches is allowed, and a stretching and strengthening program may be started as symptoms subside [23•]. Local corticosteroid injection can also be performed in certain athletes, but this is generally not required. In adolescent athletes, if there is an avulsion of the iliac apophysis with significant displacement, then open reduction and internal fixation should be considered. Operative repair may also be considered for athletes with significant muscle detachment who do not have bony fractures of the iliac wing [24]. The area should be adequately padded if an early return to contact sports is allowed.

Anterior thigh
Quadriceps contusion

Quadriceps femoris contusions typically result from blunt trauma to the anterior, medial, or lateral thigh during contact sports participation. The injury usually occurs in the layer directly in contact with the femur and this damage can range from intracellular

edema to muscle fiber disruption, small capillary damage, and subsequent hemorrhage [25,26].

At the initial time of injury, the patient commonly experiences acute thigh pain at the contusion site. In mild or moderate injuries, the athlete may be able to continue to play. With more severe injuries, the athlete will have pain that persists with increasing swelling of the anterior thigh compartment, loss of knee motion, and possibly ipsilateral knee effusion.

A landmark article by Jackson and Feagin [27] reviewed quadriceps injuries in U.S. Military Academy cadets. The authors were able to classify quadriceps contusions as either mild, moderate, or severe based primarily on the loss of knee flexion at 48 hours. Mild contusions had knee motion of at least 90°, whereas moderate contusions had knee motion at less than 90°; severe contusions resulted in knee motion of less than 45°.

Treatment

Most recent treatment protocols have the same general principles [28,29]. During the first 24 hours after the injury, the athlete should be immobilized in full knee flexion with ice, and elevation should be used to limit the amount of hemorrhaging. The patient should be reevaluated after this initial period of immobilization and adjustments can be made as needed. After the initial 48 hours, the patient begins self-paced, gentle, active flexion and extension exercises until there is greater than 90° of knee motion and good quadriceps control. The patient should be allowed progressive weight bearing during this time. When normal gait and knee motion of greater than 90° has been obtained, a progressive resistance-exercise program may be initiated. Contact sports are allowed when the athlete has 120° of pain-free motion at the knee and full strength. Athletes who return to contact sports should be protected from reinjury by the use of a football-type girdle with hard thigh pads for a period of 3 to 6 months. The time required for athletes to return to full participation in sports varies depending on the severity of the injury. With moderate quadriceps contusions, return to full participation may be as early as 2 to 4 weeks after the injury. For more severe injuries, the length of disability can be up to 8 to 10 weeks or longer [30,31].

Complications

In a follow-up evaluation of the U.S. Military Academy experience, the most often seen residual complication was loss of knee flexion and this loss of motion significantly delayed return to unrestricted activities [32].

Two other complications can also occur after blunt trauma to the thigh. Heterotopic ossification (myositis ossificans traumatica) can form in the scar of the inflammatory repair process. Also, if there is significant initial hemorrhage and edema of the anterior thigh compartment, the possibility of compartment syndrome of the anterior thigh must be considered. These two possibilities will be discussed in further detail in the next two sections.

Heterotopic ossification

Studies have shown that heterotopic ossification (myositis ossificans traumatica) is a common complication that can occur after quadriceps contusion [29–33]. The true incidence of myositis ossificans is not known, the Jackson and Feagin [27] found it to be 20% in cadets with quadriceps contusions. The incidence of myositis ossificans increases with the severity of the injury and also with repeated episodes of reinjury.

Typically, the athlete presents with a firm mass after a quadriceps contusion that does not seem to resolve over time. There may be loss of knee motion and persistent tenderness at the site. This heterotopic ossification usually occurs in the muscles adjacent to the bone from a process where the damaged connective tissue develops chondroid and osteoid matrix instead of the normal fibroblastic scar tissue [34]. At 2 to 4 weeks following the quadriceps contusion, plain radiographs may show a soft tissue mass containing calcified densities [31]. This mass may appear identical to fracture callus formation and may be confused with an osteosarcoma. In heterotopic ossification, the osteoid matrix is initially deposited in the peripheral aspect of the lesion where it gradually converts to lamellar bone. This maturation to lamellar bone progresses from the periphery into the center of the lesion. This is in contrast to osteogenic sarcoma, which initially calcifies in the center of the lesion and progresses to the periphery [24,35,36].

Treatment

Most myositis ossificans can be treated nonoperatively. The goal should be to limit the formation of heterotopic ossification by early and determined management of quadriceps contusions. If the patient develops a mass large enough to restrict knee range of motion or function, surgical excision is an option

(Fig. 5.3) [1,24,29,35,36]. After 6 to 12 months, the lesion should be mature. If conservative treatment fails, surgical excision may be offered, which should allow most athletes to return to full activity.

Compartment syndrome of the thigh

Acute thigh compartment syndrome is relatively rare. It usually is caused by high-velocity trauma, but it has also been reported to occur in sports injuries [37–41]. The diagnosis of compartment syndrome in the thigh may be more difficult than in the lower leg because the findings are often similar to those associated with a severe quadriceps contusion. Therefore, compartment pressure monitoring has been advocated to evaluate this problem [42•].

Treatment

The treatment of anterior thigh compartment syndrome remains somewhat controversial. Most reports recommend emergent fasciotomy if the anterior thigh compartment pressures are elevated greater than 30 to 45 mm Hg or within 10 to 30 mm Hg of the diastolic pressure [37–40]. Robinson *et al.* [41], however, reviewed complications associated with surgical decompression of the anterior thigh and concluded that this was not a benign procedure. Furthermore, the authors reported successfully treating patients with confirmed thigh compartment pressures in excess of 50 mm Hg with a nonsurgical treatment program. Therefore, it is difficult to recommend the exact treatment regimen for any athlete with this problem.

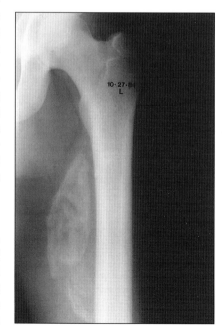

FIGURE 5.3

Radiograph of extensive myositis ossificans (heterotopic ossification) in the thigh musculature. The ossification may need to be excised if it interferes with function.

In general, however, nonoperative treatment for acute thigh compartment syndrome may be possible in athletes without accompanying wounds or fractures. Initial treatment should include ice packs, bed rest, elevation of the thigh to heart level, and immobilization of the knee in full flexion. Neurovascular status, thigh circumference, and compartment pressures should be measured on admission and at regular intervals during the initial 24 to 48 hours. If the patient can not be properly monitored, the athlete's symptoms worsen, or the physician is uncomfortable with this treatment protocol, then operative fasciotomy should be considered. Whether nonoperative or surgical management of anterior thigh compartment syndrome has been used, athletes have been reported able to return to full sporting activities with minimal functional limitations [24,37,39–41].

Medial thigh

The muscles injured along the medial side of the thigh are usually the hip adductors. Contusions are rare, whereas strains are common in this region. The patient may complain of pain in the medial thigh or the groin. The most commonly injured muscles are the adductor longus and magnus. The usual site of injury is the musculotendinous junction [43]. If the athlete complains of pain along the symphysis pubis or inferior pubic rami, in addition to a palpable mass, then the possibility of an avulsion fracture must also be considered. Plain radiographs or bone scanning can normally distinguish these avulsion fractures from pure muscle/tendon injuries.

Treatment

As for most muscle injuries, initial treatment of adductor musculature injuries consists of conservative measures [44,45]. Rest, ice, compression, and elevation followed by a regular stretching program is usually curative. Deep heating or ultrasound may increase intramuscular bleeding and should be avoided. Muscle strengthening, which prevents healing of the muscle in a shortened position, may begin when full range of motion has been regained by the athlete. In very unusual or chronic cases, surgical management has been necessary to return the patient to sporting activities. This may involve excision of scar or granulation tissue within the involved tendon. Tenotomies can also be performed if no abnormal tissue can be found within the ten-

dons [45–47]. Postoperative rehabilitation stresses range-of-motion exercises and slowly increasing muscle strengthening. The return to sports may take 3 to 6 months after surgery.

Osteitis pubis

If the athlete complains of persistent groin pain that radiates into the pubis, then osteitis pubis must also be considered. Symptoms are often nonspecific, thereby delaying diagnosis and treatment. Usually on examination there will be tenderness over the pubis, tightness of the adductor muscles, and pain with resisted adduction of the leg. Plain radiographs and bone scan can also aid in the diagnosis of osteitis pubis [29,48•,49].

Treatment

Recommended treatment for osteitis pubis normally is conservative. It includes rest, ice, and adductor stretching as described for muscle strains. The problem is that the resolution of symptoms may require prolonged rest and ultimately take 3 to 9 months [50]. A new report by Holt *et al.* [48•] on college athletes suggests that corticosteroid injection into the symphysis pubis may allow them a more rapid return to intercollegiate athletics. Patients were able to return to activity free of pain only 3 weeks after corticosteroid injection.

Posterior thigh

The posterior thigh musculature is composed of the hamstring muscles. Because the hamstrings (except for the short head of the biceps) cross both the hip and the knee, they are more vulnerable to injury during sporting activities. In many athletes, the hamstrings are weaker than the quadriceps musculature, which is believed to result in an increased risk of injury [29,44]. Activities involving rapid hamstring contraction or hip hyperflexion when the knee is in full extension most commonly cause hamstring strains [51]. The athlete often experiences a sudden pain in the posterior thigh and may report an audible "pop" during the injury. Palpation with the patient in the prone position usually can identify the region of maximal tenderness or a palpable defect.

Plain radiographs are useful to determine the amount of displacement if an avulsion fracture is present. Magnetic resonance imaging (MRI) has not been routinely used in evaluating these injuries, but in one recent study in professional athletes, MRI was found to be useful in determining the extent of muscle damage. For those athletes with greater than 50% cross-sectional muscle involvement, the time to return to sports was usually longer than 6 weeks [52].

Treatment

Most hamstring injuries can again be managed conservatively with rest, ice, and a physical therapy program that emphasizes stretching and strengthening. The goals of stretching and strengthening should not only be the return of the athlete to sporting activities but also the prevention of reinjury. Therefore, effort should be made to increase the strength of the hamstrings relative to the quadriceps. A program of specific stretching prior to athletic activity may also decrease the incidence of these injuries. Thermal or neoprene pants are often worn by players to prevent these muscle injuries, and one recent report suggests that they may be helpful [53].

Although most hamstring injuries can be managed nonoperatively, proximal bony avulsion fractures, which usually occur in children and adolescents, may require surgical repair or resection if the bony fragment becomes prominent (Fig. 5.4). One recent report suggests that complete ruptures of the proximal origin of the hamstring muscles in adults, even without bony avulsion, may require a surgical repair or reconstruction to restore athletic function. The authors state that the best results are seen if surgery is performed within the first few days after injury [54].

CHRONIC OVERUSE INJURIES
Stress fractures

Although stress fractures were typically first recognized in the feet of military recruits, as distance running became more popular, reports of stress fractures in athletes became more prevalent [55–57]. Overall, in individuals who sustain a stress fracture, femoral involvement is reported to be as low as 4% in the general population, up to 10% in the average runner, and as high as 43% in military recruits. There is a higher incidence of femoral neck stress fractures as compared with femoral shaft stress fractures in both athletic and nonathletic populations [44]. The exact cause for stress fractures has yet to be elucidated. In general, the concept of fatigue failure of normal bone in response to excessive stress was first suggested by Hartley [58]. Roub [59] modified

Hartley's model by suggesting that the term stress fracture be used to describe a disruption of normal bone remodeling in response to stress. Bone responds to Wolf's law, meaning that during the remodeling phase, if the bone is continually stressed from either cyclic overloading or a dramatic increase in the muscular forces applied across their bony attachments, the bone may become temporarily weakened. This remodeling process can proceed until the cortex is disrupted, causing symptoms in the athlete. To fit the diagnostic criteria, a stress fracture must occur in an otherwise normal bone in healthy individuals who have no history of specific injury to the area.

The major presenting symptom associated with stress fractures is usually pain with weight bearing that seems to increase with activities. Initially the pain only occurs with strenuous activities, but as the stress continues, the athlete may experience discomfort even with daily life. The pain is often poorly localized and patients typically present with an antalgic gait. The pain is normally described as an aching sensation that subsides after cessation of activity [60–62].

Radiographic evaluation

In addition to a detailed history and physical examination, initial evaluation of an athlete suspected of a stress fracture should include standard AP, lateral, and oblique radiographs of the area in question. The initial radiographs may typically be unremarkable because stress fractures only become evident on plain radiographs during the reparative phase. After 2 to 4 weeks, plain radiographs may show the onset

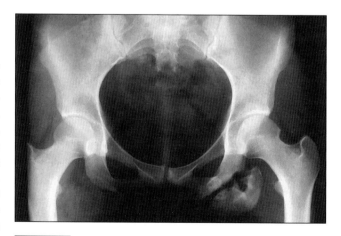

FIGURE 5.4

With this type of posterior hamstring injury the bony prominence may be painful during sitting. Repair or excision of the mass may be indicated in this situation.

of periosteal callus or endosteal hypertrophy in the region of the stress fracture [55,63]. Therefore, plain radiographs are helpful for the late diagnosis of stress fracture. The gold standard for early detection of clinically suspected stress fractures is radionuclear scanning using technetium polyphosphate (^{99}Tc), which has the ability to concentrate in the areas of enhanced metabolic rate and increased blood flow [64,65]. Bone scans should be abnormal 24 to 72 hours after the onset of stress fracture (Fig. 5.5A). This may be as early as 3 weeks prior to the appearance of changes on plain radiographs. Positive radionuclear bone scans show areas of increased uptake within the bone at the sites suspected of stress fracture. Although bone scanning is much more sensitive, plain radiographs are still important because they can determine the exact area involved and the true biologic nature of the bone abnormalities [66]. Although unusual, bone scans have also been reported to be falsely negative [67,68]. In those cases where there is still a high clinical suspicion of stress fracture, CT and MRI have been reported to be helpful as further diagnostic techniques [61,69] (Fig. 5.5B). MRI demonstrates edema within the medullary cavity as well as loss of signal with disruption of the trabecular pattern and cortex at the suspected fracture site.

General considerations

Any athlete who is diagnosed with a stress fracture must be counseled to prevent recurrence. Typically, training errors—especially in runners—are the most common reason for the development of stress fracture. Athletes must be cautioned about the hazards of rapidly increasing mileage, the importance of proper shoe wear, and the influence of various running surfaces as they relate to the magnitude of repetitive stress seen in the lower extremity. Also, any female athletes with a history of amenorrhea or oligomenorrhea should have a complete workup prior to resuming activities because they have a much higher risk of development of stress fractures due to their reduction in bone density [62].

Femoral neck stress fractures

Athletes with femoral neck stress fractures usually present with pain and persistent groin discomfort that seems to be increased with physical activity.

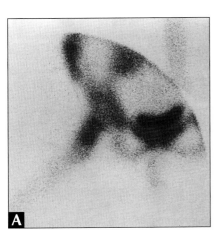

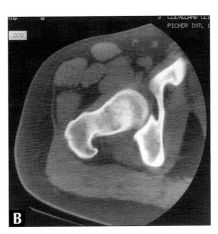

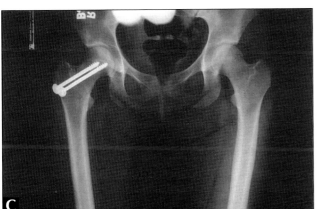

FIGURE 5.5

A, Bone scan showing a lesion of the femoral neck region suspected to be a stress fracture in a runner. **B,** Computed tomography scan of this femoral neck lesion confirms stress fracture. Magnetic resonance imaging may also be used to delineate this type of lesion. **C,** Placement of percutaneous screws through the femoral neck to prevent displacement of the stress fracture.

The pain may also be centered over the anterior thigh or knee. There may be more hip pain with internal rotation or with extremes of hip rotation. Initial radiographs will usually be negative unless the symptoms have been present for 2 to 4 weeks [70]. Bone scan, as described previously, is highly sensitive in detecting these types of lesions of the femoral neck (*see* Fig. 5.5*A*).

Treatment

The treatment decisions for athletes have normally been based on the radiographic appearance of the fracture pattern. Devas [71] reported a classification system that divided femoral neck stress fractures into two types based on their location and pattern. The first type of fracture is a transverse fracture involving the superior portion of the femoral neck. This fracture occurs on the tension side of the femoral neck and has a high likelihood of displacement with continued stress. Internal fixation is usually recommended for these types of femoral neck stress fractures before displacement occurs (Fig. 5.5*C*). The second type of stress fracture of the femoral neck is seen along the inferior medial portion. It has been described as a compression type of stress fracture. These types of fractures are more common in younger patients, and they rarely become displaced with continued stress. Therefore, treatment for a compression type of stress fracture of the femoral neck is usually nonsurgical with protected weight bearing until there is radiographic evidence of healing. Range-of-motion exercises and nonimpact loading and conditioning are allowed with this type of femoral neck stress fracture. If a compression-type femoral neck stress fracture becomes a complete nondisplaced fracture or continues to cause symptoms in the athlete after an adequate course of nonsurgical treatment, the patient may also require internal fixation to stabilize this fracture. Hardware, in general, may be removed approximately 1 year after the surgery if the patient's femoral neck stress fracture is healed and the athlete is symptom free. Obviously any type of displaced femoral neck fracture is a surgical emergency and requires immediate anatomic reduction and internal fixation to prevent long term complications for the patient.

Complications

Whether treated nonoperatively or surgically, most femoral neck stress fractures have relatively few complications if they are diagnosed early before displacement. Complications usually occur in the ath-

letes who go on to have a displaced femoral neck stress fracture that then requires more major surgery. Therefore, femoral neck stress fractures must be treated aggressively. Early diagnosis with a high index of suspicion in a symptomatic athlete is necessary to assure good long-term results. A study of femoral neck stress fractures has shown that up to 50% of patients have a decreased level of activity after treatment compared with their preinjury level. All elite athletes decreased their activity to a recreational level after diagnosis of a femoral neck stress fracture [24]. Therefore, even in the absence of complications, femoral neck stress fractures can threaten the careers of elite athletes and cannot be considered a benign condition.

Femoral shaft stress fractures

Femoral shaft stress fractures can also be very difficult to diagnose. They demand a high index of suspicion in a symptomatic athlete. Patients normally complain of anterior thigh pain that is increased with activity and may also present with an antalgic gait and limp. On physical examination, the pain may radiate from the thigh into the groin or knee. The Fulcrum test is an excellent physical examination test. It places stress on the femoral fracture site and reproduces the pain the athlete normally experiences during activities (Fig. 5.6) [72●●].

Again, plain radiographs may typically be negative unless the pain has been present for a long time. If the plain radiographs show new periosteal bone formation and callus along the femoral shaft or a longitudinal fracture line in the cortex, the diagnosis can be established. Bone scanning, however, is the most sensitive test. Plain radiographs are useful for late confirmation of the diagnosis and are a means of following the extent of the healing process.

Most femoral shaft stress fractures are seen along the proximal and middle thirds of the medial side where the highest stresses are concentrated in the femur [44]; however, they can occur at any anatomic location.

Treatment

In comparison to femoral neck stress fractures, most femoral shaft stress fractures can be treated nonsurgically because there seems to be less risk of displacement [61,72●●]. The treatment program consists initially of protected touch-down weight bearing of the involved extremity with the patient using crutches. When the patient is off crutches and pain free, low-impact training can begin within the range the patient's symptoms allow. The athlete should advance slowly into progressive resistive exercises and increased impact loading until able to return to normal activities. Most athletes are able to return to activities between 8 and 14 weeks after onset of their injury.

Snapping hip syndrome

A variety of distinct entities, both intra- and extra-articular in origin, have been identified with the snapping hip syndrome. The athlete will typically complain of a snapping sensation in the hip that may be painful. This snapping sensation can usually be reproduced with certain distinct motions of the hip joint [5•]. The most common cause is irritation of the greater trochanteric bursa by the overriding iliotibial band. This results in a trochanteric bursitis and the snapping and discomfort may be reproduced during hip flexion and extension with the leg in internal rotation [24].

Other extra-articular causes of snapping hip syndrome can result from tenosynovitis of the iliopsoas tendon near its insertion at the lesser trochanter and the snapping of the iliopsoas tendon as it passes over the iliopectineal eminence [73]. In these athletes, hip abduction and external rotation may reproduce their symptoms.

Rarer causes of snapping hip syndrome include the iliofemoral ligaments riding over the femoral head and the snapping of the long head of the biceps femoris over the ischial tuberosity. Intra-articular pathology (*eg,* labral tears, loose bodies,

and synovial chondromatosis) can also cause snapping hip syndrome [5•].

Treatment

For trochanteric bursitis caused by irritation from the iliotibial band, treatment generally consists of a nonsurgical program of rest, nonsteroidal anti-inflammatory medications, strengthening of the gluteal muscles, and stretching the iliotibial band. Occasionally, local corticosteroid injection may be necessary to relieve the symptoms of trochanteric bursitis. In very rare cases that do not respond to nonoperative measures, surgical release of the iliotibial band may be performed [24].

Again, in athletes with tenosynovitis of the iliopsoas tendon, a nonsurgical program of anti-inflammatory medication and stretching exercises seems to relieve the snapping sensation. Surgical release or lengthening of the iliopsoas tendon has been described, but is rarely needed.

If intraarticular pathology of the hip can be identified and the athlete's symptoms do not respond to conservative measures, then surgical intervention may be required. This can be accomplished through either hip arthroscopy or formal arthrotomy, depending on the exact lesion present and the experience of the orthopedic surgeon.

Iliotibial-band friction syndrome

The iliotibial band (ITB) can cause symptoms in the proximal thigh at the greater trochanter of the hip. In general, problems with the ITB are usually

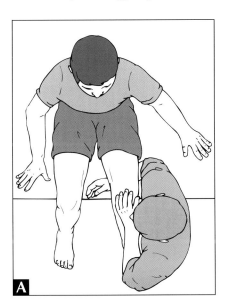

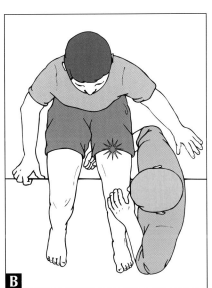

FIGURE 5.6

A The fulcrum test as described by Johnson *et al.* initially begins with the examiner's forearm under the distal thigh as gentle downward pressure is applied to the top of the knee. **B,** As the examiner's forearm is moved proximally, pain is felt by the patient when the arm is directly under the region of stress fracture of the femoral shaft. In our experience this seems to be a fairly sensitive test. (*From* Johnson *et al.* [72]; with permission.)

seen at its distal extent along the lateral aspect of the knee. This is an overuse condition seen in long-distance runners and other athletes who participate in sports requiring repetitive knee flexion. When the knee is extended, the ITB lays anterior to the lateral epicondyle of the femur. As the knee is flexed, the ITB passes over the condyle to lie posteriorly. This can cause irritation and inflammation of the bursa between the ITB and the lateral femoral condyle [74].

Athletes with this condition typically present with pain along the lateral aspect of the knee during activities. The pain is normally localized over the lateral epicondyle, which is proximal to the lateral joint line. These patients have pain with active or passive motion of the knee but have a full range of motion in relation to the contralateral knee. There should be minimal pain along the joint line itself.

Tightness of the ITB seems to be the most common cause of this condition. Since this is a chronic overuse injury, it usually results from rapid changes in training, especially from emphasis on hill training in runners, cyclists, and other long-distance athletes. Radiographs are usually normal.

Treatment

The most effective treatment strategy seems to be prevention of the problem, if possible [75]. Most athletes will respond to a nonoperative treatment regimen consisting of ITB stretching, anti-inflammatory medications, ultrasound, application of ice, and alterations in their training schedule. If symptoms persist, local corticosteroid injections may also be used. Assessment of the athlete's biomechanics, foot pronation, running shoes, and shoe modifications may all help prevent this ITB syndrome in runners. For cyclists, adjustments to the seat and peddle of the bicycle and changes in their training program may be beneficial. If the conservative treatment program fails and the athlete continues to be symptomatic, surgical intervention may be indicated [76]. These procedures involve removing a portion of the ITB or the prominent lateral ridge of the femur or may be procedures that effectively lengthen the ITB itself.

REFERENCES AND RECOMMENDED READING

Recently published papers of particular interest have been highlighted as:
* •   Of special interest
* ••   Of outstanding interest

1. O'Donoghe DH: *Treatment of Injuries in Athletes.* Philadelphia: WB Saunders; 1970.

2. Walsh ZT, Micheli LJ: Hip dislocation in a high school football player. *Phys Sports Med* 1989, 17:112–120.

3. Sim FH, Scott HG: Injuries of the Pelvis and Hip in Athletes. In *The Lower Extremity and Spine in Sports Medicine.* Edited by Nicholas JA, Hershmann EB. St. Louis: CV Mosby; 1986.

4.•• Gross ML, Nasser S, Finerman, GAM: Hip and pelvis. In *Orthopaedic Sports Medicine.* Edited by DeLee JC, Drez D. Philadelphia: WB Saunders; 1994.
Superb chapter on the diagnosis and treatment of athletic injuries of the hip and pelvis.

5.• Paletta GA, Andrish, JT: Injuries about the hip and pelvis in the young athlete. *Clin Sports Med* 1995, 14:591–628.
Review of injuries of the hip and pelvic region that can occur in young athletes.

6. Cooper DE, Warren RF, Barnes R: Traumatic subluxation of the hip resulting in aseptic necrosis and chondrolysis in a professional football player. *Am J Sports Med* 1991, 19:322–324.

7. Epstein HC: *Traumatic Dislocation of the Hip.* Baltimore: Williams and Wilkins; 1980.

8. Lieberman JR, Altchek DW, Salvati EA: Recurrent dislocation of a hip with a labral lesion: treatment with a modified Bankart-type repair. *J Bone Joint Surg Am* 1993, 75A:1524–1527.

9. Koval KJ: Hip: Trauma. In *OKU 5 Home Study Syllabus.* Edited by Kasser JR. Rosemont: American Academy of Orthopaedic Surgeons; 1996.

10. Dreinhofer KE, Schwarzkopf SR, Haas NP, *et al.*: Isolated traumatic dislocation of the hip: long-term results in 50 patients. *J Bone Joint Surg Br* 1994, 76:6–12.

11. Canale, ST, King EK: Pelvic and Hip Fractures. In *Fractures in Children.* Edited by Rockwood CA, Wilkins KE, King R. Philadelphia: JB Lippincott; 1991.

12. Waters PM, Millis MB: Hip and pelvic injuries in the young athlete. *Clin Sports Med* 1988, 7:513–526.

13. Finby N, Begg CF: Traumatic avulsion of ischial epiphysis simulating neoplasm. *N Y State J Med* 1967, 67:2488–2490.

14. Metzmaker JN, Pappas AM: Avulsion fractures of the pelvis. *Am J Sports Med* 1985, 13:349–358.

15. Sundar M, Carty H: Avulsion fractures of the pelvis in children: a report of 32 fractures and their outcome. *Skeletal Radiol* 1994, 23:85–90.

16. Veselko M, Smrkolj V: Avulsion of the anterior-superior iliac spine in athletes: Case Reports. *J Trauma* 1994, 36:444–446.

17. Schlonsky J, Olix ML: Functional disability following avulsion fracture of the ischial epiphysis: report of two cases. *J Bone Joint Surg Am* 1972, 54A:641–644.

18. Wootton JR, Cross MJ, Holt KW: Avulsion of the ischial apophysis: the case for open reduction and internal fixation. *J Bone Joint Surg Br* 1990, 72B:625–627.

19. Dimon JH: Isolated fractures of the lesser trochanter of the femur. *Clin Orthop* 1972, 82:144–148.

20. Frost A, Bauer M: Skier's Hip: A new clinical entity? *J Orthop Trauma* 1991, 5:47–50.

21. Davidson BL, Weinstein SL: Hip fractures in children: a long-term follow-up study. *J Pediatr Orthop* 1992, 12:355–358.

22. Gross ML, Wolff A, Distefano M: Hip fractures in children. *Orthop Grand Rounds* 1986, 3:9.

23.• Arrington ED, Miller MD: Skeletal muscle injuries. *Orthop Clin N Amer* 1995, 26:411–421.
Review of muscle anatomy, physiology, and injury and its treatment.

24. Campbell JD: Injuries to the pelvis, hip and thigh. In *OKU Sports Medicine*. Edited by Griffin LY. Rosemont: American Academy of Orthopaedic Surgeons; 1994.

25. Walton M, Rothwell AG: Reactions of thigh tissues of sheep to blunt trauma. *Clin Orthop* 1983, 176:273–281.

26. Ciullo JV, Zarins B: Biomechanics of the musculotendinous unit: relation to athletic performance and injury. *Clin Sports Med* 1983, 2:71–86.

27. Jackson DW, Feagin JA: Quadriceps contusions in young athletes. *J Bone Joint Surg Am* 1973, 55:95–105.

28. Aronen JG, Chronister R, Ove PN, *et al*: Thigh contusions: minimizing the length of time before return to full athletic activities with early immobilization in 120 degrees of knee flexion. *Orthop Trans* 1991, 15:77–78.

29. Young JL, Laskowski ER, Rock MG: Subspeciality clinics: physical medicine and rehabilitation: thigh injuries in athletes. *Mayo Clin Proc* 1993, 68:1099–1106.

30. Lipscomb AB, Thomas ED, Johnston RK: Treatment of myositis ossificans traumatica in athletes. *Am J Sports Med* 1976, 4:111–120.

31. Rothwell AG: Quadriceps hematoma: a prospective clinical study. *Clin Orthop* 1982, 171:97–103.

32. Ryan JB, Wheeler JH, Hopkinson WJ, *et al*: Quadriceps contusions: west point update. *Am J Sports Med* 1991, 19:299–304.

33. Booth DW, Westers BM: The Management of Athletes with Myositis Ossificans Traumatica. *Can J Sport Sci* 1989, 14:10–16.

34. Sawyer JR, Myers MA, Rosier RN, Puzas JE: Heterotopic ossification: clinical and cellular aspects. *Calcif Tissue Int* 1991, 49:208–215.

35. Bosse A, Wanner KF, Weber A, M ller KM: Morphological and clinical aspects of heterotopic ossification in sports. *Int J Sports Med* 1994, 15:325–329.

36. Doukas WC, Christensen KP: Surgical treatment of symptomatic, posttraumatic heterotopic ossification in the abductor mass off the pubic arch. *Orthopedics* 1996, 19:893–895.

37. Colisimo AJ, Ireland ML: Thigh compartment syndrome in a football athlete: a case report and review of the literature. *Med Sci Sports Exerc* 1992, 24:958–963.

38. Winternitz WA, Methany JA, Wear LC: Acute compartment syndrome of the thigh in sports related injuries not associated with femoral fractures. *Am J Sports Med* 1992, 20:476–478.

39. Wise JJ, Fortin PT: Bilateral, exercise-induced thigh compartment syndrome diagnosed as exertional rhabdomyolysis. *Am J Sports Med* 1997, 25:126–129.

40. Kahan JSG, McClellan RT, Burton DS: Acute bilateral compartment syndrome of the thigh induced by exercise. *J Bone Joint Surg Am* 1994, 76:1068–1071.

41. Robinson D, On E, Halperin N: Anterior compartment syndrome of the thigh in athletes: indications for conservative treatment. *J Trauma* 1992, 32:183–186.

42. Mubarak SJ, Owen CA, Hargens AR, *et al.*: Acute compartment syndromes: diagnosis and treatment with the aid of the wick catheter. *J Bone Joint Surg Am* 1978, 60:1091–1095.

43. Zarins B, Ciullo JV: Acute Muscle and Tendon Injuries in Athletes. *Clin Sports Med* 1983, 2:167–182.

44. Brunet ME, Hontas RB: The thigh. In *Orthopaedic Sports Medicine*. Edited by DeLee JC, Drez D. Philadelphia: WB Saunders; 1994.

45. Renstrˆm PAHF: Tendon and muscle injuries in the groin area. *Clin Sports Med* 1992, 815–827.

46. Åkermark C, Johansson C. Tenotomy of the adductor longus tendon in the treatment of chronic groin pain in athletes. *Am J Sports Med* 1992, 20:640–643.

47. Kälebo P, Karlsson J, Swärd L, Peterson L: Ultrasonography of chronic tendon injuries in the groin. *Am J Sports Med* 1992, 20:634–639.

48.• Holt MA, Keene JS, Graf BK, Helwig DC: Treatment of osteitis pubis in athletes: results of corticosteroid injections. *Am J Sports Med* 1995, 23:601–606.
Study finding an earlier return to athletics for athletes injected with corticosteroids for treatment of osteitis pubis.

49. Batt ME, McShane JM, Dillingham MF: Osteitis pubis in collegiate football players. *Med Sci Sports Exerc* 1995, 27:629–33.

50. Fricker PA, Taunton JE, Ammann W: Osteitis pubis in athletes: infection, inflammation or injury? *Sports Med* 1991, 12:266–279.

51. Sallay PI, Friedman RL, Coogan PG, Garrett WE: Hamstring muscle injuries among water skiers: functional outcome and prevention. *Am J Sports Med* 1996, 24:130–136.

52. Pomeranz SJ, Heidt RS: MR Imaging in the prognostication of hamstring injury. *Radiology* 1993, 189:897–900.

53. Upton PAH, Noakes TD, Juritz JM: Thermal pants may reduce the risk of recurrent hamstring injuries in rugby players. *Br J Sports Med* 1996, 30:57–60.

54. Orava S, Kujala UM: Rupture of the ischial origin of the hamstring muscles. *Am J Sports Med* 1995, 23:702–705.

55. Fullerton LR: Femoral neck stress fractures. *Sports Med* 1990, 9:192–197.

56. Hershman EB, Lombardo J, Bergfeld JA: Femoral shaft stress fractures in athletes. *Clin Sports Med* 1990, 9:111–119.

57. Clement DB, Amman W, Taunton JE, *et al.*: Exercise-induced stress injuries to the femur. *Int J Sports Med* 1993, 14:347–352.

58. Hartley JB: "Stress" or fatigue fractures of bone. *Br J Radiol* 1943, 16:255–267.

59. Roub LW, Gumerman LW, Hanley EN, *et al.*: Bone stress: a radionuclide imaging perspective. *Radiology* 1979, 132:431–438.

60. Sterling JC, Edelstein DW, Calvo RD, Webb, R: Stress fractures in the athlete: diagnosis and management. *Sports Med* 1992, 14:336–346.

61. Monteleone, GP: Stress fractures in the athlete. *Orthop Clin North Am* 1995, 26:423–432.

62. Reeder MT, Dick BH, Atkins JK, Pribis AB, Martinez JM: Stress fractures: current concepts of diagnosis and treatment. *Sports Med* 1996, 22:198–212.

63. Savoca CJ: Stress fractures: a classification of the earliest radiographic signs. *Radiology* 1991, 100:519–534.

64. Martire JR: The role of nuclear medicine bone scans in evaluating pain in athletic injuries. *Clin Sports Med* 1987, 6:713–737.

65. Zwas ST, Elkanovitch R, Frank, G: Interpretation and classification of bone scintigraphic findings in stress fractures. *J Nucl Med* 1987, 28:452–457.

66. Prather JL, Nusynowitz ML, Snowdy HA, *et al.*: Scintigraphic findings in stress fractures. *J Bone Joint Surg Am* 1977, 59:869–874.

67. Sterling JC, Webb RF, Meyers MC, Calvo RD: False negative bone scan in a female runner. *Med Sci Sports Exerc* 1993, 179–185.

68. Keene JS, Lash EG: Negative bone scan in a femoral neck stress fracture. *Am J Sports Med* 1992, 20:234–236.

69. Shin AY, Morin WD, Gorman JD, Jones SB, Lapinsky AS: The superiority of magnetic resonance imaging in differentiating the cause of hip pain in endurance athletes. *Am J Sports Med* 1996, 24:168–176.

70. Fullerton LR, Snowdy HA: Femoral neck stress fractures. *Am J Sports Med* 1988, 16:365–377.

71. Devas MB: *Stress Fractures*. New York, Churchill Livingstone, 1975.

72.•• Johnson AW, Weiss CB, Wheeler DL: Stress fractures of the femoral shaft in athletes: more common than expected. *Am J Sports Med* 1994, 22:248–256.
Excellent physical examination test to aid in the diagnosis of femoral shaft stress fracture.

73. Cardinal E, Buckwalter KA, Capello WN, Duval N: US of the snapping iliopsoas tendon. *Radiology* 1996, 198:521–522.

74. Cox JS, Blanda JB: The knee. In *Orthopaedic Sports Medicine*. Edited by DeLee JC, Drez D. Philadelphia: W.B. Saunders; 1994.

75. Firer P: Aetiology and treatment of iliotibial band friction syndrome abstract. *J Bone Joint Surg Br* 1990, 72:742.

76. Martens M, Libbrecht P, Burssens A: Surgical treatment of the iliotibial band friction syndrome. *Am J Sports Med* 1989, 17:651–654.

KNEE LIGAMENT PROBLEMS

Paul J. Schreck and Douglas W. Jackson

Ligament stability of the knee joint depends primarily on the anterior cruciate ligament (ACL), the posterior cruciate ligament (PCL), the medial collateral ligament (MCL), and the posterolateral ligamentous complex (PLC), which includes the lateral collateral ligament (LCL), arcuate ligament, popliteofibular ligament, and popliteus tendon. If injury to the knee compromises one or several of these structures, altered knee kinematics can lead to functional instability and further compromise of the meniscus and articular cartilage and can predispose to further degenerative changes. The goal of diagnosis and effective treatment is to restore normal knee kinematics and permit return to the preinjury activity level.

HISTORY AND PHYSICAL EXAMINATION

The preinjury knee status as well as the mechanism of the current injury may provide useful clues to diagnosis. The most common mechanisms causing ACL injuries are either valgus-rotation or hyperextension. Another potential mechanism is a backward fall in skiing with associated sudden and maximal quadriceps contraction. The patient sustaining an ACL disruption often reports a characteristic audible "pop," the onset of rapid swelling, and the inability to continue play.

Isolated PCL injury is typically related to a posterior force on the anterior tibia of a flexed knee. This can occur with dropping to the knees with a plantar-flexed ankle in sports or a dashboard injury in a motor vehicle accident. A valgus stress may create an isolated MCL injury, but with high-energy injury and rotation of the tibia, a combined ACL and MCL or PCL and MCL injury can result. Varus knee displacement with rotation or a blow to the anteromedial tibia is a typical element of LCL and PLC injury.

A sideline examination immediately following injury permits knee ligament assessment before swelling, joint effusion, and muscle spasm have set in. If initial assessment is limited because of pain, guarding, and spasm, sequential examinations are warranted to establish a more accurate diagnosis. Aspiration of the knee joint effusion may confirm a hemarthrosis or fat globules, which suggest osteochondral fracture. A lidocaine injection following the aspiration is considered by some to allow a more comfortable and reliable examination.

Ligamentous stability testing should always involve comparison with the contralateral limb. Lachman anterior laxity testing and assessment of the presence of a pivot shift are an essential part of the routine examination. Particularly for subtle findings and for quantitation of the degree of laxity, instrumented measurement may be helpful. We have used the KT-1000 (Medmetric, San Diego, CA) instrumented measurement device. Placing a thigh bolster or the examiner's knee under the patient's thigh often allows the patient to relax the hamstrings, which is necessary for an accurate examination (Fig. 6.1).

Assessment of the PCL is best done with a posterior drawer maneuver with the knee flexed at 90°. The normal step-off of the anteromedial tibial in relation to the femur at 90° is approximately 1 cm anterior. If the tibia is flush with the medial femoral condyle or posterior to it, this is consistent with a grade II or III injury, respectively. The quadriceps active test is useful to confirm the posterior tibial step-off when other examination findings are subtle. To perform the quadriceps active test, the patient places the heel on the bed with the knee flexed at 90°. The patient is asked to slide his heel distally on the bed, which fires the quadriceps muscle. In a PCL-deficient knee, the tibia is visibly subluxed anteriorly from a posteriorly sagging position.

Determination of an MCL or LCL injury is performed by a valgus or varus stress test, respectively, with the knee in 30° of flexion. Pain with a stress maneuver without significant difference in the side-to-side opening, focal tenderness, and swelling are consistent with a grade I injury. Increased opening compared with the contralateral side with a good endpoint represents a grade II injury. A lack of a definitive endpoint with stress usually reflects a grade III injury. Increased opening with a stress maneuver in full extension suggests disruption of either the ACL or the PCL, as

these act as secondary restraints to a varus or valgus moment. To evaluate for posterolateral complex injury, the patient is placed prone and an external rotation force applied to the feet with the knees first at 30 flexion and then at 90° flexion. An increase of 15° of rotation on the involved compared with the uninjured side is an abnormal finding. If there is increased rotation at 30°, the posterolateral complex (the popliteus tendon, arcuate complex, and the LCL) is injured. If there is increased rotation at 30° and even greater increased rotation at 90°, the PCL and the posterolateral complex are compromised. A positive reverse pivot shift is also typically present with a posterolateral complex injury.

IMAGING

We prefer to obtain plain radiographs in four views as part of the initial evaluation. Anteroposterior, lateral, tunnel, and Merchant views are taken. Secondary conditions such as degenerative changes and previous injury are evaluated. The lateral capsular avulsion fracture, or Segond fracture, may be seen with acute ACL tears. Particular attention is made to avulsion-type injuries with bony fragments seen at ligamentous insertion sites.

A magnetic resonance imaging (MRI) scan is an elective study that can provide a significant amount of information in terms of prognosis and treatment planning. Ligamentous injury can be confirmed

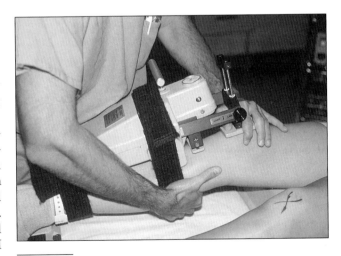

FIGURE 6.1

The degree of anteroposterior laxity is measured using an instrumented measurement device and compared with the uninjured side.

with MRI and can define meniscal pathology and osteochondral injuries, which could affect treatment decisions and preoperative patient counseling [1]. With an acute ACL tear, MRI often shows anterior lateral femoral condyle and posterior lateral tibial plateau bone bruising on gradient-echo sequencing. This is an almost pathognomonic finding of an acute ACL tear [2] (Fig. 6.2).

ANTERIOR CRUCIATE LIGAMENT

Treatment approach

The initial approach to the acute ACL injury is to limit swelling and to initiate therapy with an emphasis on attaining a full range of motion coupled with isometric quadriceps and hamstring exercises.

Factors considered in the determination of treatment include the degree of knee laxity, the associated ligamentous or meniscal injuries, and the patient's functional demand and expectations [3••]. Sports that require frequent changes in direction and speed are most likely to cause "giving way" episodes in the ACL-deficient knee and are considered high-risk activities. High-risk activities include basketball, soccer, football, volleyball, and skiing. Conversely, cycling, jogging, and swimming are considered low-risk activities and may be better tolerated in a patient with an ACL-deficient knee.

Overall, approximately one third of patients with an ACL tear will be satisfied with their knee function after appropriate rehabilitation is completed. Another one third of patients will experience problems primarily with athletic activity. Some of these patients can be treated nonoperatively. However, if the patient is not interested in activity modification and wishes to continue involvement in high-risk activities, reconstruction of the ACL is recommended. Another one third of patients will have difficulty with even minimal activity and will not be able to successfully cope with the knee instability without surgical reconstruction.

Advanced patient age alone is not a contraindication to ACL reconstruction. The majority of ligamentous reconstructions are performed on patients in their teens, 20s, and early 30s who are unwilling to modify their activity after ACL injury. A higher percentage of patients in their 40s and above are willing to discontinue high-risk activities. We have performed over 300 reconstructions in patients over 40 years of age who demonstrated disabling functional instability with their sports interests and who did not wish to modify their activities. If their primary complaint is instability, these patients have realized success with ACL reconstruction similar to the success achieved in younger patients.

Operative technique

Examination under anesthesia

A preoperative side-to-side ligamentous knee examination is performed under anesthesia. In addition, we recommend that an instrumented measurement be performed with emphasis on the manual maximum displacement prior to surgery. If the patient demonstrates an asymmetric pivot shift examination and a measured increase in anterior laxity of 5 mm on the injured side, the proce-

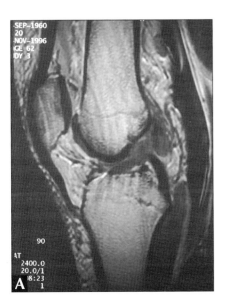 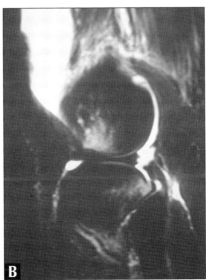

FIGURE 6.2

Magnetic resonance imaging (MRI) of an acute anterior cruciate ligament (ACL) tear. **A,** MRI demonstrates increased signal intensity within the ligament consistent with ACL tear. **B,** MRI using gradient echo sequence demonstrates the characteristic bone contusions of the posterior lateral tibial plateau and the anterior lateral femoral condyle.

dure would begin with the harvest of the autograft. Otherwise, diagnostic arthroscopy is performed prior to harvesting the graft.

Preparation

We preinject the incision and the portals with 15 to 20 mL of 0.25% bupivicaine with epinephrine to help decrease bleeding as well as for postoperative analgesia. Gravity inflow is used and a tourniquet is typically not necessary [4]. An arthroscopic pump can also be used, although it is not our preference.

Graft harvest: selection and technique

Autograft tissue such as bone-patellar tendon-bone (BPTB) or semitendinosis–gracilis hamstring (HS) tendon is our choice of graft. The majority of patients were treated with BPTB in the past because of superior graft fixation, reliable incorporation of the bone plugs, and excellent clinical results. Currently, improved fixation techniques have been developed for HS graft and essentially equivalent clinical results have been shown in recent studies [5••,6,7]. A quadrupled HS graft provides more collagen and has been shown to be even stronger than BPTB graft (Hecker *et al.*, Paper presented at the AOSSM Specialty Day conference, San Francisco, 1997). Additionally, some authors have reported an equally or more rapid rehabilitation with HS graft [8••], fewer patellofemoral problems, and a

smaller incision is used. The issue of anterior knee pain as related to graft selection is controversial and may be related to data obtained historically when patients were immobilized postoperatively or dissimilar rehabilitation was used. We will typically recommend HS graft, however, if there are premorbid patellofemoral symptoms.

Reconstruction using an allograft still has a role in ACL reconstruction [9]. Allograft disadvantages include a slower and less robust graft incorporation, a higher risk of failure, and a potential for disease transmission. Advantages include a lack of donor site morbidity, a smaller incision, and the availability of graft material particularly for simultaneous multiple ligament reconstructions [10]. We currently use allografts in cases of multiple ligament reconstructions, if there is a lack of donor site tissue, or at patient request. Fresh-frozen allografts are used after appropriate screening and testing is complete.

The central one third of the patellar tendon, usually 10 mm in width, is harvested with a double scalpel. An oscillating bone-plug harvester (Stryker, Kalamazoo, MI) is used to harvest the bone plugs. By selecting the appropriate-diameter bone-plug harvester to match the tunnel size, minimal trimming of the graft is necessary, which adds to the efficiency of this method. A #2 nylon passage suture and three #5 braided distal tensioning sutures are

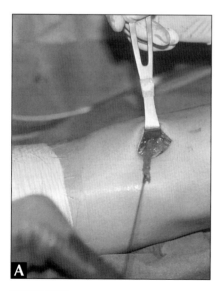
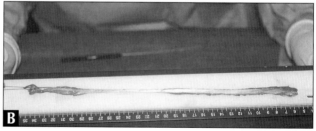
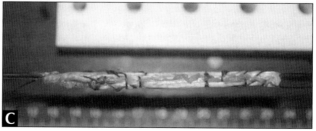

FIGURE 6.3

Hamstring graft. **A,** Semitendinosus tendon harvest through longitudinal skin incision, which will also be used for tibial bone tunnel site. Note the slightly distal anteromedial arthroscopic portal for this technique. **B,** Harvested semitendinosus tendon prior to preparation. **C,** Prepared quadrupled semitendinosus-gracilis graft. The graft is gathered with whip-stitch and proximal end marked at depth of insertion (30 mm).

placed. The graft is kept moist and held under tension until passage.

Hamstring graft harvest is done through a 2- to 3-cm incision medial to the tibial tubercle at the insertion of the palpable pes anserinus tendons. The same incision will be used for the tibial tunnel. Typically both the semitendinosus and the gracilis are harvested and doubled over for a quadruple strand graft. A closed tendon harvester is used. If the semitendinosus tendon is long and robust, it can potentially be tripled or even quadrupled and the gracilis spared. Preparation of the HS graft depends on planned fixation technique. Our preference is interference screw fixation using the Donjoy RCI screw (Smith-Nephew DonJoy, Carlsbad, CA). The quadrupled graft is then gathered at its proximal and distal ends with a #2 ethibond whip-stitch suture. A #2 nylon passage suture proximally and #2 braided nonabsorbable tensioning sutures distally are placed. The proximal graft is marked at 30 mm, which will be the depth of the femoral tunnel and the level of insertion (Fig. 6.3). The graft diameter is then measured with a graft sizer to assess the minimum diameter tunnel through which the graft will pass.

Several excellent alternative techniques of hamstring graft fixation have been developed and demonstrated, including a two-incision suture post-fixation and a single-incision Endobutton (Acufex Microsurgical, Mansfield, MA) fixation technique. We have found the Endobutton to be particularly useful in younger patients to avoid placement of hardware across open physeal plates. Further clinical study is needed to evaluate the outcomes of the various fixation methods.

Arthroscopy and notchplasty

A diagnostic arthroscopy is performed while an assistant simultaneously prepares the graft. All treatable chondral and meniscal pathology is addressed. If there is a repairable meniscal tear, meniscal sutures are placed and tied, or meniscal arrows (Bionix, Inc., Malvern, PA) are used, and then the ligament reconstruction is completed.
If there is significant notch stenosis, a notchplasty is performed [11•]. A small curved osteotome is used to open the anterior notch and the bone fragments are removed with a grasper. The notch is tapered from anterior to posterior with an arthroscopic burr or resector (Fig. 6.4). Care should be taken to not remove excessive articular cartilage. A probe should be used to confirm identification of the over-the-top position. Awareness of the normal ridge at the origin of the anterior cruciate ligament should prevent inadvertent anterior femoral tunnel placement. Additionally, we prefer an over-the-top guide (Stryker), which will provide a 1- to 2-mm wall posterior to the femoral tunnel.

Femoral tunnel

Many of the early failures of ACL reconstruction were likely related to poor tunnel placement. Too anterior of a femoral tunnel causes the knee to be tight in flexion and the graft at risk for rupture. Reproducible and accurate tunnel placement is critical regardless of the method used.

We prefer to guide the femoral tunnel placement using the posterior aspect of the notch with an over-the-top guide. Once the diameter of tunnel is determined, a guide with appropriate offset is selected to leave a 1- to 2-mm rim of bone posterior to the tunnel (Figs. 6.5 and 6.6) This technique maintains an intact posterior cortex for interference fixation and prevents placement of the femoral tunnel anteriorly. After the notchplasty is performed, the guidewire position is marked using the over-the-top guide in the 10:30 or 1:30 position (for a right or left knee,

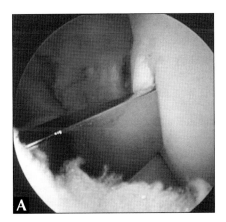
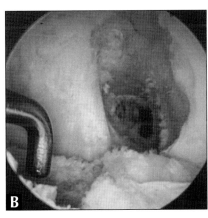

FIGURE 6.4

A, A small curved osteotome is used to open the anterior notch. **B,** An arthroscopic burr is then used to taper the notch anterior to posterior.

respectively). This location is checked visually and the posterior wall palpated with a probe to confirm correct positioning.

With the BPTB technique, typically a 10-mm tunnel is drilled over a guidewire through the tibial tunnel, once it has been created. The tunnel is made 3 to 5 mm deeper than the leading bone plug (25 mm for a 20-mm bone plug).

If the HS technique is used, the femoral tunnel is marked as above and then the knee is brought nearly into maximal flexion. This degree of knee flexion is easily reproduced by appropriately positioning a footrest under the drapes preoperatively (Fig. 6.7). Next, a guidewire is passed through the anteromedial portal into the femur at the marked point and then passed out the anterolateral thigh. The femoral tunnel is drilled through the anteromedial portal for two reasons. First, a specialized stepped router (Smith & Nephew, Donjoy, Carlsbad, CA) is used that cannot pass through the tibial tunnel because of its shape, which matches the interference screw with a countersink for the RCI screw head. Second, the interference screw is thus able to be placed through the anteromedial portal in the same degree of knee flexion, resulting in precise collinearity with the tunnel.

A cannulated 4.5-mm drill is passed over this guidewire to just breach the lateral femoral cortex and then it is withdrawn. The tunnel is then drilled with the stepped router. The size router selected and thus the tunnel diameter created is determined by selecting the smallest diameter through which the prepared HS graft can pass. The guide pin has an eyelet that is used to pass a doubled strand of heavy suture through the anteromedial portal and out the femoral tunnel, with the free ends out of the anterolateral thigh. The ends of this suture are clamped together and the suture is later retrieved for graft passage.

Tibial tunnel

Proper tibial tunnel placement is as critical as proper femoral tunnel placement [12]. If the tibial tunnel is placed too far anteriorly, graft impingement on the roof of the notch can occur. This is manifest clinically in the postoperative period by difficulty in obtaining full extension, a persistent effusion, and, potentially, graft failure. The tibial tunnel is positioned centrally within the footprint of the ACL adjacent to the posterior border of the anterior horn of the lateral meniscus. The PCL is also a good landmark and the drill guide tip should be about 7 mm anterior to the PCL base. When properly placed, the ACL touches and deviates slightly around the PCL.

For a BPTB graft, the length of the tibial tunnel is easily determined by subtracting 50 mm (an estimate of femoral tunnel depth and intra-articular distance) from the total graft length [13]. This should prevent protrusion of the bone plug from the tibial tunnel. Once the guidewire is appropriately positioned, a cannulated coring reamer with a diameter 1 mm greater than the bone plug diameter is used for easy graft passage. The coring reamer removes the ACL tibial stump and provides a source of bone graft for the plug harvest sites. The femoral tunnel is now created with a calibrated cannulated acorn drill over a guidewire through the tibial tunnel with the knee in about 90° flexion. The guidewire is only advanced about 1 cm to avoid cutting the wire with the drill. Any loose fragments of bone in the joint are removed at this time. The integrity of the posterior wall is confirmed with a probe.

For a HS graft, a standard cannulated reamer of the smallest diameter that the graft will pass through is used. The tunnel is made 50 mm in length. There is always excess graft when the tendons are doubled over, so it is not likely that the tunnel could be made

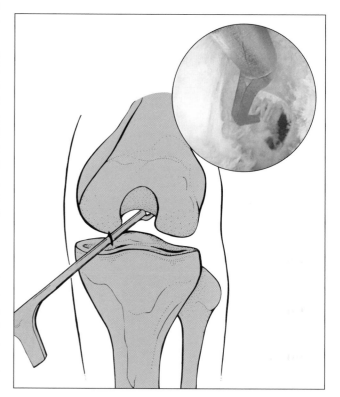

FIGURE 6.5

The over-the-top guide is positioned along the posterior aspect of the notch in the 10:30 or 1:30 position (right or left knee, respectively) and the center of the femoral tunnel is marked.

too long. However, if a single tendon graft is used in a tripled manner, the tunnel length may need to be shortened. There is no need to create a countersunk area at the tibial tunnel because a nonheaded soft tissue interference screw will be used. It is important to clear away the soft tissue from the anterior tibial entrance site with an elevator so the graft does not bind up during passage. Additionally, the entrance of the tunnel into the joint should be smoothed with a rasp or shaver to avoid a sharp edge on which the graft could abrade.

Graft implantation

For the BPTB technique, a Beath pin (guide pin with eyelet) is passed retrograde through the tibial and femoral tunnels and out the anterolateral thigh. The nylon passage suture on the graft is threaded through the eyelet and pulled out proximally. If the bone plug size allows, the graft is usually reversed with the tibial plug placed in the femoral tunnel (Fig. 6.8). We advance the graft until the bone plug

is flush with or recessed slightly beyond the tunnel opening. The femoral plug should be positioned so the collagen is posterolateral in the tunnel. A clamp or grasper is used to maintain the proper orientation of the graft as it is advanced into the tunnel.

For the HS technique, the previously placed #2 nylon suture is retrieved through the tibial tunnel using an arthroscopic grasper. The graft passage sutures are threaded through the looped end of the #2 nylon suture and passed retrograde through the tunnels. The graft itself is then advanced with a snug graft to tunnel fit but without excess resistance. The graft must advance to the previously marked level of 30 mm. If the graft does not advance easily, residual soft tissue at the anterior tibial tunnel entrance may need to be cleared.

Graft fixation

For the BPTB technique, a 7 mm × 20 mm interference screw is passed over a guidewire that has been positioned anteromedially in the tunnel against the

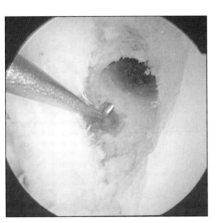

FIGURE 6.6
After drilling, a 1- to 2-mm rim of bone remains posterior to the femoral tunnel.

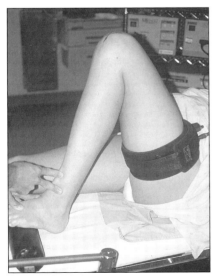

FIGURE 6.7
When performing the hamstring anterior cruciate ligament technique, the heel is placed on a foot positioner located under the drapes to accurately reproduce the knee flexion angle for tunnel drilling and interference screw fixation.

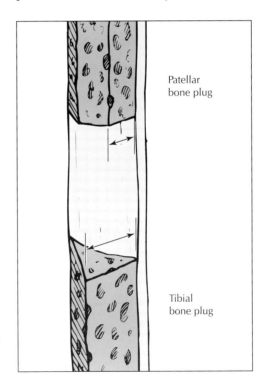

Patellar bone plug

Tibial bone plug

FIGURE 6.8
Added offset of cancellous bone to graft provides greater protection from cutting of the graft at the femoral tunnel with the interference screw. Thus the tibial bone plug typically is used in the femoral tunnel.

cancellous surface of the bone plug (Fig. 6.9). The knee is flexed at approximately 110° while the screw is advanced to avoid divergence of the graft and screw [14]. The screw is advanced until it is flush with the end of the bone plug. The integrity of the femoral fixation is then tested by firmly pulling the distal tension sutures with the knee still in flexion.

Traction is then applied to the tibial graft sutures and the knee is cycled through a range of motion with a finger on the tip of the tibial bone plug. If correctly placed, the graft will shorten by a millimeter or so when the knee is brought into full flexion. By palpation, it should be noted that the distal bone plug is able to move freely in the tibial tunnel to allow graft tensioning. With the knee in 25° to 30° of flexion and a slight posterior displacement force on the proximal tibia, manual traction is applied to the

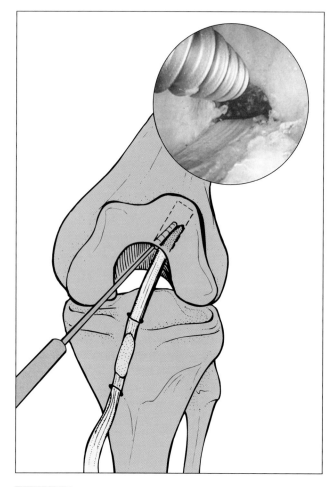

FIGURE 6.9

An interference screw is passed over a guidewire positioned anteromedially in the femoral tunnel against the cancellous surface of the bone plug.

graft. A 9 mm × 25 mm interference screw is inserted over a guidewire between the plug and the tunnel wall. The graft and screw should not extend beyond the tibial cortex or they could cause irritation of the overlying skin and soft tissue. The knee is again cycled to ensure a full range of motion. A "pop" or "click" palpated during cycling is suggestive of fixation failure. A Lachman test is performed to confirm knee joint stability

With the HS graft, the fixation technique is very similar with several exceptions. The femoral RCI interference screw (Smith & Nephew, Donjoy, Carlsbad, CA) is inserted over a guidewire through the anteromedial portal with the knee in the same degree of flexion as when the femoral tunnel was drilled. A fixed footrest under the drapes provides a simple reproducible method to reproduce the knee flexion angle (*see* Fig. 6.7). To engage the screw, the screwdriver is tapped with a mallet. The screw is advanced until the head seats firmly within the countersunk bone. The graft fixation is tested as above and the knee ranged. Tibial fixation proceeds as with the BPTB technique but using a soft tissue interference screw (Smith & Nephew; Donjoy, Carlsbad, CA). The rounded head of the RCI screw decreases its potential as a stress riser as it abuts the midgraft in the femoral tunnel, but the RCI is not required on the tibial side because of the location at the end of the graft. The range of motion and stability are tested similar to the BPTB technique. If satisfactory, the excess graft is cut distally and the passage sutures removed.

Bone graft and closure
The arthroscope is reintroduced into the joint to confirm there is no graft impingement on full extension and to perform a final inspection for any loose debris.

With the BPTB technique, the patellar and tibial defects each are filled with half of the tibial tunnel bone core, which is trimmed to fit the defects. The bone grafts are held in place by suturing the overlying soft tissue. The patellar defect is loosely approximated with interrupted suture and the peritenon is then meticulously repaired with a running 2.0 absorbable suture. With the HS technique, the sartorius fascial layer is reapproximated with absorbable suture. The subcutaneous tissue and skin is closed in layers and steristrips applied to the wound.

The joint is injected with 20 mL of 0.25% bupivicaine with 1:200,000 epinephrine and 4 mg of intra-articular morphine preparation [15] for postoperative pain control. This intra-articular analgesic protocol has facilitated performance of ACL reconstruction surgery at our facility on an outpatient basis. A postoperative manual maximum KT-1000 arthrometer testing is performed. If the side-to-side difference is greater than 2 mm, the graft fixation and tension as well as tunnel placement must be reassessed. A sterile dressing, compressive stocking, and knee immobilizer are then applied and the patient discharged to home when comfortable.

Rehabilitation

The postoperative courses and rehabilitation programs for both the BPTB and HS graft reconstructions are identical. Immediate weight-bearing as tolerated with crutches and a knee immobilizer is permitted. The knee is kept immobilized in extension during sleep and weight-bearing for the first 4 weeks. The brace is discontinued after 4 weeks or when the patient has adequate quadriceps control, full extension, and minimal joint effusion. Range of motion and quadriceps strengthening exercises as instructed by physical therapy are begun within days. An emphasis is placed on early symmetric knee extension [16].

Progression with the rehabilitation program and advancement toward sports activities is highly individualized. Patients are encouraged to use a stationary bike at 3 weeks and progress to a stair-climbing machine. Typically, patients are able to jog in the pool within 2 months and jog on the road by 3 months. Return to agility and sport-specific drills is permitted at 4 to 5 months. Return to high-risk activities may be allowed as early as 6 months and is based on a full and painless range of motion with quadriceps and hamstring strength within 10% of the contralateral limb. Most individuals take longer to heal, however, and will reach their maximum improvement at 1 to 2 years. Although there is little evidence supporting the effectiveness of functional braces, most of our patients involved in high-risk activities use one for the first year or so during sports.

MEDIAL COLLATERAL LIGAMENT

Isolated MCL injuries typically occur with a valgus loading force to the knee. Combined ACL and MCL injuries can occur with a blow to posterolateral leg, causing valgus, flexion, and internal rotation of the femur on the tibia.

Isolated MCL injuries, including grade III injuries, are treated nonoperatively. Clinical studies have demonstrated that MCL injuries treated nonsurgically regain motion and strength faster than those treated surgically with no difference in stability [17,18]. The initial treatment program includes rest, ice, anti-inflammatory drugs, and elevation. A knee immobilizer and crutches, used initially for comfort, are discontinued as symptoms allow after a few days. Physical therapy is initiated with an emphasis on early motion. Ligaments subjected to stress during healing may be stronger, have better collagen alignment, and heal faster than those treated with immobilization [19]. Rehabilitation of the quadriceps and the lower extremity musculature is advanced as the symptoms allow. We allow return to full activities when the patient is free of pain. Grade III injuries may require 2 to 3 months to return to unrestricted activities.

Particularly in athletes involved in high-risk activities, combined ACL and MCL injuries do poorly if treated nonoperatively [20]. We treat combined injuries with nonoperative management of the MCL [21•]. After an initial brief period of rest and immobilization, an emphasis is placed on restoration of a full range of motion. Once swelling has diminished and motion regained, reconstruction of the ACL proceeds with the technique described. Postoperatively, the knee is rehabilitated similar to the manner described for ACL reconstruction of an isolated ACL injury [22•].

POSTERIOR CRUCIATE LIGAMENT

Posterior cruciate ligament injuries are much less common than ACL injuries. A common mechanism of PCL injury in the athlete is pretibial trauma with a flexed knee, such as occurs when dropping to the knee with the foot in plantar flexion. Forced knee hyperflexion is also a common mechanism of injury of the PCL. Compared with ACL injury, an audible pop is not typically experienced and subsequent swelling develops more slowly. On examination there may be minimal or no detectable postinjury effusion. Most athletes are able to bear weight on the knee after an acute injury but perceive the knee as feeling abnormal. Because many PCL injuries are overlooked, routine careful screening for PCL injury is advised. MRI scan may be used as an adjunct to the examination by an experienced clinician and can often confirm the diagnosis and identify associated injuries. Whereas MRI can be helpful in evaluating the integrity of the PCL with acute injury, the MRI appearance of the PCL can be equivocal in cases of chronic PCL insufficiency.

Making treatment decisions

Nonoperative management of isolated PCL injuries has been shown to produce variably satisfactory results in up to 80% of patients [23,24]. Conversely, when there is associated ligamentous injury, a less-desirable functional result is likely [25]. Despite return to full activity in many cases, significant symptoms and degenerative changes from the injury seem to increase with time [26]. The degenerative changes occur predominately in the medial and patellofemoral compartments.

Results with reconstructive techniques in posteriorly unstable knees have been encouraging. However, some residual posterior laxity, grade I or even grade II, occurs postoperatively in a disconcerting number of cases. This may reflect persistent laxity or stretching out of the graft due to undiagnosed or unaddressed torn secondary stabilizing structures (combined injury) or shortcomings in current reconstructive techniques. New surgical methods are currently being developed to improve current techniques using multiple-strand reconstruction or open posterior–onlay grafting [27•]. Surgical reconstruction techniques have improved with added knowledge of anatomic and biomechanical factors [28,29]. If a single-bundle reconstructive technique is used, we believe that the PCL anterolateral bundle should be reconstructed as it is most functional in knee flexion.

Indications for surgery

As with ACL injuries, the treatment decision must be individualized. Our surgical indications for PCL reconstruction are somewhat narrower than those for the ACL. We will consider reconstruction in cases of isolated grade III posterior instability in high-demand athletes and in those patients who remain symptomatic despite rehabilitative therapy. We will also treat PCL injuries when combined with other ligamentous injuries such as posterolateral instability patterns. With combined ACL and PCL injuries, there are proponents of reconstructing only the ACL or only the PCL versus reconstructing both either simultaneously or in a staged manner. This injury represents a knee dislocation, and thus neurovascular assessment and appropriate intervention takes priority in the work-up. Symptomatic chronic PCL insufficiency is often associated with some degree of posterolateral instability. Both the PCL as well as the posterolateral corner, which is composed of the LCL, popliteal tendon, and arcuate ligament (arcuate complex), should be addressed. In patients with a varus knee deformity, a proximal tibial osteotomy should be considered to reduce the stress on the reconstructed complex postoperatively.

Operative technique

The goal of PCL reconstruction is to restore the anterior tibial step-off at 90° of flexion. We perform PCL reconstruction using an arthroscopically assisted technique. Patient positioning and examination under anesthesia are performed similar to that described for ACL reconstruction.

In the past we primarily used Achilles tendon allograft to reconstruct the PCL. Achilles tendon provides a long graft with excellent strength and there is abundant bone available to shape the plug with a conical taper to allow for press-fit fixation in the femoral tunnel. Because of concerns with allograft tissue, we currently prefer autologous BPTB graft for primary, isolated PCL reconstruction. However, with combined ligament injury and revision surgery, we still use allograft tissue for reasons of tissue availability.

Tibial tunnel preparation

The posterior tibial attachment of the PCL is debrided with a combination of curved elevators and curettes. Soft tissue is stripped 2 to 3 cm distally along the proximal tibial sulcus posteriorly. Good visualization and adequate debridement may require use of a 70° arthroscope and a posterior medial portal. Caution must be taken not to damage the neurovascular structures posteriorly.

A tibial PCL drill guide (Acufex, Mansfield, MA) is inserted through the anteromedial portal with the knee in 90° of flexion. The tip of the drill guide is hooked over the tibial plateau with the tip at the junction of the middle and distal thirds of the posteriorly sloping proximal tibial sulcus at the PCL insertion (Fig. 6.10). Distally, we prefer to position the drill guide just medial and distal to the tibial tubercle, or, alternatively, within the BPTB bone plug harvest defect. The tunnel can also be placed lateral to the tibial tubercle with elevation of the musculature, although this is not our preference. With combined ACL and PCL reconstruction, an adequate bone bridge must be created between tunnels. At the selected position, a longitudinal skin incision is made and dissection is carried down to bone.

The posterior neurovascular structures are most at risk during drilling of the tibial tunnel [30]. A guide pin is drilled up to but not through the posterior cortex. The guide pin position is confirmed with fluoroscopy and the pin is gently tapped through the cortex. A 10-mm cannulated reamer with a rounded rather than a square shoulder is used to lessen the chance of early posterior cortical break-out and subsequent neurovascular damage. A curette is held over the tip of the guidewire during reaming as well. The reamer should be visualized as

it cuts through the cortex of the tibia. A correctly placed tunnel will exit at the anatomic center of the PCL attachment in the tibial fossa. A curette is then used to round the tunnel edge to lessen the chance of graft abrasion.

Femoral tunnel preparation

The femoral drill guide is positioned so that the center of the femoral tunnel is in the anterior half of the footprint of the PCL approximately 8 to 10 mm proximal to the articular edge of the medial femoral condyle. This approximates the 10:00 position for a left knee and the 2:00 position for a right knee (Fig. 6.11). A 2-cm longitudinal skin incision is made midway between the medial femoral epicondyle and the articular margin. The vastus medialis obliquus is retracted superiorly and the medial femoral epicondyle is exposed. The

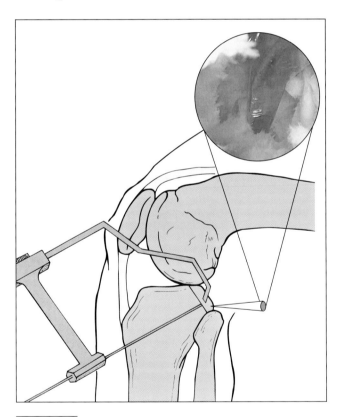

FIGURE 6.10

The tip of a posterior cruciate ligament tibial drill guide is hooked over the tibial plateau with the tip at the junction of the middle and distal thirds of the posteriorly sloping proximal tibial sulcus, with the knee in 90° of flexion.

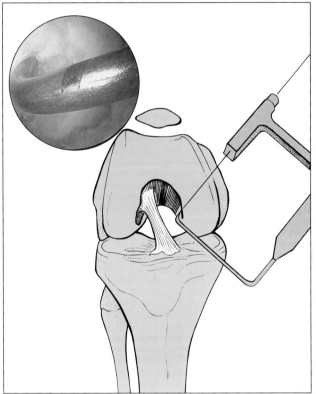

FIGURE 6.11

Intra-articularly, the posterior cruciate ligament (PCL) femoral drill guide tip is positioned 8- to 10-mm proximal to the articular margin at the 10:00 or 2:00 position (left or right knee, respectively) in the anterior half of the residual PCL footprint. Extra-articularly, the drill guide is positioned between the medial femoral epicondyle and the trochlea 5 to 8 mm from the articular margin.

femoral drill guide is positioned medially approximately 5 to 8 mm from the articular cartilage of the trochlea and the pin is advanced. The pin is thus angled slightly distal to proximal as it courses toward the notch, which will decrease the angle of the graft as it exits the tunnel. The tunnel is drilled with a 10-mm cannulated drill bit with a curette over the tip of the guidewire to protect intra-articular structures. Placing the tunnel too close to the articular surface may cause avascular necrosis and collapse. The tunnel entrance into the joint is smoothed with a curette and the reamings debrided from the joint.

Graft preparation

If an Achilles allograft is used, it is thawed in an antibiotic saline solution and then trimmed to shape. The bone plug is shaped conically, tapering from 12 to 10 mm to allow for press-fit fixation in the femoral tunnel. The collagenous portion of the tendon is gathered on itself and whip-stitched with a #2 ethibond suture. If an autologous BPTB graft is used, it is harvested and passage sutures placed in a similar manner to that described with ACL reconstruction. If desired, press-fit fixation of the BPTB graft at the femoral tunnel can be performed by shaping the tibial bone plug with a conical taper.

Graft implantation

A rubber catheter is passed retrograde through the tibial tunnel and out the femoral tunnel. Our preference is to use the catheter to pass a Gore Smoother (WL Gore and Associates., Inc., Flagstaff, AZ) into the joint. This instrument is used as a rasp to smooth the edges of the tunnel entrances and then can be used to feed graft passage suture through the joint.

Antegrade graft passage through the joint and around the steep angle at the intra-articular entrance to the tibial tunnel is facilitated in several ways. The leading portion of graft can be inserted into the end of the Gore Smoother before it is removed from the joint and the graft thus advanced as this device is removed. A hemostat or other smooth curved instrument can be used as a pulley over which the graft will turn to negotiate the angle and prevent abrasion of the graft. Additionally, the leading portion of graft can be lubricated with sterile lubrication jelly.

Graft fixation

The graft is first fixed into the femoral tunnel. Either the graft is tamped in to form a good press-fit or it is fixed with an interference screw once the graft position is determined along the length of the tunnels. The press-fit fixation can also be augmented if necessary with an interference screw. The graft is then tensioned and the graft visualized, assuring there is no impingement while the knee joint is cycled. The graft length should remain constant or shorten slightly with knee flexion.

The knee is brought up to 90° of flexion and the graft tensioned with an anterior drawer force applied [31]. Appropriate graft tension should restore the normal 1 cm step-off of the medial tibial plateau. The graft is fixed in the tibial tunnel with an interference screw for BPTB graft. For Achilles allograft, a screw and soft-tissue washer are placed through the graft and secured. The knee is ranged and stability checked. There should be a negative posterior drawer and normal tibial step-off. The wounds are closed in layers and the patient placed in a knee immobilizer.

Rehabilitation

Elevation and ice are used to minimize swelling and pain. Weight-bearing as tolerated is allowed with crutches in a knee immobilizer. The knee is kept immobilized in extension during sleep and weight-bearing for the first 4 to 6 weeks. The brace is discontinued after 6 weeks if the patient has adequate quadriceps control, full extension, and a nonantalgic gait.

Straight leg raises and quadriceps sets are performed with avoidance of open-chain hamstring exercises. Passive range-of-motion exercises are initiated with the goal of reaching 110° of flexion by the 12-week mark. It is imperative that anteriorly directed support be maintained under the posterior proximal tibia during range-of-motion activities. Posterior tibial sagging could potentially cause stretching out of the graft.

Return to agility and sport-specific drills is individualized. Patients are encouraged to use a stationary bike at 4 to 6 weeks and progress to a stair-climbing machine. Pool jogging can resume within 3 months and jogging on the road by 4 to 5 months. The return to normal sports activities is based on a full and painless range of motion with quadriceps and hamstring strength within 10% of the contralateral limb. Return to sports may be allowed at 8 to 12 months.

LATERAL COLLATERAL LIGAMENT AND POSTEROLATERAL COMPLEX

Isolated acute injury of the structures of the PLC, LCL, arcuate ligament, popliteofibular ligament, and popliteus tendon is uncommon. Treatment of PLC injuries is controversial and there are few reports available on the results of posterolateral repairs and reconstructions [32,33,34•]. Controversy also exists as to which anatomic structures should be the focus of reconstruction for posterolateral instability. Recent attention has focused on the popliteofibular ligament as a central element of posterolateral stability [35].

We manage acute isolated LCL injuries nonoperatively with a rehabilitation program similar to that with MCL injuries. Patients with grade I and II injuries usually return to sports within 3 to 6 weeks if they are free of pain and they have a full range of motion. Those with grade III injuries may require a hinged knee brace and an extended period of rehabilitation. Persistent symptoms usually indicate a combined injury such as a PLC and PCL injury, and operative intervention may be required.

A PCL injury associated with greater than 10 mm of posterior laxity suggests a combined ligamentous injury. In the case of PLC and PCL combined injury, the PCL is reconstructed first. If significant lateral instability persists after PCL graft fixation is performed, the posterolateral structures are explored intraoperatively. In our experience with cases of symptomatic chronic PCL and posterolateral injury, the PCL is the cornerstone of the reconstruction.

If varus alignment exists with posterolateral instability, we first perform a high tibial osteotomy to eliminate the varus moment, which could stretch out a ligamentous repair. This procedure alone may eliminate the symptomatic varus thrust and thus be therapeutic. If symptoms persist after recovery, ligamentous reconstruction is then performed.

Combined ACL-LCL injuries are managed with ACL reconstruction and then the lateral stability is assessed intraoperatively with stress testing. The ACL reconstruction typically provides sufficient stability to then treat the LCL component of the injury nonoperatively. If significant lateral laxity persists after fixation of the ACL graft, we explore and repair the lateral and posterolateral structures. The anatomy of the posterolateral structures is more easily defined during the acute period and thus repair of the posterolateral structures is more feasible. We prefer to address combined ACL and LCL injuries in the acute period because our results are better than if the combined injuries were treated after a 3- to 6-week delay.

Operative technique

For acute repair of the posterolateral structures, a midlateral incision is made from the level 2 cm above the patella to the level of Gerdy's tubercle. The peroneal nerve is located and protected throughout the procedure. Preoperative examination should carefully document the status of the nerve function as it may have sustained a significant stretch at the time of knee injury. The iliotibial band and biceps femoris tendons and their insertions are inspected and can be repaired at the conclusion of the procedure if avulsed [36]. Through the interval between these structures, access to the LCL and the posterolateral capsular structures is obtained. If needed the iliotibial band may be mobilized and retracted anteriorly.

If the popliteus tendon is torn, it is repaired first. When avulsed from its femoral insertion, it is reattached to bone with suture anchors. The torn LCL is repaired primarily if possible. Nonabsorbable suture is used if it is torn in the midsubstance; suture anchors are used if it is avulsed. If the ligamentous tissue is insufficient for repair, the LCL is reconstructed. Multiple techniques have been described, but our preference is Achilles tendon allograft prepared with a 6-mm bone plug. A tunnel is drilled longitudinally in the proximal fibula taking care to identify and protect the peroneal nerve. The bone plug is fixed in the tunnel with an interference screw. The proximal graft is positioned at the LCL origin and the knee ranged to assure appropriate positioning and graft tension prior to fixation. It is fixed with a low-profile screw and soft-tissue washer. The arcuate ligament if torn is repaired at this time with nonabsorbable sutures. The iliotibial band and biceps femoris are repaired and the wound closed. A hinged knee brace is initially locked in extension prior to beginning supervised range-of-motion exercises with physical therapy.

CONCLUSION

Knee ligament injuries are very common in athletes. Accurate diagnosis is made with knowledge of the injury mechanism, a careful physical examination, and selected studies. The goal of treatment is to restore knee biomechanics and maximize function, including return to desired sports activity in athletes. Certain injuries, such as MCL sprains, can be treated by nonoperative means with a high likelihood of return to premorbid activity. Other injuries, such as an ACL tear, will not typically heal and may poten-

tially cause permanent symptomatic knee instability despite adequate attempts at nonoperative therapy. Thus, surgical reconstruction of knee ligaments such as the ACL is often indicated to restore knee stability and return patients to their desired activity level. An appropriate postoperative rehabilitation program should follow to facilitate attaining this goal.

REFERENCES AND RECOMMENDED READING

Recently published papers of particular interest have been highlighted as:

- Of special interest
- • Of outstanding interest

1. Spindler KP, Schils JP, Bergfeld JA, *et al.*: Prospective study of osseous, articular, and meniscal lesions in recent anterior cruciate ligament tears by magnetic resonance imaging and arthroscopy. *Am J Sports Med* 1993, 21:551–557.

2. Speer KP, Spritzer CE, Bassett FH III, *et al.*: Osseous injury associated with acute tears of the anterior cruciate ligament. *Am J Sports Med* 1992, 20:382–389.

3.•• Daniel DM, Stone ML, Dobson BE, *et al.*: Fate of the ACL-injured patient: a prospective outcome study. *Am J Sports Med* 1994, 22:632–644.
Clinical follow-up of 292 patients with acute traumatic hemarthrosis at mean of 64 months after injury. Factors that correlated with surgical reconstruction of the ACL after injury were preinjury hours of sports participation, degree of knee laxity, and patient age.

4. Arciero RA, Scoville CR, Hayda RA, Snyer RJ: The effect of tourniquet use in anterior cruciate ligament reconstruction: a prospective randomized study. *Am J Sports Med* 1996, 24:758–764.

5.•• O'Neill DB: Arthroscopically assisted reconstruction of the anterior cruciate ligament. *J Bone Joint Surg Am* 1996, 78:803–813.
Three ACL reconstruction techniques were assessed in a prospective, randomized study with follow-up of 125 patients at least 2 years after surgery. There was no significant difference in overall outcome among groups, which included two-incision semitendinosus-gracilis graft, two-incision patellar tendon graft, and endoscopic patellar tendon graft.

6. Maeda A, Shino K, Horibe S, *et al.*: Anterior cruciate ligament reconstruction with multistranded autogenous semitendinosus tendon. *Am J Sports Med* 1996, 24:504–509.

7. Marder RA, Raskind JR, Carroll M: Prospective evaluation of arthroscopically assisted anterior cruciate ligament reconstruction: patellar tendon versus semitendinosus and gracilis tendons. *Am J Sports Med* 1991, 19:478–484.

8.•• Howell SM, Taylor MA: Brace-free rehabilitation, with early return to activity, for knees reconstructed with a double-looped semitendinosus and gracilis graft. *J Bone Joint Surg Am* 1996, 78:814–825.
Forty-one patients underwent return to unrestricted activities at 4 months after ACL reconstruction with a double-looped semitendinosus and gracilis graft. Ninety percent of patients had an absent pivot shift and less than 3 mm of increased side-to-side laxity, with no deterioration in stability nor in functional results at 2 years postoperatively.

9. Noyes FR, Barber-Westin SD: Reconstruction of the anterior cruciate ligament with human allograft. *J Bone Joint Surg Am* 1996, 78:524–537.

10. Shapiro MS, Freedman EL: Allograft reconstruction of the anterior and posterior cruciate ligaments after traumatic knee dislocation. *Am J Sports Med* 1995, 23:580–587.

11.• LaPrade RF, Burnett QM II: Femoral intercondylar notch stenosis and correlation to anterior cruciate ligament injuries: a prospective study. *Am J Sports Med* 1994, 22:198–203.
A 2-year prospective study was performed on intercollegiate athletes in pivoting and cutting sports. The radiographic notch-width index, a ratio that measures the width of the anterior outlet of the intercondylar notch divided by the total condylar width at the level of the popliteal groove, was measured for each knee. There were seven ACL tears in 213 athletes. There was a correlation between femoral intercondylar notch stenosis and noncontact ACL injuries.

12. Jackson DW, Gasser SI: Tibial tunnel placement in ACL reconstruction. *Arthroscopy* 1994, 10:124–31.

13. Kenna B, Simon TM, Jackson DW, *et al.*: Endoscopic ACL reconstruction: a technical note on tunnel length for interference fixation. *J Arthroscopy* 1993, 9:228–230.

14. Lemos MJ, Jackson DW, Lee TQ, Simon TM: Assessment of initial fixation of endoscopic interference femoral screws with divergent and parallel placement. *Arthroscopy* 1995, 11:37–41.

15. Joshi GP, McCarroll SM, *et al.*: Intra-articular morphine for pain relief after knee arthroscopy. *J Bone Joint Surg Br* 1992, 74:749–751.

16. Shelbourne KD, Trumper RV: Preventing anterior knee pain after anterior cruciate ligament reconstruction. *Am J Sports Med* 1997, 25:41–47.

17. Shelbourne KD, Porter DA: Anterior cruciate ligament-medial collateral ligament injury: nonoperative management of medial collateral ligament tears with anterior cruciate ligament reconstruction. A preliminary report. *Am J Sports Med* 1992, 20:283–286.

18. Weiss JA, Woo SL, Ohland KJ, *et al.*: Evaluation of a new injury model to study medial collateral ligament healing: primary repair vs. nonoperative treatment. *J Orthop Res* 1991, 9:516–528.

19. Gomez MA, Woo SL, Amiel D, *et al.*: The effect of increased tension on healing medial collateral ligaments. *Am J Sports Med* 1991, 19:347–354.

20. Anderson C, Gillquist J: Treatment of acute isolated and combined ruptures of the anterior cruciate ligament: a long-term follow-up study. *Am J Sports Med* 1992, 20:7–12.

21.• Hillard-Sembell D, Daniel DM, Stone ML, *et al.*: Combined injuries of the anterior cruciate and medial collateral ligaments of the knee. *J Bone Joint Surg Am*1996, 78:169–176.
Sixty-six patients with a combined ACL and MCL injury were retrospectively evaluated an average of 45 months after treatment. There was no difference in clinical nor stress radiographic findings of valgus instability between patients who had ACL reconstruction and MCL repair versus those with ACL reconstruction only or those treated nonoperatively. The authors conclude there is no need to repair an injured MCL after this combined ligament injury.

22.• Shelbourne KD, Patel DV: Management of combined injuries of the anterior cruciate and medial collateral ligaments. *J Bone Joint Surg Am* 1995, 77:800–806.
Review of treatment approach to combined ACL and MCL injuries and associated meniscal pathology.

23. Fowler PJ, Messieh SS: Isolated posterior cruciate ligament injuries in athletes. *Am J Sports Med* 1987, 15:553–557.

24. Parolie JM, Bergfeld JA: Long-term results of nonoperative treatment of isolated posterior cruciate ligament injuries in the athlete. *Am J Sports Med* 1986, 14:35–38.

25. Torg JS, Barton TM, Pavlov H, Stine R: Natural history of the posterior cruciate ligament-deficient knee. *Clin Orthop* 1989, 246:208–216.

26. Keeler PM, Shelbourne KD, McCarrol JR, *et al.*: Nonoperatively treated isolated posterior cruciate ligament injuries. *Am J Sports Med* 1993, 21:132–136.

27.• Berg EE: Posterior cruciate ligament tibial inlay reconstruction. *Arthroscopy* 1995, 11:69–76.
A technique is described that uses a popliteal arthrotomy to fix the graft to the tibia. This method avoids the acute angle the graft makes at the tibial tunnel when an arthroscopic reconstruction is performed, which may be a source of graft abrasion.

28. Markolf KL, Slauterbeck JR, Armstrong KL, *et al.*: A biomechanical study of replacement of the posterior cruciate ligament with a graft: Part I. Isometry, pre-tension of the graft, and anterior-posterior laxity. *J Bone Joint Surg Am* 1997, 79:375–380.

29. Markolf KL, Slauterbeck JR, Armstrong KL, *et al.*: A biomechanical study of replacement of the posterior cruciate ligament with a graft: Part II. Forces in the graft compared with forces in the intact ligament. *J Bone Joint Surg Am*1997, 79:381–386.

30. Jackson DW, Proctor CP, Simon TM: Arthroscopic assisted PCL reconstruction: a technical note on potential neurovascular injury related to drill bit configuration. *Arthroscopy* 1993, 9:224–227.

31. Burns WC, Draganich LF, Pyevich M, Reider B: The effect of femoral tunnel position and graft tensioning technique on posterior laxity of the posterior cruciate ligament-reconstructed knee. *Am J Sports Med* 1995, 23:424–430.

32. Fanelli GC, Giannotti BF, Edson CJ: Arthroscopically assisted combined posterior cruciate ligament/posterior lateral complex reconstruction. *Arthroscopy* 1996, 12:521–530.

33. Noyes FR, Barber-Westin SD: Surgical restoration to treat chronic deficiency of the posterolateral complex and cruciate ligaments of the knee joint. *Am J Sports Med* 1996, 24:415–426.

34.• Noyes FR, Barber-Westin SD: Treatment of complex injuries involving the posterior cruciate and posterolateral ligaments of the knee. *Am J Knee Surg* 1996, 9:200–213.
Review of evaluation and treatment of lateral and posterolateral complex knee injuries.

35. Maynard MJ, Deng X, Wickiewicz TL, Warren RF: The popliteofibular ligament: rediscovery of a key element in posterolateral stability. *Am J Sports Med* 1996, 24:311–316.

36. Terry GC, LaPrade RF: The biceps femoris muscle complex at the knee: its anatomy and injury patterns associated with acute anterolateral-anteromedial rotary instability. *Am J Sports Med* 1996, 24:2–8.

OTHER KNEE PROBLEMS AND INJURIES

Dipak V. Patel, Michael J. Pagnani, and Russell F. Warren

THE MENISCUS
Meniscectomy and meniscal repair

The menisci contain both free nerve endings and corpuscular mechanoreceptors. Thus, they may act as a source of proprioceptive information for muscular tone and coordination [1]. A deficiency in this proprioceptive input may contribute to articular cartilage degeneration after loss of meniscal tissue.

A group of investigators qualitatively examined fluid washout before an arthroscopic examination of the knee [2]. When clear fluid was obtained, only 6.3% of the patients had meniscal pathology. In contrast, 68% of patients with abnormal fluid had meniscal lesions. The authors suggested that analysis of synovial fluid may be useful as a screening test to reduce the number of negative arthroscopies.

Several long-term follow-up studies have shown that meniscectomy (either total or partial) commonly initiates degenerative changes in the knee [3–7]. Patients with malalignment or large body mass appear to be at an increased risk for the development of osteoarthritis. Currently, most surgeons agree that every attempt should be made to preserve as much of the meniscal tissue as possible to minimize the risk of subsequent osteoarthritis developing in the knee.

Meniscal repair is generally performed in younger patients with a peripheral meniscal injury large enough to create an unstable fragment. Partial tears or tears less than 1 cm in length are abraded but are not repaired if stable. Before meniscal repair is performed, the site of tear is identified and probed. Tears in the middle zone of the meniscus are unlikely to heal and are generally not repaired. Tears in the outer third of the meniscus with good-quality tissue are considered suitable for repair.

Over the years, various techniques have been developed for repair of a meniscal tear. These include the "open," "inside-out," "outside-in," and "all-inside" techniques. The choice of technique is based on factors such as site of the tear and surgeon's preference.

DeHaven *et al.* [8••] reported the long-term clinical and radiographic results of open meniscal repair in 30 consecutive patients (33 repairs). The mean postoperative follow-up was 10.9 years (range, 10.1 to 13 years). Seven meniscal retears (21%) were documented (six demonstrated by repeat arthroscopy and one suspected on clinical evaluation). Three of 21 (14%) acute repairs (performed within 6 weeks of injury) retore, compared with four of 12 (33%) chronic repairs. None of the 12 menisci in stable knees sustained retears, compared with seven of 21 (33%) menisci in unstable knees. Standing radiographs showed no degenerative changes in 22 of 26 (85%) compartments with successful repairs as compared with three of seven (43%) compartments with retorn menisci. The authors concluded that the long-term survival rate of repaired menisci was 79% and that increased retear rates were seen in unstable knees.

In recent years, various authors have reported on the results of meniscal repair using the arthroscopic inside-out technique [9,10••,11•,12,13]. Eggli *et al.* [10••] evaluated the results of meniscal repair in 52 patients with anterior cruciate ligament (ACL)–stable knees, at an average follow-up of 7.5 years. In 40 patients, the meniscal repairs had not failed and these patients were examined clinically and radiographically. In their study, significantly more failure occurred when the rim width of the tear was greater than 3 mm and when the tear was repaired with resorbable sutures. The following factors were found to favorably influence meniscal healing: time from injury to surgery less than 8 weeks, patient age less than 30 years, tear length less than 2.5 cm, and tear in the lateral meniscus. The overall failure rate after 7.5 years was 27% (14 of 52); 64% (nine of 14) of the failures occurred in the first 6 months after repair. The clinical and radiographic evaluation of the successfully repaired knees showed that 90% (36 of 40) had normal knee function; the remaining 10% had nearly normal knee function.

Horibe *et al.* [11•] treated 278 torn menisci in 264 patients using an arthroscopically assisted inside-out technique. A total of 132 meniscal repairs in 122 patients were evaluated by second-look arthroscopy. At review, only nine patients had

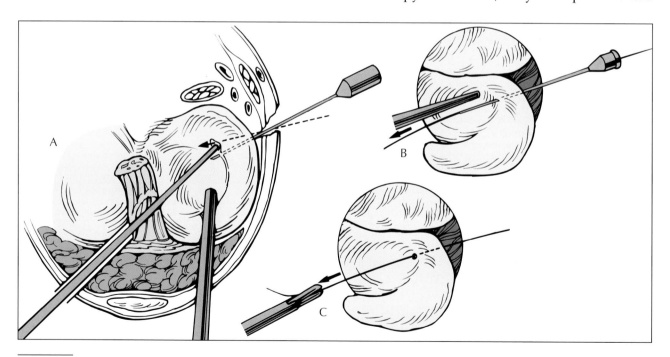

FIGURE 7.1

The "outside-in" technique of meniscal repair. **A,** An 18-gauge spinal needle is placed across the tear. **B,** Sutures are passed through the needle. **C,** The sutures are pulled out through an anterior portal.

meniscal symptoms, such as locking, swelling, or pain. Ninety-seven (73%) menisci had healed completely at the repair site, but there were new tears in different areas of 21 menisci, some of which had complete healing at the repair site. Incomplete healing, seen in 23 (17%) menisci, was frequently near the popliteus tendon, most commonly where there had been an associated ACL injury. They concluded that arthroscopically assisted meniscal repair seems to be a reliable procedure, but some clinically successful cases had either incomplete healing at the repair site, a newly formed tear in the meniscal body, or both. These lesions may cause meniscal symptoms to appear at a later date.

Recently, Rodeo and Warren [14] reported their experience with the outside-in meniscal repair technique. The authors reviewed 90 arthroscopic meniscal repairs performed by Dr. Warren, using the outside-in technique after a minimum follow-up of 2 years. In their series, 86% of the patients had a successful outcome. Sixty-seven percent of the patients were asymptomatic and had objective evidence of complete healing, whereas 19% of the patients were minimally symptomatic and had objective evidence of partial healing. There was a 14% failure rate indi-

cated by the presence of significant symptoms or objective evidence of the meniscal tear's failure to heal. The failure rate was 15% (five of 33) in patients with a stable knee and 38% (five of 13) in patients with an unstable knee. The rate of failure was only 5% (two of 38) in patients undergoing concomitant ACL reconstruction.

We prefer to use the outside-in technique for tears in the anterior or middle portions of the meniscus (Fig. 7.1), and the inside-out technique for repairing tears of the posterior segment of the lateral meniscus (Fig. 7.2).

Morgan [15] reported an all-inside arthroscopic technique for a meniscal repair. The arthroscopic all-inside meniscal suturing technique offers the arthroscopist a way of placing vertically oriented sutures through peripheral posterior horn tears (located posterocentrally) without the risks of nerve, vessel, or posterior capsular entrapment inherent in both the outside-in and the inside-out arthroscopic methods. This technique introduces new instrumentation that allows the surgeon to both place sutures and tie suture knots intra-articularly under arthroscopic control. This method of arthroscopic meniscal repair is technically demanding and requires considerable arthroscopic skills and experience.

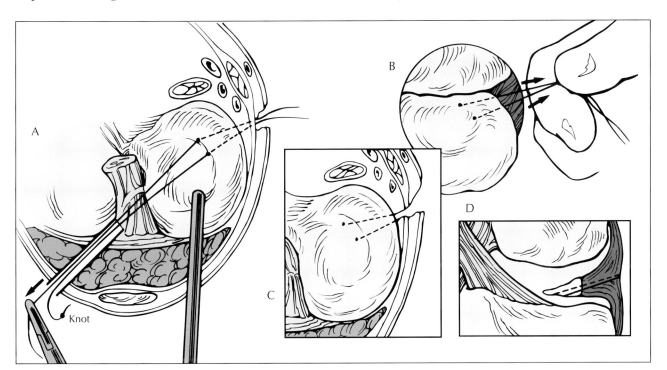

FIGURE 7.2

The "inside-out" technique of meniscal repair. **A**, Sutures are passed by directing a long, flexible needle through a cannula placed through the anterior portal. The sutures are then recovered through a small, posterior incision. **B**, The sutures are pulled flush to approximate the edges of the meniscal tear. **C** and **D**, The sutures are tied.

Recently, an endoscopic meniscal repair technique using the T-Fix suture device (Acufex Microsurgical, Inc., Mansfield, MA) was reported by Barrett *et al.* [16]. This method of meniscal repair allows ease of suture placement for meniscus stability without the problems associated with ancillary incisions, such as the risk of neurovascular injuries. It is ideal for the central posterior horn tears that are difficult to repair using conventional techniques. Vertical tears, bucket-handle tears, flap tears, and horizontal tears can be approached using a temporary "anchor stitch" to stabilize the meniscus before T-Fix repair. Barrett and Treacy [17] have also reported the use of T-Fix suture anchor in fascial sheath reconstruction for complex meniscal tears. The repair rate for complex meniscal tears can be increased with the use of fascial sheaths in combination with an exogenous blood clot. In recent years, biodegradable meniscal arrows (Bionx Implants, Inc., Malvern, PA) have also been developed for the treatment of meniscal tears that are suitable for repair.

Meniscal healing in the avascular zone may be enhanced by the use of an exogenous fibrin clot [18]. Use of a fibrin clot (Fig. 7.3) is recommended in conjunction with isolated repair of the meniscal tears. Animal studies have also investigated the use of a degradable, porous polyurethane polymer and the combination of fibrin sealant and endothelial cell growth factor in stimulating meniscal repair [19,20]. Although these studies are preliminary, they offer exciting glimpses of possible future developments in the effort to retain meniscal tissue.

Few authors have evaluated the role of arthroscopic meniscectomy and limited debridement for meniscal tears in older patients [21,22]. The results of two studies showed that moderate or severe radiographic degenerative changes and full-thickness cartilage loss correlated with poorer results. It appears that arthroscopic debridement is useful if osteoarthritis has not progressed to malalignment.

In an interesting study, Mohr and Henche [23] found that the loss of a resected meniscal fragment during surgery did not affect outcome in most patients. Despite the fact that these fragments were up to 4 cm in length, only three of 23 patients with an irretrievable fragment were dissatisfied and required a repeat surgery. The authors found that the loose piece of meniscal tissue tended to adhere to a location where it did not become a mechanical hindrance.

Abnormalities in limb motion and muscle activation may persist for as long as 8 weeks after arthroscopic partial medial meniscectomy [24]. Although rapid motor recovery is generally assumed to occur after this "minor procedure," a supervised rehabilitation program may provide some benefits in restoring motor recovery.

Meniscal tears in anterior cruciate ligament–deficient knees

The menisci of active patients with knee instability fare poorly. Irvine and Glasgow [25] performed arthroscopic examinations of 100 consecutive patients with ACL insufficiency at an average of 3 years after injury. In their study, only 14 patients had intact menisci, and 57 patients had full-thickness tears. Full-thickness meniscal tears were associated with a longer time interval between the injury and operation.

The development of osteoarthritis after meniscectomy appears to be related to the condition of the ACL [5]. French investigators performed a long-term follow-up study of patients who had undergone a partial meniscectomy [7]. Radiographic evidence of

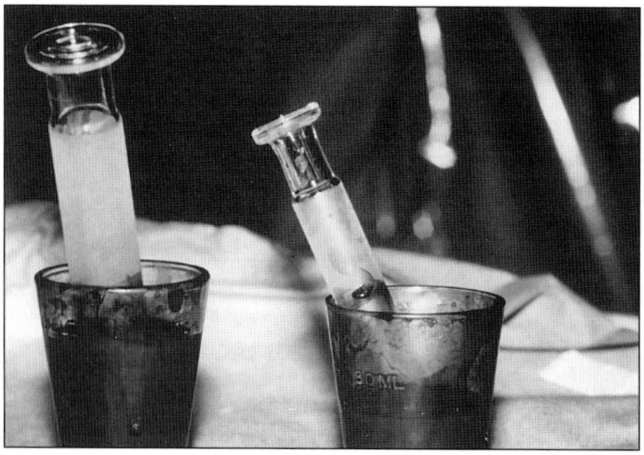

FIGURE 7.3

A fibrin clot is prepared using the barrel of a glass syringe.

osteoarthritis was found in 86% of patients with ACL-deficient knees observed for 30 years, compared with 50% of patients in whom the ACL was intact.

If the ACL is reconstructed in conjunction with a meniscal repair, a favorable effect on meniscal healing is noted. Cannon and Vittori [26] found that the success rate of meniscal repair was much greater (93% versus 50%) in patients who had a concomitant reconstruction of the ACL than in patients with stable (ACL intact) knees. The rim width of the meniscus was similar in the two groups. The increase in the healing rate was attributed to two factors: 1) reduction in the anterior tibial translation after ACL reconstruction that protected the meniscus, and 2) increased intra-articular bleeding and fibrin clot formation after ACL reconstruction. We urge reconstruction of the ACL-deficient knee when a reparable lesion of the meniscus is noted. In our experience, only 5% of meniscal repairs performed concomitantly with ACL reconstruction have failed at 4 years. In contrast, the failure rate is approximately 40% if the ACL is deficient and not reconstructed.

Meniscal replacement

The development of osteoarthritis after meniscal resection has led to a search for a method of meniscal regeneration or replacement. Two preliminary animal studies illustrate this continuing quest. Sommerlath and Gillquist [27] implanted a Dacron meniscal prosthesis with a polyurethane coating into rabbit knees. Synovial tissue ingrowth was noted in 93% of the prostheses. The prosthesis decreased joint stiffness to values that approached normal, but it was ineffective in dissipating energy under load. It was associated with a high incidence of osteophyte formation and severe synovial reaction.

Stone *et al.* [28] implanted absorbable, copolymeric, collagen-based meniscal scaffolds in dog stifle joints. Substantial meniscal regeneration was noted in 63% of the knees. By 9 to 12 months after implantation, the "successfully regenerated" menisci resembled the normal canine meniscus on histologic and biochemical examination. The authors concluded that the scaffolds support meniscal fibrochondrocyte ingrowth and may provide an avenue to complete meniscal regeneration.

Meniscal allografts

As the development of a synthetic meniscus or a meniscal scaffold has evolved, surgeons have become interested in meniscal transplantation using allograft tissue. Basic science work has helped to identify some inherent difficulties of meniscal transplantation. Arnoczky *et al.* [29] deep froze dog menisci in liquid nitrogen to kill all cells within the menisci, which were then reimplanted. The menisci were found to be repopulated with cells that seemed to originate from the adjacent synovium. The phenotype of these cells was unclear, but they resembled meniscal fibrochondrocytes. The cells migrated over the superficial surface of the meniscus and began to invade its deeper portions. However, the central core of the meniscus remained acellular even 6 months after reimplantation. In addition, there were mild histologic alterations in the normal collagen architecture. The authors believed that this finding was consistent with a remodeling phenomenon that accompanies cellular repopulation, and they cautioned that similar processes may render the allograft menisci more susceptible to injury.

Jackson *et al.* [30] analyzed autografts and both fresh and cryopreserved allografts after meniscal transplantation in a goat model. There were few gross and microscopic differences between transplanted and control menisci. The viability of the autograft menisci approached 100%, whereas that of the allografts was found to be 71% to 83%. Analysis of the water and proteoglycan content of the allograft menisci (both fresh and cryopreserved) revealed substantial changes in their biochemical makeup. The authors expressed their concern over the long-term function of meniscal allografts.

In a follow-up study using the same goat model, Jackson *et al.* [31] found that viable cells in meniscal allografts do not survive transplantation. Instead, the meniscus is repopulated entirely by host cells. The authors suggested that grafts containing living cells may not offer any advantages over those in which the cells are killed. The cost and risks for disease transmission are also greater when measures are taken to prevent cell death.

Further highlighting the problem of disease transmission, Asselmeier *et al.* [32] described an incident in which multiple tissues were obtained from a seronegative donor apparently infected with HIV. Several recipients of these tissues tested HIV-positive and included a patient who received a fresh-frozen patellar tendon allograft. Three patients who received freeze-dried soft-tissue allografts tested negative. There exists a "window" of seronegativity after HIV infection during which currently available HIV antibody tests may not detect the virus in potential allograft donors, despite their being infectious. In the future, the refinement of HIV-antigen testing may help to close this window. In recent years, polymerase chain reaction (PCR) testing has facilitated the early detection of HIV infection and decreased the risk of disease transmission.

A detailed review on the indications, operative techniques, results, and complications of meniscal allograft transplantation in humans has been reported by Veltri *et al.* [33]. The experimental nature and the risks for disease transmission should be carefully explained to patients who are candidates for the meniscal allograft surgery. We have used meniscal allografts to treat patients with a meniscal deficiency and evidence of articular surface degeneration. Most of our patients have had a concomitant ACL instability. Loss of the meniscal tissue appears to add a component of varus–valgus rotational instability in some patients. Replacing both menisci can dramatically reduce this abnormal varus–valgus motion. If clinical results prove satisfactory, the indications for meniscal transplantation may be extended to patients with minimal cartilage deterioration. This latter group of patients would seem most likely to benefit from the procedure.

When a meniscal allograft is to be transplanted, radiographs of the knee should be provided to the tissue bank to ensure proper sizing of the meniscus. Meniscal transplantation may be performed by an open or an arthroscopic technique. The arthroscopic technique is technically demanding, particularly if the anterior and posterior horns of the meniscus are left attached to the bone plugs. Our technique involves drilling 6-mm holes from the anteromedial tibia to the anatomic insertions of the meniscal horns. A standard ACL-tibial drill guide and guidewire are used to facilitate hole placement. The meniscal allograft is usually prepared by passing heavy, nonabsorbable sutures through bone plugs attached to the horns. The sutures are first passed into the posterior drill hole, and then the posterior horn of the meniscus is pulled through an enlarged arthroscopic portal. The posterior bone plug is reduced into the posterior drill hole. The remainder of the meniscus is then introduced into the knee, and the anterior sutures are used to reduce the anterior horn. After the meniscal horns are satisfactorily aligned, the meniscus is reduced, and its peripheral attachments are fixed with additional sutures. Either an outside-in or an inside-out technique may be used.

Generally, we elect to use bone plugs at the horn attachments (Fig. 7.4). Recently, Chen *et al.* [34•]

performed a cadaveric study to determine if secure attachment of the horns of the lateral meniscus during transplantation affects the load-bearing function of the meniscus. Six knee joints were loaded in compression (310 N) and the interarticular contact pressure in the joint was measured using a pressure-sensitive film inserted into the joint. Each knee was tested first with the original intact meniscus and then tested again after each of the following surgical procedures involving the original lateral meniscus: 1) total meniscectomy, 2) meniscal transplantation with a tibial bone bridge, 3) meniscal transplantation with neither horn secured, 4) meniscal transplantation with the anterior horn secured, 5) meniscal transplantation with the posterior horn secured, and 6) meniscal transplantation with both horns secured. The results were as follows. The joint with an intact meniscus gave the largest contact area and the smallest peak contact pressure. The joint with the total meniscectomy gave the smallest contact area and the largest peak contact pressure. A meniscal transplantation with either a tibial bony bridge or with both horns secured gave results similar to those for the joint with an intact meniscus. A meniscal transplantation with only one horn secured gave results somewhere in between those for the intact joint and those for the joint without a meniscus. And a meniscal transplantation with neither horn secured gave results similar to those for a joint without a meniscus. This study has shown the importance of attachment of both horns during a lateral meniscal transplantation.

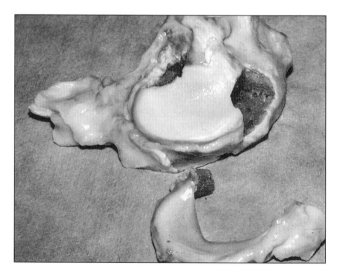

FIGURE 7.4

A meniscal allograft is harvested with bone plugs.

When both the medial and lateral menisci and the ACL are deficient, we have used an open technique in which the meniscal horns are left attached to a 2-cm-wide section of the intercondylar eminence of the allograft tibia (Fig. 7.5). A slot is created in the native tibial intercondylar eminence, and the allograft is press-fitted into the slot. The bony portion of the allograft may be fixed with a cancellous screw oriented longitudinally in the tibia. The peripheral attachments of the menisci are attached to the capsular tissue and the proximal tibia with the aid of suture anchors. An allograft patellar tendon may be placed through the bony portion of the meniscal allograft to reconstruct the ACL.

Our preliminary results have demonstrated that most menisci show evidence of healing. Second-look arthroscopic examinations reveal a striking resem-blance to normal menisci in many cases. The most conspicuous clinical finding at early follow-up has been a decrease in mediolateral laxity. The true results of this procedure may not be known for many years. The goal is to decrease the risk of artic-ular surface degeneration, which may take 20 to 30 years to manifest itself.

Imaging

Magnetic resonance imaging (MRI) can be extremely helpful in the diagnosis of meniscal injury. However, the reliability of MRI may be affected by patient age. Hodler *et al.* [35] investigated the use of MRI to evaluate the menisci of elderly cadaveric knees. They found that degenerative meniscal changes often mimicked tears, and that the specifici-

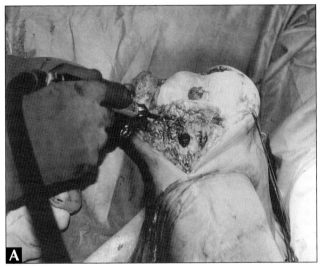

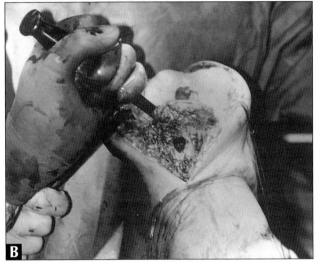

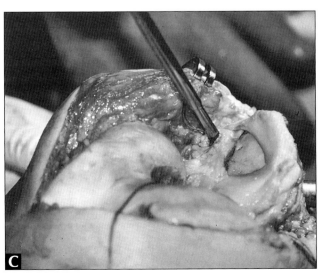

FIGURE 7.5

Open technique for replacement of both medial and lateral menisci. **A**, A slot is cut in the native intercondylar emi-nence. **B**, The eminence is removed with an osteotome. **C**, The allograft menisci (still attached to the allograft tibia) are press-fitted into the recipient tibia and fixed with a cancel-lous screw.

ty, sensitivity, and accuracy of MRI were reduced in this population. They recommended that grade 3 signals be described as "degenerated with a high probability of a tear" when seen in elderly patients. Gerngross and Sohn [36] reported that use of a 7.5-Hz head with a real-time ultrasonographic scanner permitted accurate detection of meniscal lesions.

Potter *et al.* [37••] reported a study on MRI of meniscal allografts and correlated the findings with clinical, arthroscopic, and histologic examination. Twenty-four patients (29 menisci) underwent MRI after meniscal transplantation. Nineteen patients had arthroscopy, and the peripheral capsular attachment, degenerative areas, or both were sampled for biopsy. They found that MRI enabled accurate assessment of allograft attachments. Fragmentation and frank extrusion of the meniscus were associated with full-thickness chondral loss. Degeneration of the meniscal allograft (indicated by an increase in the signal intensity on MRI) was seen with moderate and severe chondral wear. Clinical results were worse in patients with meniscal extrusion, with complaints of locking. Patients with mild fragmentation of the meniscus reported pain without locking. Histologic examination of excised allografts revealed myxomatous degeneration without immunologic reaction. They concluded that MRI can help assess placement of the meniscal allograft, evaluate the articular cartilage, and enable differentiation of meniscal fragmentation from meniscal extrusion. Preoperative assessment of the articular cartilage is important in order to identify patients who may be at risk for failure.

KNEE ARTHROSCOPY
Complications

Infections after knee arthroscopy are usually noted within 2 weeks of the index procedure. Clinical characteristics include mild to moderate elevation of temperature, moderate to severe knee pain, erythema, swelling, warmth, and drainage from the arthroscopic portal wound. It is worth noting that these signs are not uniformly present. Aspiration of the synovial fluid generally yields purulent material if the infection is caused by coagulase-positive staphylococci; however, frank purulence may be absent if the offending organism is coagulase-negative. Cellular analysis of the fluid usually reveals more than 90% polymorphonuclear leukocytes. Gram's stains may be negative with coagulase- or gram-negative species; blood cultures may reveal

the organism. The serum leukocyte count may be elevated but often is not. Erythrocyte sedimentation rates are usually elevated. If there is any suspicion of infection, fluid should be sent for culture, and the culture results should be closely monitored.

Treatment options include needle aspiration, arthroscopic debridement, or arthrotomy. Generally, we have avoided treatment by needle aspiration and prefer arthroscopic treatment, unless the extent or location of the infectious process dictates that arthrotomy is required. Empiric broad-spectrum antibiotic coverage is modified as culture and sensitivity data become available. Measurement of serum bacteriocidal titers and antibiotic peak and trough levels (when appropriate) are helpful in ensuring proper antibacterial coverage. Antibiotics are administered intravenously for a minimum of 2 to 6 weeks.

Armstrong *et al.* [38] noted several risk factors associated with subsequent infection after knee arthroscopy. Intra-articular injection of corticosteroid agents correlated significantly with infection. Infection was also believed to be associated with longer operative times, previous surgical procedures on the knee, and the performance of chondroplasty or soft-tissue debridement.

In the past few years, mechanical fluid irrigation systems have become popular. These infusion pumps use pressure-sensitive devices to maintain joint distension by controlling the inflow and the outflow from the joint. However, these devices can cause extravasation of fluid, with potentially catastrophic results.

Bomberg *et al.* [39] reported on two patients who required fasciotomy for the treatment or prevention of extravasation-induced compartment syndrome. Early recognition of the extravasated fluid and prompt discontinuation of the mechanical pump were advised. Synovial rupture may occur without an audible "pop" and should be considered when the pump cannot maintain joint distension or when excessive flow is required to distend the knee. Generally, if capsular tears are suspected, the pump should be avoided or pressures kept low. If extensive extravasation is noted, compartment-pressure monitoring is indicated. The fluid may be resorbed rapidly, but vascular compromise mandates immediate surgical release of the compartment. Using a gravity-fed system, Arangio and Kostelnik [40] found that the minimum pressure allowing adequate visualization of the knee was related to the diastolic but not systolic blood pressure.

Recently, Ekman and Poehling [41] reported an

experimental study (using 12 live-pig hind limbs and, as shams, three additional limbs) to objectively evaluate the risk of compartment syndrome as a complication during arthroscopy, particularly with the use of mechanical infusion systems. This study showed that, when elevated compartment pressures occur, extravasated fluid dissipates quickly, minimizing the risk of compartment syndrome and subsequent neuromuscular damage.

Pain management

In a randomized study, the postoperative intra-articular injection of morphine after knee arthroscopy resulted in lower pain scores and less need for systemic analgesics [42]. Randomized trials have also supported an analgesic effect of nonsteroidal anti-inflammatory drugs (NSAIDs) in the immediate postoperative period; however, the conclusions of these studies differed regarding the effect of NSAIDs on eventual functional recovery after arthroscopy. One group found that NSAID administration was associated with an earlier return to work [43]. Another study concluded that these medications did not hasten functional recovery from arthroscopy [44].

When bupivacaine hydrochloride (a local anesthetic) is injected intra-articularly for postoperative analgesia, the drug is absorbed systemically. The risk for approaching toxic serum levels can be reduced by adding epinephrine to the agent or by administering the anesthetic after tourniquet inflation [45].

Highgenboten *et al.* [46] examined 10-day pain profiles after arthroscopic surgery on the knee and found that most patients had low levels of analgesic use and low perceived-pain levels by the fourth postoperative day. The postoperative administration of corticosteroids did not affect pain profiles. As mentioned previously, corticosteroid use has been associated with septic arthritis after knee arthroscopy. We have found that a single intramuscular dose of ketorolac (Toradol; Syntex Laboratories, Palo Alto, CA) is very effective in reducing pain and analgesic use after knee arthroscopy.

OSTEOCHONDRAL LESIONS

In a histologic study of articular cartilage lesions in rabbit knees, Shapiro *et al.* [47] offered some interesting insights into the repair of articular cartilage defects. In their study, excellent reconstitution of cartilage was noted as early as 4 weeks after creation of the defect, with further maturation from 6 to 12 weeks. Initially, a fibrinous arcade appeared at the surface edge of the defect. This arcade is believed to act as a "scaffold" that directs mesenchymal cells (derived from marrow) to produce a fibro-cartilaginous matrix at the surface edge. Deeper mesenchymal cells differentiate into chondroblasts. These chondroblasts in the deeper portion of the defect synthesize a cartilaginous matrix that is indistinguishable from normal articular cartilage. The deepest layers of the defect usually mature to form a subchondral bone plate with a typical tidemark. If the defect does not traverse subchondral bone, the marrow cells cannot contribute to the repair process. Cartilage cells in the adjacent residual cartilage do not participate in repair. In some cases, the investigators noted gaps between the new and adjacent cartilage, suggesting a lack of firm physical interdigitation between the old and repaired cartilage. The authors postulated that micromotion may result when mechanical stresses are applied to the new cartilage and that this motion may be related to the eventual development of arthritic change.

Using a dog model, Paletta *et al.* [48] found that packing a full-thickness cartilage defect with exogenous fibrin clot led to a more organized and advanced healing response than was seen in control defects during the first 8 weeks of the process. At 12 and 24 weeks, this difference in healing was less pronounced. The clot-filled defects tended to heal more uniformly and with less surface depression, particularly if they were located in an unloaded site on the knee.

Other investigators have examined the effects of growth factors and hyaluronic acid derivatives on articular cartilage [49,50]. These substances may protect cartilage against biochemical injury and stimulate its repair.

In an animal study investigating the fate of articular cartilage after cryopreservation and transplantation, Schachar *et al.* [51] concluded that cryopreserved osteoarticular allografts retain their metabolic and biochemical activity after 1 year of implantation. However, the authors observed that the long-term potential of autograft tissues appear to be superior to that of the allografts.

The treatment of osteochondral defects of the knee can be difficult and unrewarding. Marandola and Prietto [52] reported a case in which an undetached, osteochondral, patellar lesion was fixed arthroscopically with a retrograde Herbert screw, thereby avoiding the need for arthrotomy. We have used a similar technique for lesions of the femoral condyle and have also performed arthroscopic fixation using absorbable pins. Japanese investigators reported an arthroscopic case in which bone pegs taken from the lateral wall of the patellar groove (outside the patellofemoral joint) and from the intercondylar area were transplanted to a large osteochondral defect in the medial femoral condyle (press-fit fixation), with excellent results at 3-year follow-up [53].

Abrasion chondroplasty with drilling of the subchondral bone has been advocated for articular cartilage defects, despite evidence that the fibrocartilaginous tissue resulting from this treatment has inferior biomechanical properties. Galloway and Noyes [54] reported a case in which a subchondral cyst developed in a patella after chondroplasty and drilling. The authors attributed this unusual lesion to the infusion of synovial fluid through the defect in the subchondral plate.

Beaver *et al.* [55] think that patients with posttraumatic defects fare better than patients with osteochondritis dissecans, osteoarthritis, or osteonecrosis after repair with fresh osteochondral allografts. The authors recommend this treatment in relatively young and active patients. Joint alignment should be corrected with osteotomy. Survivalship analysis revealed a success rate of 75% at 5 years and 63% at 14 years.

Garrett *et al.* [56] observed 27 adult patients with

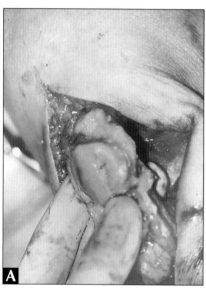

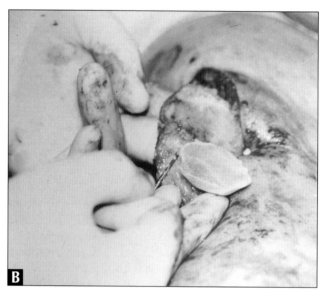

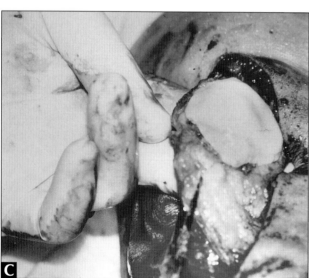

FIGURE 7.6

Treatment of refractory chondral defect of the patella using an osteochondral allograft. **A**, Native patella showing grade 4 osteoarthrosis. **B**, The patella is prepared, and the osteochondral allograft is shown. **C**, The allograft is fixed using retrograde Herbert–Whipple screws.

a diagnosis of osteochondritis dissecans of the lateral femoral condyle. The authors noted that such lesions were rare and tended to be larger and more fragile than lesions of the medial femoral condyle. They concluded that the adult form of osteochondritis dissecans of the lateral femoral condyle carries a dismal prognosis regarding progressive degenerative changes in the knee. And they also recommended abrasion chondroplasty for small lesions (< 2 cm) but advocated allograft osteochondral transplantation for larger defects. Schenck and Goodnight [57] wrote an excellent review on osteochondritis dissecans involving the knee, elbow, and talus.

We have used osteochondral allografts (fixed with a retrograde Herbert–Whipple screw) for the treatment of refractory cartilage defects of the patella (Fig. 7.6). We have also used a "microfracture technique" (Steadman, Personal communication) in which arthroscopic "picks" are used to create punctate defects that communicate with subchondral bone. This technique avoids the potential damage to surrounding cartilage cells and subchondral bone that may result from the thermal effects of drilling. Patients treated with the microfracture technique should avoid weight-bearing activity for 6 weeks after the procedure to eliminate the risk of an insufficiency fracture. In recent years, filling of the chondral defects using autogenous chondrocyte transplantation (popularly known as the "cell culture technique") has been attempted [58]. However, at this time, the long-term outcome of such a procedure is unclear. Prospective, randomized, controlled studies are required to clarify the role of autogenous chondrocyte transplantation in the treatment of chondral and osteochondral defects.

THE PATELLA
Patellar instability

A report from Finland concluded that the vastus medialis inserts more proximally in patients with patellar dislocations than in normal patients [59]. The authors recommend that surgeons consider advancing the vastus medialis in combination with other realignment procedures to accentuate the medial pull of the quadriceps.

Recurrent patellar instability that does not respond to rehabilitative measures may be treated by proximal realignment of the extensor mechanism (Fig. 7.7). Generally, the procedure is open, with release of the lateral patellar retinaculum and reefing plus advancement of the medial patellar retinaculum and vastus medialis obliquus (VMO). Anteromedial transposition of the tibial tubercle (Fulkerson's technique) is often necessary to obtain proper patellar tracking. We recommend such distal realignment (Fulkerson's technique) when proximal realignment fails to reduce the Q angle to less than 20°. Simmons and Cameron [60] suggested transposition of the patellar tendon distally, without medialization or recessing, when recurrent patellar dislocation is associated with patella alta.

Although short-term outcome of these open procedures has generally been satisfactory, they tend to leave a large and unsightly scar. Recently, some surgeons have described arthroscopic techniques for soft-tissue realignment [61,62]. The results of these procedures are preliminary, and it is unclear whether their indications can be extended to patients with grossly abnormal anatomy. In time, however, arthroscopic techniques may provide an alternative method of treating recurrent patellar instability.

FIGURE 7.7
A computerized arthrotomogram showing lateral subluxation of the patella.

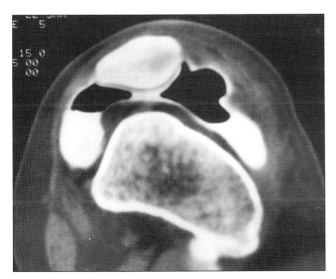

The long-term results of realignment procedures for patellar instability are not well documented in the literature, but a recent clinical study offered sobering statistics. Arnbjornsson *et al.* [63] studied 21 patients who had a unilateral operation for bilateral recurrent dislocation of the patella. The procedures included proximal realignments, distal realignments, and combinations of these techniques. At a mean follow-up of 14 years, the operated knees were clinically worse, with a higher incidence of patellofemoral osteoarthrosis (75%) than the nonoperated knees (29%). Six of the operated and four of the nonoperated knees still had recurrent dislocations of the patella. The authors concluded that although these procedures may have short-term benefits, long-term results are poor.

Patellar pain and tendonitis

An electromyographic study of patients with patellofemoral pain syndrome revealed no significant differences in quadriceps activity compared with the control group [64]. The authors did find that patients with the largest Q angles demonstrated smaller VMO activity than did the control group and patients with smaller Q angles. They suggested VMO strengthening with the knee in 90° of flexion to minimize shear forces on the patella. Another report found a strong relationship between iliotibial band (ITB) tightness and a reduction in the medial glide of the patella in patients with patellofemoral dysfunction [65].

Doucette and Goble [66] found that 84% of patients with a diagnosis of lateral patellofemoral compression syndrome were asymptomatic after an 8-week course of physical therapy that included VMO strengthening, ITB stretching, and patellar taping and mobilization. They also noted a significant decrease in Merchant's congruence angle in patients who improved, suggesting that exercise can alter patellar tracking. O'Neill *et al.* [67•] found that an exercise program tended to improve Merchant's congruence angles in skeletally immature individuals, but such improvement was unusual in adults.

The differential diagnosis of patellofemoral pain should include lesions of the patellar tendon and patellar stress fractures. Karlsson *et al.* [68] used ultrasonography to evaluate 91 partial ruptures of the patellar tendon. They found that the lesion length could be predicted by ultrasonography and that larger lesions were more likely to require surgical intervention. Scranton and Farrar [69] reported

on six athletes with chronic, disabling, anterior knee pain. Standard conservative treatment did not alleviate pain, and operative exploration revealed mucoid cystic degeneration in the patellar tendon. Mucoid degeneration should be suspected in patients with focal, unremitting, infrapatellar pain and a history of trauma. MRI may provide a clue to this unusual and difficult diagnosis.

Recently, two studies have reported the use of MRI in patients with patellar tendonitis [70,71]. McLoughlin *et al.* [70] studied 15 patients with a clinical diagnosis of patellar tendinitis who underwent gadolinium-enhanced MRI of the knee. The purpose of this study was to characterize the MRI features of patellar tendinitis. Grades of patellar abnormality, based on findings in the enthesial region at MRI, correlated with signs of increasing fibrovascular repair: grade 1 (four patients), enhanced area adjacent to patellar apex with marginal zone of intermediate signal intensity, and a patellar apical chondral-bone avulsion; grade 2 (five patients), same findings as in grade 1 but without avulsion; grade 3 (six patients), homogeneous, nonenhancing area of intermediate signal intensity adjacent to the patellar apex seen on all images. Changes were most obvious posteriorly and involved the central and medial thirds of the tendon. Chronic injury to the medial retinaculum was a common associated finding. The authors concluded that patellar tendinitis demonstrates a consistent spectrum of changes at MRI that can help understanding of the origin and treatment of damage.

Johnson *et al.* [71] reviewed the radiographic and MRI appearances of 24 knees with patellar tendinitis resistant to conservative therapy. The purpose was to identify the characteristic MRI appearance and to determine if the patellar morphology was abnormal. A significant thickening of the patellar tendon was found in all cases; this was a more reliable diagnostic feature than a high signal within the superior posterior and central aspect of the tendon at its proximal attachment. The site of the lesion shown by MRI is more compatible with impingement of the inferior pole of the patella against the patellar tendon than a stress overload of the tendon. In this study, when the patellar morphology was compared with that of a matched control group, there were no significant differences in the length of the patella, inferior pole, or length of the articular surface.

Teitz and Harrington [72] described two cases of stress fracture of the patella, an unusual injury that appears to be caused by bending stresses to the patella during knee flexion. These fractures are generally associated with repetitive low loading, particularly prolonged isometric quadriceps contraction with the knee in 30° to 45° of flexion. The development of acute pain may be accompanied by an audible "pop." Clinical examination reveals tenderness over the distal portion of the patella and an effusion. The diagnosis may be confirmed by radiographs or bone scan. Treatment initially consists of long-leg cast immobilization for nondisplaced fractures and open reduction and internal fixation for displaced fractures.

OSGOOD–SCHLATTER DISEASE

Osgood–Schlatter disease, commonly termed "traction apophysitis of the tibial tubercle," occurs secondary to repetitive stress on the extensor apparatus (Fig. 7.8). The condition is often associated with jumping sports. Treatment is generally conservative, and surgery is rarely required for persistent pain. Binazzi *et al.* [73] found that superior results were obtained when the prominent tibial tubercle was removed in addition to the loose, intratendinous ossicles. Other techniques, including bone grafting and drilling of the tibial tubercle, were less satisfactory. We have noted that in young patients (about 20 years of age), a loose ossicle may be found beneath the insertion of the patellar tendon into the tibial tuberosity. Excision of this ossicle may be required if the patient has persistent symptoms despite conservative measures. Generally, in our experience, excision of the prominent tibial tuberosity is not necessary.

BLEEDING DISORDERS

Several recent articles have discussed knee arthroscopy in patients with bleeding disorders. Barber and Prudich [74] reported on two men who developed acute hemarthroses of the knee after an episode of trauma. Both were noted to have stable knees. After arthroscopy, the patients experienced persistent bleeding that required erythrocyte and component replacement. Investigations revealed that both men had mild hemophilia A. The authors cautioned that patients with persistent unresolving hemarthroses should be evaluated for coagulation disorders before operative intervention.

Triantafyllou *et al.* [75] found that both open and arthroscopic synovectomies of the knees reduced bleeding episodes in patients with classic hemophilia. Motion of the knee was much better and the need

for coagulation factor VIII replacement was reduced in patients who had undergone an arthroscopic procedure. Neither type of procedure halted the eventual development of hemophilic arthropathy.

Cohen *et al.* [76] described an unusual case in which an HIV-positive patient with hemophilia presented 19 months after arthroscopic synovectomy with increasingly frequent hemarthroses and a palpable thrill over the knee. The patient was found to have an arteriovenous fistula of the medial superior genicular artery that communicated with the popliteal artery. The authors thought the fistula was caused by an intraoperative injury to the medial superior genicular artery when a sharp trocar was used to introduce the arthroscope. The patient was successfully treated by surgically ligating the bleeding vessels.

Wiedel [77•] prospectively evaluated 10- to 15-year results of arthroscopic synovectomy of the knee in patients with hemophilia. Nine knees (eight patients) with severe hemophilia A and one patient with hemophilia B underwent arthroscopic synovectomy. One complication occurred immediately postoperatively in a 8-year-old boy who developed a severe hemarthrosis that required arthroscopic evacuation. His postoperative recovery was compromised, and he suffered significant loss of motion of the knee. In this series, recurrent hemarthroses developed in only one patient after an injury to the knee. A second arthroscopic synovectomy was performed 45 months after the initial procedure. Other

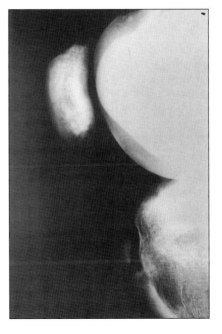

FIGURE 7.8

Lateral view of the knee showing Osgood–Schlatter disease.

than the patient who lost motion after the postoperative complication, all patients initially regained or improved their range of motion. The latest follow-up, however, showed several patients losing motion, which correlated with clinical and radiographic evidence of progressive changes of hemophilic arthropathy. The one patient with coagulation factor IX deficiency required a total knee replacement 8 years after synovectomy. The authors concluded that arthroscopic synovectomy was effective in reducing recurrent hemarthroses and maintaining range of motion. Joint deterioration, however, continued to occur, although probably at a slower rate.

PIGMENTED VILLONODULAR SYNOVITIS

Pigmented villonodular synovitis (PVNS) is a benign, proliferative, etiologically undetermined disease of the synovium. It may involve tendon sheaths, bursae, or joints, with the latter occurring as diffuse involvement or a localized nodule. It is characterized by deposition of hemosiderin within an overgrowth of villous processes. PVNS usually affects a single joint, the knee being most commonly involved. Schwartz *et al.* [78] reviewed 99 patients who had PVNS affecting large joints and found that the knee was involved in 75% of the patients, with the diffuse type being most common. The pathologic synovial tissue may be found in the intercondylar notch area, the medial and lateral gutters of the knee, or both.

The disease commonly affects patients in their middle years of life. Patients usually present with a long history of symptoms, including joint pain, swelling, palpable masses, stiffness, and occasionally locking. At times, the clinical presentation of PVNS can mimic that of a meniscal tear. Van Meter and Rowdon [79] reported a case of a localized PVNS presenting as a locked, bucket-handle tear of the lateral meniscus in an otherwise healthy 27-year-old man. Plain radiographs are usually normal during the early course of the disease but may show joint effusion and faint calcification in some cases. In the later part of the disease, the proliferative synovium can cause erosive, cystic, or sclerotic changes in adjacent bone. MRI is helpful for making a diagnosis of PVNS, and the MRI findings of PVNS have been reported recently by Bravo *et al.* [80]. Because of the large amount of hemosiderin present, there are focal areas of marked signal loss on T_2-weighted

MRIs. The presence of bony erosions on both sides of a large joint, a joint effusion, and focal areas of signal void on MRI is highly characteristic of PVNS.

There are no specific systemic or joint-fluid laboratory tests for PVNS. On histological examination, a variety of cell types are evident among a loose fibrous stroma, including histiocytes, giant cells, foam cells, and synoviocytes. Hemosiderin deposits are almost always present but may vary widely in quantity, depending on the amount of bleeding in the affected synovial tissue.

The treatment of PVNS consists of excision of the lesion. Localized lesions generally respond well to arthroscopic excision of the nodule. The recurrence rate after excision of a localized nodule is low. In patients with diffuse PVNS, partial synovectomy (by arthroscopic or open techniques) is associated with a high rate of recurrence, as much as 56% (five of nine cases) in a series reported by Ogilvie-Harris *et al.* [81]. Therefore, a total synovectomy (by arthroscopic or open techniques) is indicated for patients with diffuse PVNS. The authors also reported a low recurrence rate (one of 11 patients) and minimal joint stiffness in knees treated by arthroscopic total synovectomy, but they emphasized the importance of both anterior and posterior portals to perform complete synovectomy. Open techniques of total synovectomy also have low recurrence rates but more commonly result in joint stiffness [82].

Radiation therapy has been used in the past with mixed results and is complicated by joint stiffness and wound-healing problems in surgical patients. Intra-articular radiation with ^{90}Y has also been used for patients with PVNS. The material is injected directly into the joint to give a concentrated localized dose. Franssen *et al.* [83] reported a clinical improvement in four of eight knees in patients with diffuse form of PVNS who were treated by intra-articular injection of 185 MBq ^{90}Y silicate. Arthroscopy was performed both prior to and 6 months after each ^{90}Y silicate treatment. In all cases, areas of persistent synovitis were found after the ^{90}Y silicate injection; this finding was confirmed both by histological examination and ^{99m}Tc=uptake measurements. Wiss [84] reported a case of a 40-year-old woman who suffered from recurrent PVNS of the knee that was successfully treated with ^{90}Y radiocolloid. Side effects of ^{90}Y therapy are few, predictable, and for the most part, avoidable. These side effects include radionecrosis of soft tissue, needle-tract pigmentation, injection site tenderness, pyrexia, and lymphocyte chromosomal abnormalities. In patients with advanced disease and bone destruction, a total-knee arthroplasty or arthrodesis of the knee may be indicated.

ILIOTIBIAL BAND–FRICTION SYNDROME

Iliotibial band–friction syndrome is an overuse injury caused by excessive friction between the ITB and the lateral femoral epicondyle. It is common in long-distance runners, cyclists, and other athletes performing repetitive knee flexion activities.

Orchard *et al.* [85•] proposed a biomechanical model to explain the pathogenesis of ITB-friction syndrome in distance runners. Their model was based on a kinematic study of nine runners with ITB-friction syndrome, a cadaveric study of 11 normal knees, and a literature review. Friction (or impingement) occurred near footstrike, predominantly in the foot contact phase, between the posterior edge of the ITB and the underlying lateral femoral epicondyle. The study subjects had an average knee flexion angle of $21.4° \pm 4.3°$ at foot strike, with friction occurring at or slightly below the $30°$ of knee flexion traditionally described in the literature. In the cadaveric knees examined, there was substantial variation in the width of the ITBs. The authors believed that this variation may affect individual predisposition to ITB-friction syndrome. The authors suggested that downhill running predisposes the runner to ITB-friction syndrome because the knee flexion angle at footstrike is reduced. Sprinting and faster running on level ground are less likely to cause or aggravate ITB-friction syndrome because, at footstrike, the knee is flexed beyond the angles at which friction occurs.

Clinically, athletes complain of pain on the lateral aspect of the knee during activity. Running downhill or climbing stairs may aggravate the symptoms because these activities usually cause excessive compression of the ITB on the lateral epicondyle of the femur. On physical examination, localized tenderness over the lateral epicondyle may be found approximately 3 cm proximal to the lateral joint line. The typical pain may be reproduced by a compression test. With the patient supine, the thumb of the examiner is placed over the epicondyle, and active flexion–extension of the knee is performed. Pain results and is usually maximum at $30°$ of knee flexion. Occasionally, soft tissue swelling, crepitus, or both are present over this area. The differential diagnoses include patellofemoral stress syndrome, lateral meniscus lesion, biceps tendonitis, or popliteus tendonitis. Murphy *et al.* [86] found that axial MRI was helpful in confirming the diagnosis of ITB-friction syndrome and in excluding other causes of lateral knee pain.

Treatment consists of altering the initiating activity and controlling the inflammatory process. Alterations in training may be useful. These include changing the duration of training activity, altering stride length, or changing direction if one is running on a circular track. Cyclists may need to change the seat height or foot position on their bicycles. A lateral-wedge orthosis may be helpful for athletes with a tight ITB, and a rigid orthosis may be useful for those with excessive pronation of the feet. Symptomatic treatment includes anti-inflammatory medications, use of ice or heat modalities, and ITB stretching exercises. Most athletes respond to nonoperative treatment. In patients with persistent, disabling symptoms despite conservative measures, surgery is indicated. This consists of resection of a triangular piece of tissue from the ITB over the lateral femoral epicondyle when the knee is in $30°$ of flexion.

Barber and Sutker [87] reported on 19 patients with ITB-friction syndrome. Most of these patients were high-mileage runners. Shoes that were worn out or had insufficient cushioning appeared to predispose to ITB-friction syndrome. All patients responded to conservative treatment. The most important aspects of treatment consisted of rest or mileage reduction, shoe modification or use of an orthosis, stretching of the ITB, and running on alternate sides of the road to avoid varus stresses to the knee. Heel lifts were thought to benefit patients with limb-length discrepancies. Operative treatment was not required in this series but may be a consideration in rare cases.

REFERENCES AND RECOMMENDED READING

Recently published papers of particular interest have been highlighted as:

• Of special interest

•• Of outstanding interest

1. Assimakopoulos AP, Katonis PG, Agapitos MV, *et al.*: The innervation of the human meniscus. *Clin Orthop* 1992, 275:232–236.

2. Royle SG, Noble J, Parkinson RW, *et al.*: The diagnostic potential of synovial effusion in meniscal pathology. *Arthroscopy* 1992, 8:254–257.

3. Fauno P, Nielsen AB: Arthroscopic partial meniscectomy: a long-term follow-up. *Arthroscopy* 1992, 8:345–349.

4. Hede A, Larsen E, Sandberg H: Partial Versus Total Meniscectomy: A prospective randomised study with long-term follow-up. *J Bone Joint Surg Br* 1992, 74:118–121.

5. Sommerlath K, Gillquist J: The long-term course of various meniscal treatments in anterior cruciate ligament deficient knees. *Clin Orthop* 1992, 283:207–214.

6. Wroble RR, Henderson RC, Campion ER, *et al.*: Meniscectomy in children and adolescents: a long-term follow-up study. *Clin Orthop* 1992, 279:180–189.

7. Neyret P, Donell ST, Dejour H: Results of partial meniscectomy related to the state of the anterior cruciate ligament: review at 20 to 35 years. *J Bone Joint Surg Br* 1993, 75:36–40.

8. •• DeHaven KE, Lohrer WA, Lovelock JE. Long-term results of open meniscal repair. *Am J Sports Med* 1995, 23:524–530.
This study reports the long-term results of meniscal repair using an open technique.

9. Tenuta JJ, Arciero RA: Arthroscopic evaluation of meniscal repairs: factors that effect healing. *Am J Sports Med* 1994, 22:797–802.

10. •• Eggli S, Wegmuller H, Kosina J, *et al.*: Long-term results of arthroscopic meniscal repair: an analysis of isolated tears. *Am J Sports Med* 1995, 23:715–720.
This study reports the long-term results of arthroscopically assisted meniscal repair for isolated meniscal tears.

11. • Horibe S, Shino K, Nakata K, *et al.*: Second-look arthroscopy after meniscal repair: review of 132 menisci repaired by an arthroscopic inside-out technique. *J Bone Joint Surg Br* 1995, 77:245–249.
This study shows evaluation of healing after meniscal repair by "second-look" arthroscopy.

12. Kimura M, Shirakura K, Hasegawa A, *et al.*: Second look arthroscopy after meniscal repair: factors affecting the healing rate. *Clin Orthop* 1995, 314:185–191.

13. Horibe S, Shino K, Maeda A, *et al.*: Results of isolated meniscal repair evaluated by second-look arthroscopy. *Arthroscopy* 1996, 12:150–155.

14. Rodeo SA, Warren RF: Meniscal repair using the outside-to-inside technique. Clin *Sports Med* 1996, 15:469–481.

15. Morgan CD: The "all-inside" meniscus repair. *Arthroscopy* 1991, 7:120–125.

16. Barrett GR, Richardson K, Koenig V: T-fix endoscopic meniscal repair: technique and approach to different types of tears. *Arthroscopy* 1995, 11:245–251.

17. Barrett GR, Treacy SH: Use of the t-fix suture anchor in fascial sheath reconstruction of complex meniscal tears. *Arthroscopy* 1996, 12:251–255.

18. Arnoczky SP, Warren RF, Spivak JM: Meniscal repair using an exogenous fibrin clot: an experimental study in dogs. *J Bone Joint Surg Am* 1988, 70:1209–1217.

19. Klompmaker J, Jansen HW, Veth RP, *et al.*: Meniscal repair by fibrocartilage? an experimental study in the dog. *J Orthop Res* 1992, 10:359–370.

20. Hashimoto J, Kurosaka M, Yoshiya S, *et al.*: Meniscal repair using fibrin sealant and endothelial cell growth factor: an experimental study in dogs. *Am J Sports Med* 1992, 20:537–541.

21. Bonamo JJ, Kessler KJ, Noah J: Arthroscopic meniscectomy in patients over the age of 40. *Am J Sports Med* 1992, 20:422–429.

22. Wouters E, Bassett FH III, Hardaker WT Jr, *et al.*: An algorithm for arthroscopy in the over-50 age group. *Am J Sports Med* 1992, 20:141–145.

23. Mohr M, Henche HR: The morbidity associated with lost or irretrievable resected meniscal fragments. *Arthroscopy* 1992, 8:84–88.

24. Durand A, Richards CL, Malouin F, *et al.*: Motor recovery after arthroscopic partial meniscectomy: analyses of gait and the ascent and descent of stairs. *J Bone Joint Surg Am* 1993, 75:202–214.

25. Irvine GB, Glasgow MM: The natural history of the meniscus in anterior cruciate insufficiency: arthroscopic analysis. *J Bone Joint Surg Br* 1992, 74:403–405.

26. Cannon WD Jr, Vittori JM: The incidence of healing in arthroscopic meniscal repairs in anterior cruciate ligament-reconstructed knees versus stable knees. *Am J Sports Med* 1992; 20:176–181.

27. Sommerlath K, Gillquist J: The effect of a meniscal prosthesis on knee biomechanics and cartilage: an experimental study in rabbits. *Am J Sports Med* 1992, 20:73–81.

28. Stone KR, Rodkey WG, Webber R, *et al.*: Meniscal regeneration with copolymeric collagen scaffolds: *in vitro* and *in vivo* studies evaluated clinically, histologically, and biochemically. *Am J Sports Med* 1992, 20:104–111.

29. Arnoczky SP, DiCarlo EF, O'Brien SJ, *et al.*: Cellular repopulation of deep-frozen meniscal autografts: an experimental study in the dog. *Arthroscopy* 1992, 8:428–436.

30. Jackson DW, McDevitt CA, Simon TM, *et al.*: Meniscal transplantation using fresh and cryopreserved allografts: an experimental study in goats. *Am J Sports Med* 1992, 20:644–656.

31. Jackson DW, Whelan J, Simon TM: Cell survival after transplantation of fresh meniscal allografts: dna probe analysis in a goat model. *Am J Sports Med* 1993, 21:540–550.

32. Asselmeier MA, Caspari RB, Bottenfield S: A review of allograft processing and sterilization techniques and their role in transmission of the human immunodeficiency virus. *Am J Sports Med* 1993, 21:170–175.

33. Veltri DM, Warren RF, Wickiewicz TL, *et al.*: Current status of allograft meniscal transplantation. *Clin Orthop* 1994, 303:44–55.

34. • Chen MI, Branch TP, Hutton WC: Is it important to secure the horns during lateral meniscal transplantation? a cadaveric study. *Arthroscopy* 1996, 12:174–181.
This cadaveric, biomechanical study shows the importance of securing both horns of the lateral meniscus during transplantation.

35. Hodler J, Haghighi P, Pathria MN, *et al.*: Meniscal changes in the elderly: correlation of mr imaging and histologic findings. *Radiology* 1992, 184:221–225.

36. Gerngross H, Sohn C: Ultrasound scanning for the diagnosis of meniscal lesions of the knee joint. *Arthroscopy* 1992, 8:105–110.

37. •• Potter HG, Rodeo SA, Wickiewicz TL, *et al.*: MR imaging of meniscal allografts: correlation with clinical and arthroscopic outcomes. *Radiology* 1996, 198:509–514.
Magnetic resonance imaging can help in the assessment of allograft placement and articular cartilage, and also enable differentiation of fragmentation of the meniscus from extrusion of the meniscus. Preoperative evaluation of the articular cartilage is important to identify patients in whom meniscal allograft surgery may fail.

38. Armstrong RW, Bolding F, Joseph R: Septic arthritis following arthroscopy: clinical syndromes and analysis of risk factors. *Arthroscopy* 1992, 8:213–223.

39. Bomberg BC, Hurley PE, Clark CA, *et al.*: Complications associated with the use of an infusion pump during knee arthroscopy. *Arthroscopy* 1992, 8:224–228.

40. Arangio G, Kostelnik KE: Intraarticular pressures in a gravity-fed arthroscopy fluid delivery system. *Arthroscopy* 1992, 8:341–344.

41. Ekman EF, Poehling GG: An experimental assessment of the risk of compartment syndrome during knee arthroscopy. *Arthroscopy* 1996, 12:193–199.

42. Joshi GP, McCarroll SM, Cooney CM, *et al.*: Intra-articular morphine for pain relief after knee arthroscopy. *J Bone Joint Surg Br* 1992, 74:749–751.

43. Nelson WE, Henderson RC, Almekinders LC, *et al.*: An evaluation of pre- and postoperative nonsteroidal antiinflammatory drugs in patients undergoing knee arthroscopy: a prospective, randomized, double-blinded study. *Am J Sports Med* 1993, 21:510–516.

44. Pedersen P, Nielsen KD, Jensen PE: The efficacy of Na-naproxen after diagnostic and therapeutic arthroscopy of the knee joint. *Arthroscopy* 1993, 9:170–173.

45. Solanki DR, Enneking FK, Ivey FM, *et al.*: Serum bupivacaine concentrations after intraarticular injection for pain relief after knee arthroscopy. *Arthroscopy* 1992, 8:44–47.

46. Highgenboten CL, Jackson AW, Meske NB: Arthroscopy of the knee: ten-day pain profiles and corticosteroids. *Am J Sports Med* 1993, 21:503–506.

47. Shapiro F, Koide S, Glimcher MJ: Cell origin and differentiation in the repair of full-thickness defects of articular cartilage. *J Bone Joint Surg Am* 1993, 75:532–553.

48. Paletta GA, Arnoczky SP, Warren RF: The repair of osteochondral defects using an exogenous fibrin clot: an experimental study in dogs. *Am J Sports Med* 1992, 20:725–731.

49. Tesch GH, Handley CJ, Cornell HJ, *et al.*: Effects of free and bound insulin-like growth factors on proteoglycan metabolism in articular cartilage explants. *J Orthop Res* 1992, 10:14–22.

50. Larsen NE, Lombard KM, Parent EG, *et al.*: Effect of Hylan on cartilage and chondrocyte cultures. *J Orthop Res* 1992, 10:23–32.

51. Schachar N, McAllister D, Stevenson M, *et al.*: Metabolic and biochemical status of articular cartilage following cryopreservation and transplantation: a rabbit model. *J Orthop Res* 1992, 10:603–609.

52. Marandola MS, Prietto CA: Arthroscopic Herbert screw fixation of patellar osteochondritis dissecans. *Arthroscopy* 1993, 9:214–216.

53. Matsusue Y, Yamamuro T, Hama H: Arthroscopic multiple osteochondral transplantation to the chondral defect in the knee associated with anterior cruciate ligament disruption. *Arthroscopy* 1993, 9:318–321.

54. Galloway MT, Noyes FR: Cystic degeneration of the patella after arthroscopic chondroplasty and subchondral bone perforation. *Arthroscopy* 1992, 8:366–369.

55. Beaver RJ, Mahomed M, Backstein D, *et al.*: Fresh osteochondral allografts for post-traumatic defects in the knee: a survivorship analysis. *J Bone Joint Surg Br* 1992, 74:105–110.

56. Garrett JC, Kress KJ, Mudano M: Osteochondritis dissecans of the lateral femoral condyle in the adult. *Arthroscopy* 1992, 8:474–481.

57. Schenck RC Jr, Goodnight JM: Osteochondritis dissecans. *J Bone Joint Surg Am* 1996, 78:439–456.

58. Brittberg M, Lindahl A, Nilsson A, *et al.*: Treatment of deep cartilage defects in the knee with autologous chondrocyte transplantation. *New Engl J Med* 1994, 331:889–895.

59. Koskinen SK, Kujala UM: Patellofemoral relationships and distal insertion of the vastus medialis muscle: a magnetic resonance imaging study in non-symptomatic subjects and in patients with patellar dislocation. *Arthroscopy* 1992, 8:465–468.

60. Simmons E Jr, Cameron JC: Patella alta and recurrent dislocation of the patella. *Clin Orthop* 1992, 274:265–269.

61. Gomes JL: Medial patellofemoral ligament reconstruction for recurrent dislocation of the patella: a preliminary report. *Arthroscopy* 1992, 8:335–340.

62. Small NC, Glogau AI, Berezin MA: Arthroscopically assisted proximal extensor mechanism realignment of the knee. *Arthroscopy* 1993, 9:63–67.

63. Arnbjornsson A, Egund N, Rydling O, *et al.*: The natural history of recurrent dislocation of the patella: long-term results of conservative and operative treatment. *J Bone Joint Surg Br* 1992, 74:140–142.

64. Boucher JP, King MA, Lefebvre R, *et al.*: Quadriceps femoris muscle activity in patellofemoral pain syndrome. *Am J Sports Med* 1992, 20:527–532.

65. Puniello MS: Iliotibial band tightness and medial patellar glide in patients with patellofemoral dysfunction. *J Orthop Sports Phys Ther* 1993, 17:144–148.

66. Doucette SA, Goble EM: The effect of exercise on patellar tracking in lateral patellar compression syndrome. *Am J Sports Med* 1992, 20:434–440.

67. O'Neill DB, Micheli LJ, Warner JP: Patellofemoral stress: a prospective analysis of exercise treatment in adolescents and adults. *Am J Sports Med* 1992, 20:151–156.

68. Karlsson J, Kalebo P, Goksor L-A, *et al.*: Partial rupture of the patellar ligament. *Am J Sports Med* 1992, 20:390–395.

69. Scranton PE Jr, Farrar EL: Mucoid degeneration of the patellar ligament in athletes. *J Bone Joint Surg Am* 1992, 74:435–437.

70. McLoughlin RF, Raber EL, Vellet AD, *et al.*: Patellar tendinitis: mr imaging features, with suggested pathogenesis and proposed classification. *Radiology* 1995, 197:843–848.

71. Johnson DP, Wakeley CJ, Watt I: Magnetic resonance imaging of patellar tendonitis. *J Bone Joint Surg Br* 1996, 78:452–457.

72. Teitz CC, Harrington RM: Patellar stress fracture. *Am J Sports Med* 1992, 20:761–765.

73. Binazzi R, Felli L, Vaccari V, *et al.*: Surgical treatment of unresolved Osgood-Schlatter lesion. *Clin Orthop* 1993, 289:202–204.

74. Barber FA, Prudich JF: Acute traumatic knee hemarthrosis. *Arthroscopy* 1993, 9:174–176.

75. Triantafyllou SJ, Hanks GA, Handal JA, *et al.*: Open and arthroscopic synovectomy in hemophilic arthropathy of the knee. *Clin Orthop* 1992, 283:196–204.

76. Cohen B, Griffiths L, Dandy DJ: Arteriovenous fistula after arthroscopic synovectomy in a patient with haemophilia. *Arthroscopy* 1992, 8:373–374.

77. • Wiedel JD: Arthroscopic synovectomy of the knee in hemophilia: 10-to-15 year follow-up. *Clin Orthop* 1996, 328:46–53.
This is a prospective long-term study (10 to 15 years of follow-up) of arthroscopic synovectomy of the knee in patients with hemophilia.

78. Schwartz HS, Unni KK, Pritchard DJ: Pigmented villonodular synovitis: a retrospective review of affected large joints. *Clin Orthop* 1989, 247:243–255.

79. Van Meter CD, Rowdon GA: Localized pigmented villonodular synovitis presenting as a locked lateral meniscal bucket handle tear: a case report and review of the literature. *Arthroscopy* 1994, 10:309–312.

80. Bravo SM, Winalski CS, Weissman BN: Pigmented villonodular synovitis. *Radiol Clin North Am* 1996, 34:311–326.

81. Ogilvie-Harris DJ, McLean J, Zarnett ME: Pigmented villonodular synovitis of the knee: the results of total arthroscopic synovectomy, partial arthroscopic synovectomy, and arthroscopic local excision. *J Bone Joint Surg Am* 1992, 74:119–123.

82. Flandry F, Hughston JC: Current Concepts Review: Pigmented villonodular synovitis. *J Bone Joint Surg Am* 1987, 69:942–949.

83. Franssen MJ, Boerbooms AM, Karthaus RP, *et al.*: Treatment of pigmented villonodular synovitis of the knee with Yttrium-90 silicate: prospective evaluations by arthroscopy, histology and ^{99m}Tc pertechnetate uptake measurements. *Ann Rheum Dis* 1989, 48:1007–1013.

84. Wiss DA: Recurrent Villonodular Synovitis of the Knee: Successful treatment with Yttrium-90. *Clin Orthop* 1982, 169:139–144.

85. • Orchard JW, Fricker PA, Abud AT, *et al.*: Biomechanics of iliotibial band friction syndrome in runners. *Am J Sports Med* 1996, 24:375–379.
This study proposes a biomechanical model to explain the pathogenesis of iliotibial band friction syndrome in distance runners.

86. Murphy BJ, Hechtman KS, Uribe JW, *et al.*: Iliotibial band friction syndrome: MR imaging findings. *Radiology* 1992, 185:569–571.

87. Barber FA, Sutker AN: Iliotibial band syndrome. *Sports Med* 1992, 14:144–148.

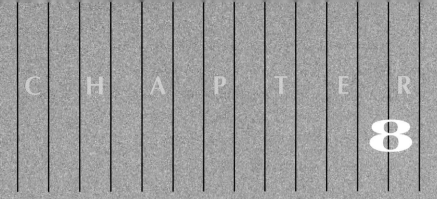

C H A P T E R

8

ANKLE AND FOOT

Paul A. Dowdy,
Mark D. Miller,
and Freddie H. Fu

Because of the increasing emphasis on fitness in our society, there has been a corresponding escalation in the number of athletic injuries, particularly to the foot and ankle. Fortunately, this trend has been matched by the enthusiastic evolution of orthopedic subspecialties in both sports medicine and foot and ankle care. Advances in this field range from a better understanding of the most common injury in sports, the ankle sprain, to diagnosis and treatment recommendations for disorders never previously described [1].

EXERTIONAL COMPARTMENT SYNDROME

Compartment syndrome, caused by elevated pressures within a confined space, has been well described in the trauma literature [2]. However, exertional compartment syndrome associated with sports participation (especially in runners) has been recognized only within the past decade [3]. It is most often chronic but rarely can be acute [4–6]. The anterior and deep posterior compartments of the leg are most frequently involved [7]. Occasionally it can involve the thigh or feet [4–6,8,9]. The typical complaint is a gradual onset of pain during exercise; the pain eventually reaches a level at which further performance is restricted [10]. Some patients may complain of numbness, tightness, or weakness, but most do not [11]. Nuclear imaging sometimes demonstrates diffuse linear uptake along the posteromedial border of the tibia, and compartment pressure measurements taken before, during, and immediately after exercise can be helpful in confirming the diagnosis [11–13]. Magnetic resonance imaging (MRI) can be a useful adjunct to the diagnosis [14]. Although there is some disagreement in the literature regarding the magnitude of pressure measurements necessary to make this diagnosis, most authors agree that resting pressures over 15 mm Hg, delay in normalization after exercise (pressure > 20 mm Hg 5 minutes following exercise), or both are consistent with chronic exertional compartment syndrome [11,15]. Nonoperative management (*eg*, activity modification and nonsteroidal medications) is sometimes successful, especially in borderline cases. One study found that compartment pressures after maximal exercise were significantly greater in runners than in cyclists [16]. The authors suggested that cycling may be an effective cross-training technique for symptomatic runners. Patients who do not respond to these measures sometimes require fasciotomies. One group of investigators reported 78% good to excellent results with surgical release [17]. Treatment of anterior and lateral compartment syndromes tends to give better out-

comes than treatment of deep posterior compartment syndrome [15,18,19]. In performing this procedure for posterior compartment syndrome, it is important to release not only the deep posterior compartment, but also the posterior tibial compartment and soleal bridge (Figs. 8.1 and 8.2) [20].

STRESS (FATIGUE) FRACTURES

Stress (or fatigue) fractures are common in athletes and represent 6% of all injuries to runners [21]. Pain, exacerbated by exercise and partially relieved by rest, is typical. Patients may relate a history of recent change in activity or training [22]. A brief menstrual history also is appropriate for female athletes

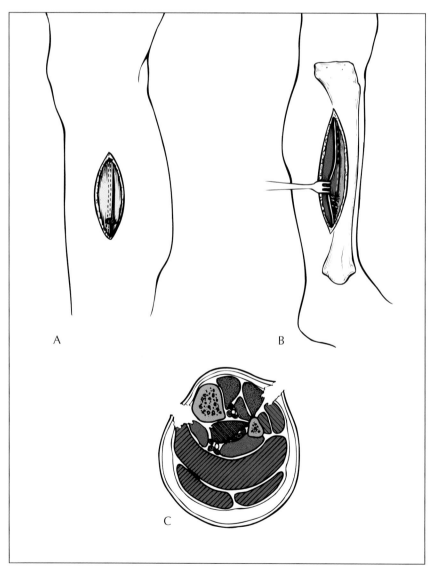

FIGURE 8.1

A, Anterolateral incision for release of anterior and lateral compartments. Care is taken to avoid the superficial peroneal nerve. **B**, Medial incision for release of superficial and deep posterior compartments. **C**, Cross-section demonstrating compartment release.

because of the association of amenorrhea and oligomenorrhea with osteoporosis [22]. One study of stress fractures in ballet dancers identified amenorrhea and heavy training schedules as predisposing factors for stress fractures [23]. Another study analyzed male and female track athletes prospectively, trying to determine the incidence of and risk factors for stress fractures [24]. They found a 21.1% incidence of stress fractures in their 53 female and 58 male athletes (mainly tibia). They could find no predictable risk factor for men, but women who had a lower bone density, history of menstrual disturbance, late menarche, less mean mass in the lower limb, a discrepancy in leg length, or a lower fat diet were predisposed to stress fracture [24]. Examination may reveal localized tenderness or induration. Radiographs may demonstrate established fractures, but nuclear imaging is most helpful in establishing the diagnosis. Computed tomography scan or tomograms can be very helpful. Stress fracture location tends to be somewhat sports specific (Table 8.1). These fractures generally resolve with activity modification and rest. One study suggested that improved shoe shock attenuation may have a preventive role in overuse injuries of the foot [25]. Recalcitrant fractures, such as transverse anterior tibial and tarsal navicular stress fractures, may require operative treatment.

The transverse anterior tibial stress fracture merits special emphasis. Persistence of the "dreaded black line," especially in light of a positive bone scan, for more than 4 to 6 months is an indication for excision and bone grafting or reamed intramedullary rod fixation (Fig. 8.3). This recom-

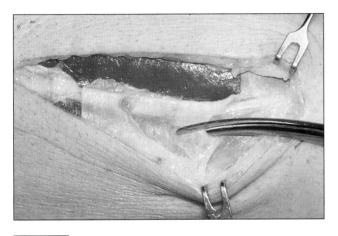

FIGURE 8.2

Case example of anterolateral compartment release. Note position of long scissors and protection of the superficial peroneal nerve.

Table 8.1	LOCATIONS OF COMMON STRESS FRACTURES ACCORDING TO TYPE OF ATHLETE
TYPE OF ATHLETE	**LOCATION OF FRACTURE**
Runners	Tibia (distal), fibula, metatarsals
Basketball players	Tarsal navicular, tibia (midshaft)
Football players	Metatarsals, first metatarsophalangeal sesamoids
Dancers	Metatarsal (base), tibia (midshaft)
Military recruits	Metatarsal (distal shaft), calcaneus, tibia (proximal)

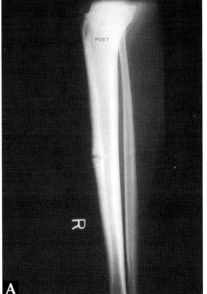

FIGURE 8.3.

Radiograph (*panel A*) and bone scan (*panel B*) of tibial stress fracture with "dreaded black line."

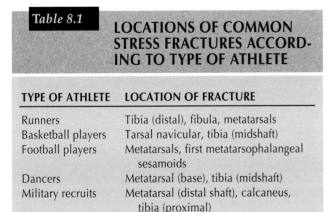

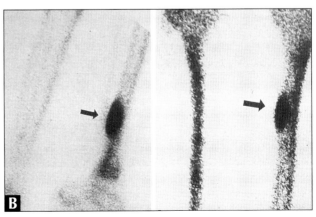

mendation is based on the results of a study in which five of six patients with anterior tibial stress fractures went on to a complete fracture [26,27]. Other authors have reported using pulsing electromagnetic fields with some success [28].

Stress fractures of the tarsal navicular can also be difficult to manage. One study emphasized the importance of immobilization and non–weight-bearing activity in the initial treatment of navicular stress fractures [29]. This treatment resulted in healing in 86% of patients versus only 26% of patients with continued weight-bearing and activity limitation. Another study recommended autologous bone grafting for complete fractures, nonunion, cysts, and incomplete fractures that did not heal with non–weight-bearing treatment [30]. The authors reported a return to the preinjury activity level within 1 year in 12 of 15 patients treated with this procedure.

Forefoot and hindfoot fractures are relatively common. Stress fractures in the forefoot most commonly involve the metatarsals, especially in the distal second and third shafts [22,31]. One group, however, reported three cases of stress fractures involving the proximal phalanx of the great toe [32]. Second metatarsal stress fractures can often be managed nonoperatively. O'Malley *et al.* [33] reviewed 61 cases of second metatarsal stress fractures occurring in ballet dancers. Excellent results were obtained in most cases by using symptomatic treatment and temporarily stopping dancing. Hindfoot fatigue fractures usually involve the calcaneus; however, talar fractures, usually involving the dome of the talus, have also been reported [34]. Patients with calcaneal stress fractures often have pain and tenderness on both sides of the heel. Radiographs may show subtle areas of increased density posteriorly, but bone scans are the most helpful. Treatment consists of activity modification with or without immobilization [22].

TENDON INJURIES
Peroneal tendon

Peroneal tendon injuries include subluxation or dislocation, tenosynovitis, and tendon splitting or rupture. Traumatic subluxation or dislocation of the peroneal tendons has been reported as being a result of various sports-related injuries. The peroneal muscles contract reflexively during the injury and break through their fibro-osseous sheath [35]. The tendons may spontaneously relocate, but if

activation of the peroneal muscles reproduces the pain or overtly dislocates the tendons, the diagnosis is confirmed [35]. Acute treatment is controversial; however, chronic, painful lesions require operative treatment. Procedures that have been advocated include soft-tissue reconstruction, bone-block techniques, tissue-transfer procedures, rerouting of the tendons, and groove-deepening procedures [10,36–38]. Tenosynovitis, tendinitis, and tendinosis of the peroneal tendons may be more common than is generally believed [39]. Longitudinal splitting of the peroneus brevis tendon has been increasingly recognized [40]. This phenomenon appears to be caused by prolonged mechanical attrition within the fibular groove following ankle trauma, and it may be associated with peroneal subluxation [40]. Bassett and Speer [41] noted in an anatomic study that the peroneal tendons contact the tip of the fibula with 15° to 25° of ankle plantar flexion, which may be a mechanism for longitudinal tears of these tendons. Repair and decompression are generally recommended for chronic lesions [10,41].

Complete tears of the peroneal tendons are unusual, especially in athletes. Primary repair is recommended if possible. However, if the tendons have retracted, anchoring the proximal tendon to the adjacent intact peroneal muscle is effective [42].

Posterior tibialis tendon

Injuries to the posterior tibialis tendon most commonly result from chronic degenerative processes in nonathletic, middle-aged women. One author noted that tendon tears occurring in younger patients are different than these typical ruptures and should be treated aggressively [43]. Another report described complete or partial posterior tibial tendon rupture in six athletic patients [44]. The authors noted that the patients described pain in the midarch region, had difficulty with push-off during running, and had a pronated, flattened longitudinal arch. The authors recommended early recognition and debridement of partial ruptures. Chronic, complete ruptures required advancement of the posterior tibialis tendon and transfer of the flexor digitorum longus tendon into the navicular. Dislocation of the posterior tibialis tendon has also been described [45,46], and treatment is similar to that of peroneal tendon dislocation, a more common disorder. Treatment consists of reduction and repair or reconstruction of the groove and retinaculum with or without reinforcement from a medial slip of the Achilles tendon detached proximally and attached to the medial malleolus [47].

Anterior tibialis tendon

Acute spontaneous rupture of the anterior tibialis tendon is uncommon but has been reported [48]. Diagnosis is confirmed by localized tenderness, inversion weakness, and a normal neurologic examination. Recommended treatment for acute rupture is surgical repair, but treatment of chronic ruptures is controversial.

Achilles tendon

Achilles tendon disorders are among the most common athletic injuries [49]. Partial ruptures of the tendon have been missed in the past but now are being recognized with increasing frequency. Because of the long-term morbidity associated with chronic partial Achilles tendon ruptures, surgical excision of scar and granulation tissue, with or without osteotomy of the calcaneal tuberosity, has been recommended. Renström [49] noted that 80% of his athletic patients returned to their former level of activity following this treatment.

Because the diagnosis of partial ruptures can be difficult, some authors have advocated special imaging modalities. A group of European investigators reported a sensitivity of 94% and specificity of 100% using ultrasonography in the diagnosis of partial ruptures [50]. Astrom *et al*. [51] compared ultrasound, MRI, and surgical findings in 27 histologically confirmed cases. All specimens revealed tendinosis histologically, whereas two of the cases were macroscopically normal. Ultrasonography was positive in 21 of 26 cases, and MRI was positive in 26 of 27 cases. The finding of abnormal MRI signal in macroscopically normal-appearing mesenchymal tissue has been shown previously in the anterior cruciate ligament [52•]. Another European group characterized Achilles tendon injuries as belonging to one of four types based on MRI: 1) inflammatory reaction, 2) degenerative change, 3) incomplete (partial) rupture, and 4) complete rupture [53].

Complete rupture of the Achilles tendon is caused by uncontrolled dorsiflexion and is classically associated with a painless "pop" that occurs after landing or jumping on the foot [54]. The Thompson test (squeezing the calf plantarflexes the foot with an intact Achilles tendon) is commonly used to diagnose Achilles tendon ruptures. A newer clinical test using a sphygmomanometer cuff is useful for both diagnosis and quantification of treatment progress [55]. Treatment of complete Achilles tendon ruptures remains controversial, but all authors agree that there is a much lower rate of rerupture with surgical treatment. Although percutaneous repair as described by Ma and Griffith [56] was initially popular, most surgeons now advocate conventional open repair [54,57]. This trend may result from reports of higher re-rupture rates and the potential for sural nerve injury associated with percutaneous repair [58,59]. We routinely perform open repair for our athletes with Achilles tendon ruptures (Fig. 8.4).

Treatment of chronic defects, particularly those with large gaps, can be challenging. Several techniques have been advocated for these cases. One European group favors pedicled muscle–tendon flaps from the triceps surae muscle transformed into free flaps or transplants [60]. Another technique, developed by Mann *et al*. [61], used the tendon of the flexor digitorum longus as a bridging graft with good to excellent results in six of seven patients.

NERVE ENTRAPMENT

Several nerve entrapment syndromes have been described on the basis of their anatomic location (Fig. 8.5). Of these, the most common entrapment syndrome in the athlete involves the superficial peroneal nerve [10]. Many nerve problems are function-

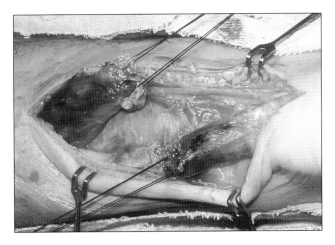

FIGURE 8.4

Mobilization of ruptured Achilles tendon before repair.

al (*ie*, the nerve is compressed only during athletic activity), and therefore special considerations in history taking, examination, and testing (*eg*, nerve conduction studies in conjunction with treadmill examination) may be necessary [62].

Saphenous nerve

The saphenous nerve can be entrapped as it pierces Hunter's canal (vastoadductor membrane). It can also be compressed as it pierces the fascia lata between the tendons of the sartorius and gracilis

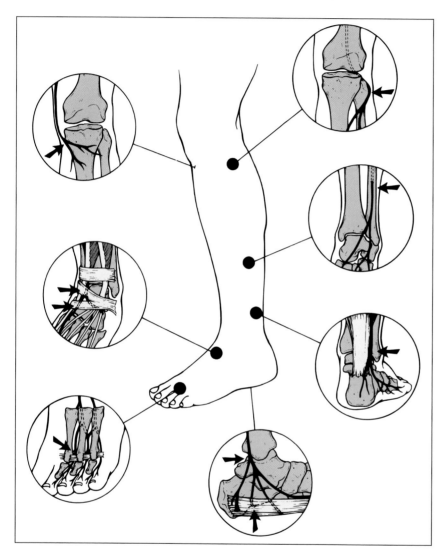

FIGURE 8.5

A, Locations of common lower extremity nerve entrapment syndromes. **B** and **C**, Surgical release of superficial peroneal nerve entrapment.

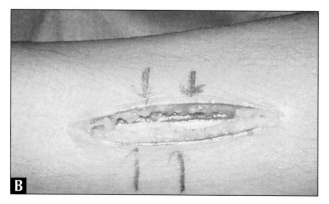

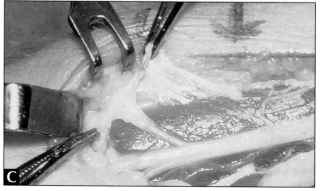

muscles. The infrapatellar branch of this nerve is commonly injured with medial approaches to the knee, sometimes resulting in a painful neuroma.

Common peroneal nerve

The common peroneal nerve can be compressed as it passes between the biceps tendon and the lateral head of the gastrocnemius muscle and behind the neck of the fibula between the two heads of the peroneus longus muscle.

It typically presents as posterolateral knee pain that radiates into the leg and foot. Electromyography studies can assist in the diagnosis. Treatment is surgical decompression.

Superficial peroneal nerve

The superficial peroneal nerve, which innervates the peroneus brevis and longus tendons, pierces the deep fascia of the anterolateral compartment approximately 12 cm proximal to the tip of the lateral malleolus. At this point, the nerve can be entrapped by fascial defects, fibrous bands, and local muscle herniation [63]. Patients may complain of pain over the lateral border of the distal calf and dorsum of the foot that is worse with activity and relieved by rest. Local tenderness, fascial defects, and provocative tests can be helpful in establishing the diagnosis. Specifically, active dorsiflexion and eversion of the foot against resistance, or passive plantarflexion and eversion, cause tenderness at the site of impingement [63]. Concomitant anterolateral compartment syndrome should be considered, and fasciotomy should be performed at the time of decompression if it is indicated. Simple exploration and decompression are usually effective.

Deep peroneal nerve (anterior tarsal tunnel)

Although the deep peroneal nerve can be compressed at several locations, the most common entrapment is under the inferior extensor retinaculum, commonly referred to as the anterior tarsal tunnel syndrome [62]. The nerve may be entrapped at the superior edge of the retinaculum, where the extensor hallucis longus tendon crosses over it [64]. Patients may complain of dorsal foot pain with occasional radiation into the first web space. Findings on examination may include localized tenderness, decreased sensation in the first web space, and weakness of the extensor digitorum brevis in more proximal entrapments. Conservative measures (eg, avoid-

ing provocative maneuvers, loosening external constraints, and modifying activity) should be tried initially. If these measures fail, exploration and surgical release of the offending structures may be indicated.

Posterior tibial nerve (tarsal tunnel)

The posterior tibial nerve can be entrapped behind the medial malleolus under the flexor retinaculum. This type of entrapment leads to what is commonly referred to as tarsal tunnel syndrome. Diagnosis may be confirmed with electrodiagnostic testing. If nonoperative treatment fails, then operative release of the retinaculum may be curative. Pfeiffer and Cracchiolo [65] cautioned that these patients often do not do as well from this operation as previously thought. Entrapment has been described distal to this point, involving the first branch of the lateral plantar nerve. This branch is entrapped between the deep fascia of the abductor hallucis longus and the medial margin of the quadratus plantae muscle [66]. Patients complain of burning pain, have tenderness along the course of the nerve, and may be unable to abduct the small toe [66]. Conservative treatment (eg, stretching, contrast baths, nonsteroidal anti-inflammatory drugs [NSAIDs], orthoses) is usually successful. In one study, surgical release of the deep fascia of the abductor hallucis was successful in 89% of cases in which extended conservative management failed [67].

Medial plantar nerve (jogger's foot)

Entrapment of the medial plantar nerve usually occurs near the area in which the flexor digitorum longus tendon crosses over the flexor hallucis longus tendon (knot of Henry). A frequent cause is external compression, eg, by the use of arch supports [62]. Symptoms may include pain radiating into the medial toes, and the patient may have localized tenderness, pain with toe-walking, and decreased sensation following activity. If conservative measures fail, surgical release is often successful.

Sural nerve

The sural nerve can be entrapped anywhere along its course. It can be irritated by injuries, ganglia, and even Achilles peritendinitis [62]. Localized tenderness can usually be elicited. Surgical release is usually effective.

Interdigital nerve

Interdigital nerve entrapment (Morton's neuroma) can occur in athletes during push-off while running.

Typically, entrapment occurs between the third and fourth metatarsals superficial to the deep transverse metatarsal ligament. Conservative management, including wider shoes, metatarsal pads, and, occasionally, anesthetic injection, steroid injection, or both can be helpful. Surgical excision of the neuroma is usually successful if these measures fail.

Plantar fasciitis

Plantar fasciitis, or inflammation of the plantar fascia in the central to medial subcalcaneal region, is difficult to diagnose and even more difficult to manage. It can be exacerbated by excessive or prolonged pronation and is best treated by rest, orthoses, and nonsteroidal medications [68]. Plantar fasciotomy has been advocated for intractable symptoms. A report of this procedure from the Mayo Clinic documented good to excellent results in 71% of 16 cases collected over a 10-year period [69]. The authors did point out, however, that the recovery was often pro-

longed, additional treatment was often required, and persistent abnormalities in foot function often remained despite satisfactory clinical results.

OS TRIGONUM

The unfused or fractured os trigonum can cause impingement in certain sporting activities, and this condition is becoming increasingly recognized, especially in ballet dancers [70]. Hedrick and McBryde [71] reported 30 cases of posterior ankle impingement. All were caused by forced plantar flexion. Most were associated with an os trigonum or posterior process fracture. Eight required excision. We recently treated a 15-year-old basketball player with posterior ankle pain that was refractory to rest, casting, NSAIDs, and other conservative measures (Fig. 8.6). Radiographs demonstrated what appeared to be a fracture of a fused os trigonum (Fig. 8.6A). Technetium bone scan demonstrated increased uptake in this area (Fig. 8.6B). Injection of

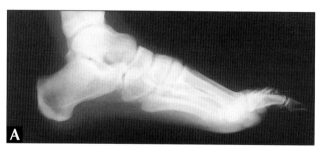

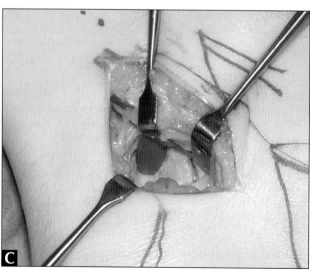

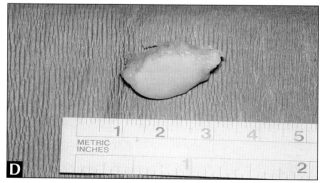

FIGURE 8.6

Symptomatic fracture of the fused os trigonum in an athlete. **A**, Lateral radiograph of symptomatic os trigonum. **B**, Bone scan demonstrates increased uptake in this area. **C**, Surgical resection of the offending bone. **D**, Surgical specimen. This patient had a successful recovery following surgery.

anesthetic in the area relieved his symptoms temporarily, and we elected to remove the offending bone surgically, with excellent relief of his symptoms (Fig. 8.6C). A similar patient with bilateral symptoms and a very large os trigonum on lateral radiography also had a positive bone scan (Fig. 8.7); she is currently improving with conservative treatment. Liu and Mirzayan [72] have reported a case of posteromedial impingement caused by soft tissue, which responded to arthroscopic resection.

ANKLE INSTABILITY

Ankle injuries are the most common joint injury seen in sports medicine, general orthopedics, and family practice [73]. The anterior talofibular ligament (ATFL) is the most commonly injured ankle ligament. Ankle sprains may be more common in larger athletes and in those with a history of an ankle sprain [74]. Patients who have ankle sprains

may be predisposed to them, either because of muscle imbalance or decreased proprioceptive characteristics [75,76]. Strain measurements have confirmed that the ATFL is most commonly injured with ankle inversion, plantar flexion, and internal rotation. Tears to the calcaneofibular ligament occur with dorsiflexion [77]. Another study confirmed that the ATFL contributed to ankle stability in plantarflexion but also suggested that the calcaneofibular ligament did so in all positions [78].

Increased emphasis has been placed on recognition of syndesmosis sprains. In one study [79], injuries to the syndesmosis were associated with a recovery time almost twice that of other patients with severe ankle sprains. The authors recommended incorporation of a "squeeze test" into the standard ankle examination to identify these patients acutely (Fig. 8.8). We also incorporate an external rotation stress to test the syndesmosis.

Studies have shown that there is a high incidence

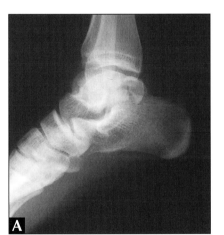

FIGURE 8.7

Radiograph (*panel A*) and bone scan (*panel B*) of a very large symptomatic os trigonum in a high school athlete.

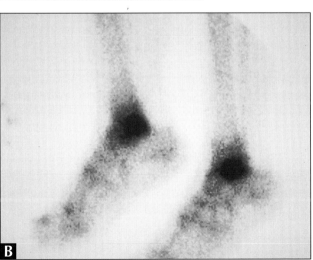

FIGURE 8.8

The "squeeze test" can identify syndesmosis injuries accurately. (*Adapted from* Hopkinson *et al.*[79]; with permission.)

of articular cartilage lesions in ankles with lateral ligament injury [80–82]. These lesions occur exclusively in chronic ankle sprains, suggesting a more aggressive approach for significant primary ankle sprains.

Several studies have confirmed that stress radiography may be of benefit in the evaluation of patients with chronic ankle instability [83,84]. Lesser degrees of anterior instability are consistent with isolated ATFL injuries, whereas greater degrees of instability may indicate combined injuries to the ATFL and the calcaneofibular ligament [84].

The effect of ankle taping on mechanical stability was found to be insignificant in one study, but helpful in another [85,86]. Another study suggested that the use of a semirigid orthosis may provide enough external support to prevent ankle sprains and to protect ligament reconstructions [87].

Currently, most authors (including ourselves) favor a modified Broström procedure for surgical treatment of ankle instability in the athlete in whom nonoperative measures have failed [88–90]. Other authors have suggested reinforcing this repair with a periosteal flap; however, we have not found this to be necessary [91]. In revision cases, and where there

is not enough local ligamentous tissue to perform a modified Broström procedure, we prefer to perform an anatomic reconstruction using a portion of the peroneus brevis or longus [92,93]. These anatomic procedures do not usually cause significant loss of subtalar motion.

ANKLE ARTHROSCOPY

Ankle arthroscopy is an effective tool in treating many ankle pathologies. Visualization is enhanced by distraction, either invasively or noninvasively [94–96,97•,98,99]. We prefer to use either no distraction (mainly for anterior lesions) or noninvasive distraction, in order to decrease the incidence of potential neurovascular or ligamentous injury seen with invasive distractors [100,101].

Indications for ankle arthroscopy have rapidly expanded from diagnostic to therapeutic procedures. Currently, arthroscopic treatment of osteochondral lesions of the talus, posttraumatic synovitis and osteoarthritis, and many other conditions of the ankle are well accepted. A long-term follow-up study of ankle arthroscopy done with various indications reported 73% good to excellent results, with

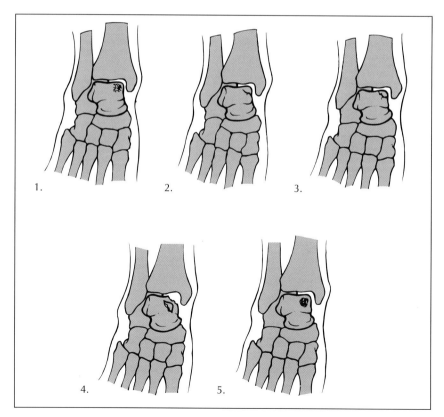

FIGURE 8.9

Fisher modification to the Berndt and Harty classification of osteochondral lesions of the talus. 1—compression; 2—partial fracture, nondisplaced; 3—complete fracture, nondisplaced; 4—displaced fracture; 5—radiolucent (fibrous) defect. (*Adapted from* Loomer *et al.* [107]; with permission.)

95% of patients indicating that they would undergo the same operation again if needed [102]. Amendola *et al.* [103••] analyzed the outcome of 79 consecutive cases of ankle arthroscopy. They found that patients with localized osteochondral talus lesions, localized bony or soft-tissue impingement, or localized lateral plica had the best results, whereas those with osteoarthritis of the ankle, posttraumatic chondromalacia or arthrofibrosis, and those patients on disability and workmen's compensation benefits did poorest.

Treatment of osteochondral lesions of the talus can often be done arthroscopically [104–106]. Loomer *et al.* [107] noted that anterior and midtalar lesions, which represent most of the lesions, can be treated arthroscopically. These authors added a fifth type to the Berndt and Harty classification scheme (Fig. 8.9). This newly described type, which was the most common variety in their series, is a radiolucent, fibrous defect in the talus. Curettage and drilling of the osteochondral lesions produced good to excellent results in 74% of their patients (Fig. 8.10). A long-term follow-up study of patients with osteochondral lesions of the talus treated with open drilling demonstrated that the initial good results of surgery deteriorated over time, with pain and swelling noted in over half the patients [108]. Nevertheless, these authors noted that only one patient in their series (18 patients) had significant pain at 9- to 15-year follow-up.

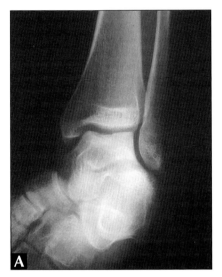

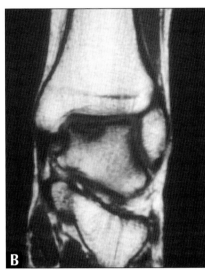

FIGURE 8.10

Surgical debridement and drilling of a symptomatic osteochondral lesion. Preoperative radiograph (*panel A*), magnetic resonance image (*panel B*), and endoscopic views (*panels C and D*) clearly demonstrate the lesion that was curetted and drilled, stimulating ingrowth of vascularized fibrocartilage.

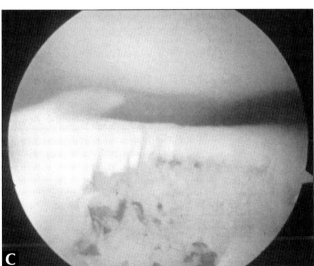

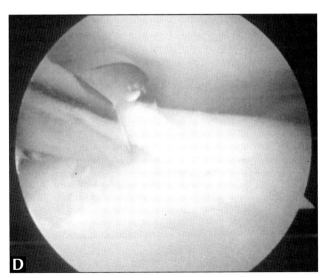

Arthroscopy is also useful in the treatment of anterior tibiotalar spurs. One study [109] noted a decreased length of hospitalization and recovery time in patients treated arthroscopically rather than with an open technique. The authors did caution, however, that patients with advanced arthritis and tibiotalar narrowing (type 4 degeneration) are not suitable candidates for arthroscopic debridement. Another study concluded that if conservative measures fail, then arthroscopic debridement of the anterior ankle compartment is effective [110].

Arthroscopy has been advocated for the treatment of anterolateral synovial impingement following injury as well [111]. One study noted excellent results in eight of nine patients treated with arthroscopic partial synovectomy [112]. A more recent series reported 90% good to excellent results following debridement of synovial thickening and scar tissue [113]. Liu *et al.* [114] reported their experience with 55 cases of anterolateral ankle impingement treated with arthroscopic resection. At an average follow-up of 2.6 years, 87% of the patients had good or excellent results, 98% were satisfied, and 84% returned to their previous sports. Unfortunately, our

experience with arthroscopic treatment in these cases has not been as remarkable. Arthroscopic treatment of talar impingement by the anteroinferior tibiofibular ligament (the Duke lesion) resulted in good to excellent results in six of seven patients following arthroscopic resection of this ligament [115]. Complications of ankle arthroscopy are relatively few, with the majority being related to damage of cutaneous nerves, especially the superficial peroneal nerve and its branches [116].

ANKLE FRACTURES

Ankle fractures are common in athletes; we treated three ankle fractures occurring in National Collegiate Athletic Association Division I football players over the past year. Interestingly, all three of these cases were pronation–external rotation injuries. Early management of ankle fractures includes acute reduction and immobilization. One study of displaced ankle fractures identified an increased incidence of skin complications in fractures that were not reduced acutely [117]. Treatment of ankle fractures does not necessarily require open reduction and

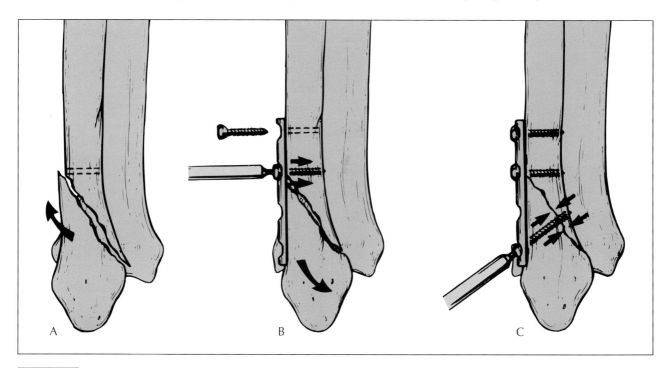

FIGURE 8.11

Technique for placement of an antiglide plate used in the fixation of lateral malleolar fractures. **A**, Type B distal fibula fracture. Note tendency of distal fragment to displace proximally. **B**, Placement of proximal screws aids in reduction of the fracture. Note that the plate is positioned posteriorly. **C**, Distal screw placement with interfragmentary screw. (*Adapted from* Winkler *et al.* [122]; with permission.)

internal fixation. A prospective study of supination–eversion type 2 injuries treated nonoperatively reported no or minimal symptoms in 45 of 49 patients at an average follow-up of 1.5 years [118].

Reports of complications associated with absorbable internal fixation necessitate judicious use of these implants. Of most concern are associated osteolysis and granulomatous reactions [119–121].

Use of the posterior antiglide plate for fixation of lateral malleolar fractures has been advocated in several studies [122,123]. This technique uses a buttress-type effect to stabilize the fracture during fixation (Fig. 8.11).

Two current studies of postoperative immobilization following open reduction and internal fixation of ankle fractures indicated there were no functional differences among a cast, an orthosis, or no cast or orthosis as long as patients were kept non–weight-bearing for 6 weeks postoperatively [124,125]. Sports activities can usually begin between the 10th and 20th weeks [125].

INJURIES TO THE GREAT TOE

Injuries to the great toe (especially "turf toe") have become increasingly frequent. This increase is probably related, at least in part, to the popularity of artificial turf [126]. The injury, which is most common in football offensive linemen and receivers, is related to severe dorsiflexion to the metatarsophalangeal joint of the great toe (Fig. 8.12). Diagnosis is made by the clinical picture of a dorsally tender, red, stiff, swollen joint [126]. The MRI appearance of turf toe has been described as a sprain or tear of the plantar metatarsophalangeal joint capsule [127]. Rehabilitation consists of range-of-motion exercises, ice, and taping. Special shoes designed for artificial turf may help reduce the incidence of these injuries. If symptoms persist, the athlete should be carefully evaluated to rule out a stress fracture of the proximal phalanx [32]. However, Clanton *et al.* [128] found a 50% incidence of persistent symptoms more than 5 years after a turf toe injury.

CONCLUSIONS

Injuries to the ankle and foot are common in athletes. Chronic or exertional compartment syndrome, if well documented, usually responds to fasciotomies. Most stress fractures do well with activity modification and other conservative measures. Certain tendon injuries, such as dislocations and ruptures, require surgical intervention. Nerve entrapment syndromes most commonly involve the

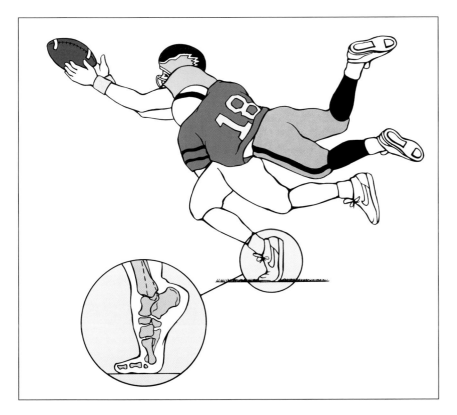

FIGURE 8.12

Mechanism of "turf toe" injury consists of severe dorsiflexion of the great toe at the metatarsophalangeal joint.

superficial peroneal nerve in athletes, and surgical release of the offending structures is often necessary. Other conditions, such as plantar fasciitis and impingement of the os trigonum, may also require surgery. Acute ankle sprains usually do well with therapy; however, chronic, recurrent ankle sprains may require surgical intervention in the form of a modified Broström procedure. Ankle arthroscopy has increased in popularity, and several studies have demonstrated good results in carefully select-

ed patients and procedures. Positive advances in ankle fracture management include emphasis on early treatment and the use of the antiglide plate. Absorbable fixation devices should be used judiciously because of reports of associated osteolysis. Injuries to the great toe are common in football, particularly on artificial turf. Increasing awareness of current trends in the diagnosis and treatment of injuries to the foot and ankle in the athlete will enhance the effectiveness of the team physician.

REFERENCES AND RECOMMENDED READING

Recently published papers of particular interest have been highlighted as:

- • Of special interest
- •• Of outstanding interest

1. Garrick JG, Requa RK: The epidemiology of foot and ankle injuries in sports. *Clin Sports Med* 1988, 7:29–36.

2. Pellegrini VD, Evarts CM: Complications. In *Rockwood and Green's Fractures and Dislocations*. Edited by Rockwood CA Jr, Green DP, Bucholz RW. Philadelphia: JB Lippincott; 1991:355–416.

3. Rorabeck CH, Bourne RB, Fowler PJ: The surgical treatment of exertional compartment syndromes in athletes. *J Bone Joint Surg Am* 1983, 65:1245–1251.

4. Blacklidge DK, Kurek JB, Soto AD, *et al.*: Acute exertional compartment syndrome of the medial foot. *J Foot Ankle Surg* 1996, 35:19–22.

5. Kahan JS, McClellan RT, Burton DS: Acute bilateral compartment syndrome of the thigh induced by exercise: a case report. *J Bone Joint Surg Am* 1994, 76:1068–1071.

6. McKee MD, Jupiter JB: Acute exercise-induced bilateral anterolateral leg compartment syndrome in a healthy young man. *Am J Orthopsychiatry* 1995, 24:862–864.

7. Martens MA, Moeyersoons JP: Acute and recurrent effort-related compartment syndrome in sports. *Am J Sports Med* 1990, 9:62–68.

8. Wise JJ, Fortin PT: Bilateral, exercise-induced thigh compartment syndrome diagnosed as exertional rhabdomyolysis: a case report and review of the literature. *Am J Sports Med* 1997, 25:126–129.

9. Middleton DK, Johnson JE, Davies JF: Exertional compartment syndrome of bilateral feet: a case report. *Foot Ankle* 1995, 16:95–96.

10. Clanton TO, Schon LC: Athletic injuries to the soft tissues of the foot and ankle. In *Surgery of the Foot and Ankle.* Edited by Mann RA, Coughlin MJ. St. Louis: Mosby-Year Book; 1993:1095–1224.

11. Eisele SA, Sammarco GJ: Chronic exertional compartment syndrome. *Instr Course Lect* 1993, 42:213–217.

12. Holder LE, Michael RH: The specific scintigraphic pattern of "shin splints in the lower leg." *J Nucl Med* 1984, 25:865–869.

13. Rorabeck CH: Exertional tibialis posterior compartment syndrome in athletes. *Clin Orthop* 1986, 208:61–64.

14. Amendola A, Rorabeck CH, Vellett D, *et al.*: The use of magnetic resonance imaging in exertional compartment syndromes. *Am J Sports Med* 1990, 18:29–34.

15. Balduini FC, Shenton DW, O'Connor KH, *et al.*: Chronic exertional compartment syndrome: correlation of compartment pressure and muscle ischemia utilizing 31P-NMR spectroscopy. *Clin Sports Med* 1993, 12:151–165.

16. Beckham SG, Grana WA, Buckley P, *et al.*: A comparison of anterior compartment pressures in competitive runners and cyclists. *Am J Sports Med* 1993, 21:36–40.

17. Jarvinen M, Aho H, Nittmmaki S: Results of the surgical treatment of the medial tibial syndrome in athletes. *Int J Sports Med* 1989, 10:55–57.

18. Abramowitz AJ, Schepsis AA: Chronic exertional compartment syndrome of the lower leg. *Orthop Rev* 1994, 23:219–225.

19. Schepsis AA, Martini D, Corbett, M: Surgical management of exertional compartment syndrome of the lower leg: long-term followup. *Am J Sports Med* 1993, 21:811–817.

20. Bourne RB, Rorabeck CH: Compartment syndromes of the lower leg. *Clin Orthop* 1989, 240:97–104.

21. James SL, Bates BT, Osternig LR: Injuries to runners. *Am J Sports Med* 1978, 6:40–50.

22. Eisele SA, Sammarco GJ: Fatigue fractures of the foot and ankle in the athlete. *Instr Course Lect* 1993, 42:175–183.

23. Kadel NJ, Teitz CC, Kronmal RA: Stress fractures in ballet dancers. *Am J Sports Med* 1992, 20:445–449.

24. Bennell KL, Malcolm SA, Thomas SA, *et al.*: Risk factors for stress fractures in track and field athletes: a twelve-month prospective study. *Am J Sports Med* 1996, 24:810–818.

25. Milgrom C, Finestone A, Shlamkovitch N, *et al.*: Prevention of overuse injuries of the foot by improved shoe shock attenuation: a randomized prospective study. *Clin Orthop* 1992, 281:189–192.

26. Green NE, Rogers RA, Lipscomb AB: Nonunions of stress fractures of the tibia. *Am J Sports Med* 1985, 13:171–176.

27. McBryde AM: Stress fractures in runners. *Clin Sports Med* 1985, 4:737–752.

28. Rettig AC, Shelbourne KD, McCarroll JR, *et al.*: The natural history and treatment of delayed union stress fractures of the anterior cortex of the tibia. *Am J Sports Med* 1988, 16:250–255.

29. Khan KM, Fuller PJ, Brukner PD, *et al.*: Outcome of conser-

vative and surgical management of navicular stress fracture in athletes: eighty-six cases proven with computerized tomography. *Am J Sports Med* 1992, 20:657–661.

30. Fitch KD, Blackwell JB, Gilmour WN: Operation for non-union of stress fractures of the tarsal navicular. *J Bone Joint Surg Br* 1989, 71:105–110.

31. Anderson EG: Fatigue fractures of the foot. *Injury* 1990, 274–279.

32. Shiraishi M, Mizuta H, Kubota K, *et al.*: Stress fracture of the proximal phalanx of the great toe. *Foot Ankle* 1993, 14:28–34.

33. O'Malley MJ, Hamilton WG, Munyak J, *et al.*: Stress fractures at the base of the second metatarsal in ballet dancers. *Foot Ankle* 1996, 17:89–94.

34. Hardaker WT Jr: Foot and ankle injuries in classical ballet dancers. *Orthop Clin North Am* 1989, 20:621–627.

35. Brage ME, Hansen ST: Tramatic subluxation/dislocation of the peroneal tendons. *Foot Ankle* 1992, 13:423–430.

36. Karlsson J, Eriksson BI, Sward, L: Recurrent dislocation of the peroneal tendons. *Scand J Med Sci Sports* 1996, 6:242–246.

37. Mason RB, Henderson JP: Traumatic peroneal tendon instability. *Am J Sports Med* 1996, 24:652–658.

38. Sammarco GJ: Peroneal tendon injuries. *Orthop Clin North Am* 1994, 25:135–145.

39. Sobel M, Bohne WHO, Markisz JA: Longitudinal attrition of the peroneus brevis tendon in the fibular groove: an anatomic study. *Foot Ankle* 1990, 11:124–128.

40. Sobel M, Geppert MJ, Olsen EJ, *et al.*: The dynamics of peroneus brevis tendon splits: a proposed mechanism, technique of diagnosis, and classification of injury. *Foot Ankle* 1992, 13:413–421.

41. Bassett FH III, Speer KP: Longitudinal rupture of the peroneal tendons. *Am J Sports Med* 1993, 21:354–357.

42. Thompson FM, Patteson AH: Rupture of the peroneus longus tendon: report of three cases. *J Bone Joint Surg Am* 1971, 71:293–295.

43. Conti SF: Posterior tibial tendon problems in athletes. *Orthop Clin North Am* 1994, 25:109–121.

44. Woods L, Leach RE: Posterior tibial tendon rupture in athletic people. *Am J Sports Med* 1991, 19:495–498.

45. Biedert R: Dislocation of the tibialis posterior tendon. *Am J Sports Med* 1992, 20:775–776.

46. Ouzounian TJ, Myerson MS: Dislocation of the posterior tibial tendon. *Foot Ankle* 1992, 13:215–219.

47. Ballesteros R, Chacon M, Cimarra A, *et al.*: Traumatic dislocation of the tibialis posterior tendon: a new surgical procedure to obtain a strong reconstruction. *J Trauma* 1995, 39:1198–1200.

48. Rimoldi RL, Oberlander MA, Waldrop JI, *et al.*: Acute rupture of the tibialis anterior tendon: a case report. *Foot Ankle* 1991, 176–177.

49. Renstrom PAFH: Mechanism, diagnosis, and treatment of running injuries. *Instr Course Lect* 1993, 42:225–234.

50. Kalebo P, Allenmark C, Peterson L, *et al.*: Diagnostic value of ultrasonography in partial ruptures of the Achilles tendon. *Am J Sports Med* 1992, 20:378–380.

51. Astrom M, Gentz CF, Nilsson P, *et al.*: Imaging in chronic Achilles tendinopathy: a comparison of ultrasonography, magnetic resonance imaging and surgical findings in 27 histologically verified cases. *Skeletal Radiol* 1996, 25:615–620.

52.• Dowdy PA, Vellet AD, Fowler PJ, *et al.*: Magnetic resonance imaging of the partially torn anterior cruciate ligament: an in-vitro animal model with correlative histopathology. *Clin J Sports Med* 1994, 4:187–191.
A study showing that magnetic resonance imaging can be so sensitive that it can visualize microscopic ligament disruption not visible to the naked eye.

53. Weinstabl R, Stiskal M, Neuhold A, *et al.*: Classifying calcaneal tendon injury according to MRI findings. *J Bone Joint Surg Br* 1991, 73:683–685.

54. Lutter LD: Hindfoot Problems. *Instr Course Lect* 1993, 42:195–200.

55. Copeland SA: Rupture of the Achilles tendon: a new clinical test. *Ann R Coll Surg Engl* 1990, 72:270–271.

56. Ma GWC, Griffith TG: Percutaneous repair of acute closed ruptured Achilles tendon: a new technique. *Clin Orthop* 1977, 128:247–255.

57. Soldatis JJ, Goodfellow DB, Wilber JH: End-to-end operative repair of Achilles tendon rupture. *Am J Sports Med* 1997, 25:90–95.

58. Bradley JP, Tibone JE: Percutaneous and open surgical repairs of Achilles tendon ruptures: a comparative study. *Am J Sports Med* 1990, 18:188–195.

59. Aracil J, Pina A, Lozano JA, *et al.*: Percutaneous suture of Achilles tendon ruptures. *Foot Ankle* 1992, 13:350–351.

60. Leitner A, Voigt CH, Rahmanzadeh R: Treatment of extensive aseptic defects in old Achilles tendon ruptures: methods and case reports. *Foot Ankle* 1992, 13:176–180.

61. Mann RA, Holmes GB, Seale DS, *et al.*: Chronic rupture of the Achilles tendon: a new technique of repair. *J Bone Joint Surg* 1991, 73:214–219.

62. Baxter DE: Functional nerve disorders in the athlete's foot, ankle, and leg. *Instr Course Lect* 1993, 42:185–194.

63. Styf J: Entrapment of the superficial peroneal nerve: diagnosis and results of decompression. *J Bone Joint Surg Br* 1989, 71:131–135.

64. Borges LF, Hallett HM, Selkoe DJ, *et al.*: The anterior tarsal tunnel syndrome: report of two cases. *J Neurosurg* 1981, 54:89–92.

65. Pfeiffer WH, Cracchiolo A III: Clinical results after tarsal tunnel decompression. *J Bone Joint Surg Am* 1994, 76:1222–1230.

66. Baxter DE, Pfeffer GB, Thigpen M: Chronic heel pain: treatment rationale. *Orthop Clin North Am* 1989, 20:563–570.

67. Baxter DE, Pfeffer GB: Treatment of chronic heel pain by surgical release of the first branch of the lateral plantar nerve. *Clin Orthop* 1992, 279:229–236.

68. Kwong PK, Kay D, Voner KT, *et al.*: Plantar fasciitis: mechanics and pathomechanics of treatment. *Clin Sports Med* 1988, 7:119–126.

69. Daly PJ, Kitaoka HB, Chao EYS: Plantar fasciotomy for intractable plantar fascitis: clinical results and biomechanical evaluation. *Foot Ankle* 1992, 13:188–196.

70. Marotta JJ, Micheli LJ: Os trigonum impingement in dancers. *Am J Sports Med* 1992, 20:533–536.

71. Hedrick MR, McBryde AM: Posterior ankle impingement. *Foot Ankle* 1994, 15:2–8.

72. Liu SH, Mirzayan R: Posteromedial ankle impingement. *Arthroscopy* 1993, 9:709–711.

73. Wilkerson LA: Ankle injuries in athletes. *Primary Care* 1992, 19:377–392.

74. Milgrom C, Shlamkovitch N, Finestone A, *et al.*: Risk factors for lateral ankle sprain: a prospective study among military recruits. *Foot Ankle* 1992, 12:26–29.

75. Baumhauer JF, Alosa DM, Renstrom PAFH, *et al.*: A prospective study of ankle injury risk factors. *Am J Sports Med* 1995, 23:564–570.

76. Lephart SM, Pincivero DM, Giraldo JL, *et al.*: The role of proprioception in the management and rehabilitation of athletic injuries. *Am J Sports Med* 1997, 25:130–137.

77. Colville MR, Marder RA, Boyle JJ, *et al.* Strain measurement in lateral ankle ligaments. *Am J Sports Med* 1990, 18:196–200.

78. Stephens MM, Sammarco GJ: The stabilizing role of the lateral ligament complex around the ankle and subtalar joints. *Foot Ankle* 1992, 12:130–134.

79. Hopkinson WJ, St Pierre P, Ryan JB, *et al.*: Syndesmosis spains of the ankle. *Foot Ankle* 1990, 10:325–330.

80. Taga I, Shino K, Inoue M, *et al.*: Articular cartilage lesions in ankles with lateral ligament injury: an arthroscopic study. *Am J Sports Med* 1993, 21:120–127.

81. Kibler WB: Arthroscopic findings in ankle ligament reconstruction. *Clin Sports Med* 1996, 15:799–804.

82. Schafer D, Hintermann B: Arthroscopic assessment of the chronic unstable ankle joint. *Knee Surg Sports Traum Arthr* 1996, 4:48–52.

83. Raatikainen T, Putkonen M, Puranen, J. Arthrography, clinical examination, and stress radiology in the diagnosis of acute injury to the lateral ligaments of the ankle. *Am J Sports Med* 1992, 20:2–6.

84. Myasa M, Amir H, Porath A, *et al.*: Radiological Assessment of a Modified Anterior Drawer Test of the Ankle. *Foot Ankle* 1992, 13:400–403.

85. Karlsson J, Andreasson GO: The effect of external ankle support in chronic lateral ankle joint instability: an electromyographic study. *Am J Sports Med* 1992, 20:257–261.

86. Leanderson J, Ekstam S, Salomonsson C: Taping of the ankle: the effect on postural sway during perturbation, before and after a training session. *Knee Surg Sports Traumatol Arthrosc* 1996, 4:53–56.

87. Lofvenberg R, Karrholm J: The influence of an ankle orthosis on the talar and calcaneal motions in chronic lateral instability of the ankle. *Am J Sports Med* 1993, 21:224–227.

88. Hamilton WG, Thompson FM, Snow SW: The modified brostrom procedure for lateral ankle instability. *Foot Ankle* 1993, 14:1–7.

89. Sobel M, Geppert M Jr.: Repair of concomitant lateral ankle ligament instability and peroneus brevis splits through a posteriorly modified Broström. *Foot Ankle* 1992, 13:224–225.

90. Hennrikus WL, Mapes RC, Lyons PM, *et al.*: Outcomes of the Chrisman-Snook and modified-Broström procedures for chronic lateral ankle instability: a prospective, randomized comparison. *Am J Sports Med* 1996, 24:400–404.

91. Sjolin SU, Dons-Jensen J, Simonser O: Reinforced anatomical reconstruction of the anterior talofibular ligament in chronic anterolateral instability using a periosteal flap. *Foot Ankle* 1991, 12:15–18.

92. Colville MR, Grondel RJ: Anatomic reconstruction of the lateral ankle ligaments using a split peroneus brevis tendon graft. *Am J Sports Med* 1995, 23:210–213.

93. Srinivasan VB, Downes EM: Split peroneus longus tenodesis for chronic lateralligamentous instability of ankle. *Injury* 1996, 27:467–469.

94. Econopouly DS, Perlman MD, Notari MA, *et al.*: The use of an ankle joint distractor in ankle arthroscopy. *J Foot Surg* 1992, 31:96–99.

95. Manderson EL, Nwaneri UR, Amin KB: The fracture table as a distraction mode in ankle arthroscopy. *Foot Ankle* 1994, 15:444–445.

96. Wright G: Technique tips: skeletal traction for ankle arthroscopy. *Foot Ankle* 1996, 17:119.

97•. Dowdy PA, Watson BV, Amendola A, *et al.*: Noninvasive ankle distraction: relationship between force, magnitude of distraction, and nerve conduction abnormalities. *Arthroscopy* 1996, 12:64–69.

The authors performed ankle distraction using a noninvasive ankle distractor in volunteers, finding that with distraction of 30 lbs for more than 1 week there were reversible nerve conduction changes. They recommend using 30 lbs or less distraction for up to 1 hour.

98. Sartoretti C, Sartoretti-Schefer S, Duff C, *et al.*: Angioplasty balloon catheters used for distraction of the ankle joint. *Arthroscopy* 1996, 12:82–86.

99. Yates C, Grana W: A simple distraction technique for ankle arthroscopy. *Arthroscopy* 1988, 4:103–105.

100. Feiwell LA, Frey C. Anatomic study of arthroscopic portal sites of the ankle. *Foot Ankle* 1993, 14:142–147.

101. Albert J, Reiman P, Njus G, *et al.*: Ligament strain and ankle joint opening during ankle distraction. *Arthroscopy* 1992, 8:469–473.

102. Feder KS, Schonholtz GJ: Arthroscopy: review and long-term results. *Foot Ankle* 1992, 13:382–385.

103.••Amendola A, Petrik J, Webster-Bogaert S: Ankle arthroscopy: outcome in 79 consecutive patients. *Arthroscopy* 1996, 12:565–573.

The authors found that localized lesions did well, whereas those patients with generalized ankle pathology or workmen's compensation benefits and disability did poorly.

104. Baker CL, Graham JM Jr: Current concepts in ankle arthroscopy. *Orthopedics* 1993, 16:1027–1035.

105. Cooper PS, Murray TF Jr: Arthroscopy of the foot and ankle in the athlete. *Clin Sports Med* 1996, 15:805–824.

106. Jaivin JS, Ferkel RD: Arthroscopy of the foot and ankle. *Clin Sports Med* 1994, 13:761–783.

107. Loomer R, Fisher C, Lloyd-Smith R, *et al.*: Osteochondral lesions of the talus. *Am J Sports Med* 1993, 21:13–19.

108. Angermann P, Jensen P: Osteochrondritis dissecans of the talus: long-term results of surgical treatment. *Foot Ankle* 1989, 10:161–163.

109. Scranton PE Jr, McDermott JE. Anterior tibiotalar spurs: a comparison of open versus arthroscopic debridement. *Foot Ankle* 1992, 13:125–129.

110. Reynaert P, Gelen G, Geens G. Arthroscopic treatment of anterior impingement of the ankle. *Acta Orthop Belg* 1994, 60:384–388.

111. Jerosch J, Steinbeck J, Schroder M, *et al.*: Arthroscopic treatment of anterior synovitis of the ankle in athletes. *Knee Surg Sports Traumatol Arthrosc* 1994, 2:176–181.

112. Thein R, Eichenblat M: Arthroscopic treatment of sports-related synovitis of the ankle. *Am J Sports Med* 1992, 20:496–499.

113. Meislin RJ, Rose DJ, Parisien S, *et al*.: Arthroscopic treatment of synovial impingement of the ankle. *Am J Sports Med* 1993, 21:186–189.

114. Liu SH, Raskin A, Osti L, *et al*.: Arthroscopic treatment of anterolateral ankle impingement. *Arthroscopy* 1994, 10:215–218. [Published erratum appears in *Arthroscopy* 1994, 10:484.]

115. Bassett FH III, Gates HS, Billys JB, *et al*.: Talar impingement by the anteroinferior talofibular ligament. *J Bone Joint Surg Am* 1990, 72:55–59.

116. Ferkel RD, Heath DD, Guhl JF: Neurological complications of ankle arthroscopy. *Arthroscopy* 1996, 12:200–208.

117. Watson JAS, Hollingdale JP: Early management of displaced ankle fractures. *Injury* 1992, 23:87–88.

118. Ryd L, Bengtsson S: Isolated fracture of the lateral malleolus requires no treatment. *Acta Orthop Scand* 1992, 63:443–446.

119. Bostman OM: Osteolytic changes accompanying degradation of absorbable fracture fixation implants. *J Bone Joint Surg Br* 1991, 73:679–682.

120. Frokjaer J, Moller BN: Biodegradable fixation of ankle fractures: complications in a prospective study of 25 cases. *Acta Orthop Scand* 1992, 63:434–436.

121. Bostman OM: Intense granulomatous inflammatory lesions associated with absorbable internal fixation devices made of polyglycolide in ankle fractures. *Clin Orthop* 1992, 278:193–199.

122. Winkler B, Weber BG, Simpson LA: The dorsal antiglide plate in the treatment of Danis-Weber type B fractures of the distal fibula. *Clin Orthop* 1990, 259:204–209.

123. Wissing JC, Van Larrhoven CJHM, Van Der Werken C. The posterior antiglide plate for fixation of fractures of the lateral malleolus. *Injury* 1992, 23:94–96.

124. Finsen V, Saetermo R, Kibsgaard L, *et al*.: Early postoperative weight-bearing in patients who have a fracture of the ankle. *J Bone Joint Surg Am* 1991, 71:23–27.

125. Chandler RW: Management of complex ankle fractures in athletes. *Clin Sports Med* 1988, 7:127–141.

126. Sammarco GJ. Turf toe. *Instr Course Lect* 1993, 42:207–212.

127. Tewes DP, Fischer DA, Fritts HM, *et al*.: MRI findings of acute turf toe: a case report and review of anatomy. *Clin Orthop* 1994, 200–203.

128. Clanton TO, Ford JJ. Turf toe injury. *Clin Sports Med* 1994, 13:731–741.

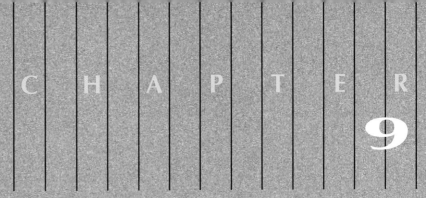

CHAPTER 9

BIOLOGY OF LIGAMENT INJURY AND REPAIR

Kevin A. Hildebrand and Cyril B. Frank

Sports medicine practices involve the diagnosis, treatment, and study of musculoskeletal soft-tissue injuries, of which ligament injuries represent a significant proportion. Exact numbers have not been compiled, but estimates indicate that around 5% to 10% of the population in North America up to age 65 suffer ligament injuries annually [1]. Knee and shoulder injuries predominate, but many other sites are "sprained," especially the spine, ankle, elbow, wrist, and hand. Because functional healing responses of damaged ligaments at various sites can be variable, many laboratory studies on ligament injury and healing have been performed. The knee ligaments have been characterized the best and have served as models for the study of the biology of ligament injury and repair. This article refers to these models, beginning with descriptions of the role of ligaments in knee joint function, normal ligament properties, and ligament healing (using the medial collateral ligament [MCL] as a model). Following that is a comparison of MCL healing with that of the anterior cruciate ligament (ACL) and a discussion of common orthopaedic treatments for ligament injuries and reconstruction of the ACL.

NORMAL LIGAMENTS

A concept of ligament function in terms of a joint as well as an understanding of normal ligament properties are important in order to discuss ligament injury and repair. This section discusses ligaments in the context of joint function followed by normal ligament biomechanical and biological properties.

Joint function

Skeletal ligaments are fibrous bands of dense connective tissue that couple bones across joints. Ligaments resist tensile loads, providing stability to a joint and helping to guide its motion. Additionally, ligaments are innervated and provide input into a proprioceptive "ligamentomuscular reflex loop." However, the exact role and relative importance of this neuromuscular mechanism in joint function remains to be investigated. Joint stability is a balance of many components that can be classified into tensile and compressive elements, and these elements can be static or dynamic (Fig. 9.1). The contributions of the various components to joint stability are dependent on the joint considered.

Biomechanical functions

The biomechanical behavior of ligaments is complex. This behavior has both time- and history-dependent loading patterns—a phenomenon termed "viscoelasticity" [2]. A ligament exposed to a constant stress (or load) will lengthen over time (or creep) (Fig. 9.2A). A ligament elongated and held at a certain length experiences a decrease in load with time; this is known as stress-relaxation (Fig. 9.2B). Both the creep and stress-relaxation become smaller over time and eventually become negligible. Creep and stress-relaxation tests are performed in the laboratory at relatively low loads, and can be termed low-load properties of the ligament. A ligament can recover from this loading, indicating that there is no damage. Viscoelasticity contributes to the perceived stiffness and laxity of ligaments in a minor way, but these properties are difficult to appreciate clinically. However, the viscoelastic properties of ligaments are important because they probably represent a very interesting fine-tuning mechanism for both ligament lengths and stresses over time.

Other biomechanical tests of ligaments in the laboratory apply a uniaxial tensile load to a bone-ligament-bone complex until it fails [2]. A load-versus-elongation curve is generated with three distinct areas: an initial toe region, a linear region, and a failure region (Fig. 9.3A). The structural properties of the bone-ligament-bone complex determined from this curve are stiffness (slope of the linear portion of the curve), ultimate load, and energy absorbed to failure (area underneath the curve). These data reflect the contribution of the entire bone-ligament-bone complex, including the insertions, in that the size of the ligament and the weakest link of this composite structure affects the magnitude of these measurements. By measuring the cross-sectional area of the ligament, the effect of size is taken into account. Dividing the load by the cross-sectional area (stress) and converting elongation to strain (the change in ligament length divided by the original ligament length) allows the determination of both a stress-versus-strain curve (Fig. 9.3B) and the material properties. These properties include the modulus (slope of the linear portion of the curve) and the ultimate tensile strength, which represent the quali-

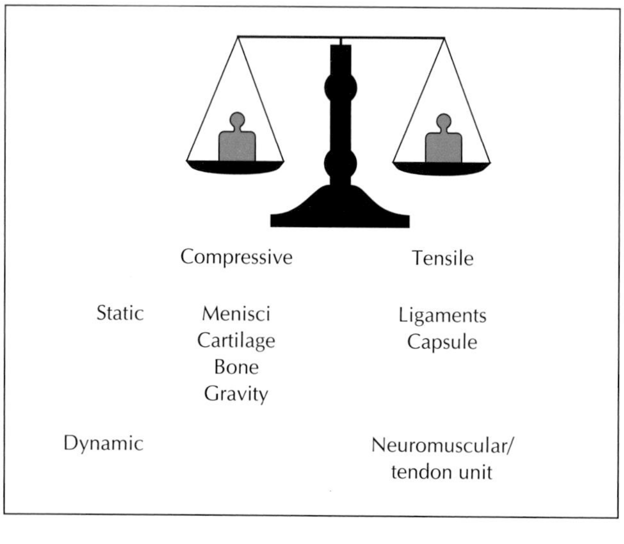

	Compressive	Tensile
Static	Menisci Cartilage Bone Gravity	Ligaments Capsule
Dynamic		Neuromuscular/ tendon unit

FIGURE 9.1

Classification of the structures contributing to joint stability: the balance of forces.

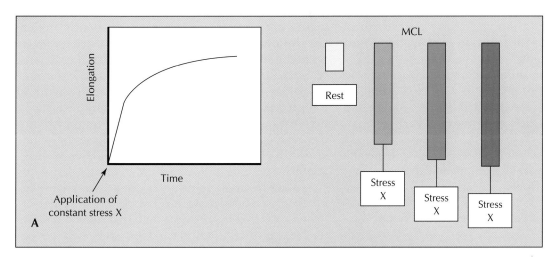

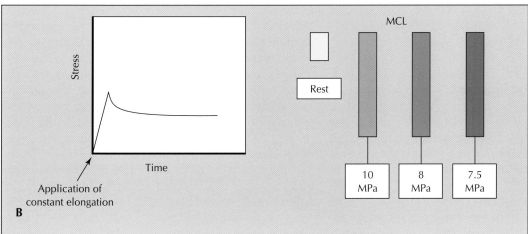

FIGURE 9.2
Viscoelastic
properties of
ligaments. **A,**
Creep. **B,** Stress-
relaxation. MCL—
medial collateral
ligament.

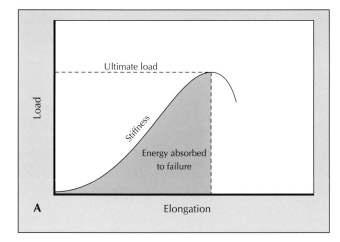

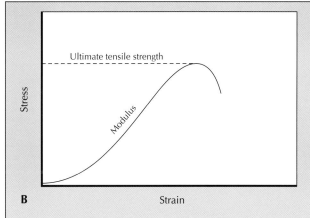

FIGURE 9.3

Load-versus-elongation curve (*panel A*) and stress-versus-
strain curve (*panel B*) obtained from uniaxial tensile test of a
bone-ligament-bone complex.

ty of the normal or healing ligament. The structural and material properties can be termed high-load properties of ligaments.

The classification of biomechanical measures into low- and high-load properties is easy to conceptualize but hard to define quantitatively because the range of in vivo loads in ligaments is unknown. Presumably, most daily activities occur at lower loads, for it appears that ligaments recover from the repetitive loads applied to them without any evidence of damage. However, clinical and laboratory interests have focused on high-load properties. Thus, because of the complex properties of the ligament during joint function, we believe that both low- and high-load properties need to be considered in order to fully characterize a normal ligament or to evaluate ligament healing.

Biologic description

Ligaments are hypocellular structures that are composed of roughly 70% water by weight (Fig. 9.4). Water is an incompressible spacer, contributes to the viscoelasticity of ligaments, and potentially serves as a transport medium [3]. The solid matrix represents the rest of the ligament, of which collagen is the overwhelming majority component. Type I collagen accounts for approximately 85% to 90% of total collagen, and is the primary, tensile, load-carrying substance in ligaments. Other matrix components include collagen types III, V, and VI as well as proteoglycans, elastin, fibronectin, and laminin [3–5]. The roles of these "minor" collagens and other

matrix components in ligaments are poorly understood; however, it is evident that they are involved with the interaction between cells and matrix and with the organization of the matrix itself. For example, some of these molecules (type V collagen and the proteoglycan decorin) regulate fibrillogenesis in other collagenous tissues [6,7]. By altering the diameters of fibrils in ligaments, levels of these molecules may affect the biomechanical properties of ligaments.

Studies of cross-sections of extra-articular knee ligaments performed with a transmission electron microscope (Fig. 9.5) have shown that ligament fibrils tend to be distributed in a wide range with a spectrum of both smaller (< 100 nm) and larger (> 100 nm) fibrils [8]. Some authors have suggested that this distribution is important to the biomechanical properties of musculoskeletal soft tissue such as ligaments [9]. This theory states that smaller fibrils are important for resisting creep or plastic deformation and that larger fibrils resist high stresses. Whereas these speculations have yet to be proven, it is likely that the proper distribution of fibril diameters is important. In both the healing MCLs (where all fibrils are smaller than normal) or in the skin and tendons of genetically modified mice (where all fibrils are much larger than normal), the tissues are weaker or fragile when compared with normal tissues [10•,11,12].

LIGAMENT INJURIES

Ligaments can be damaged by different causes [13–15], trauma being most common (Table 9.1). A

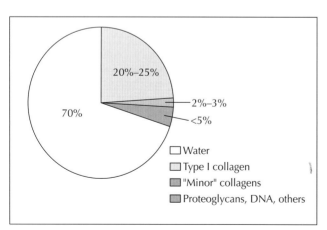

FIGURE 9.4

Biochemical composition of ligaments. The numbers represent the approximate percentages of the total ligament (wet weight).

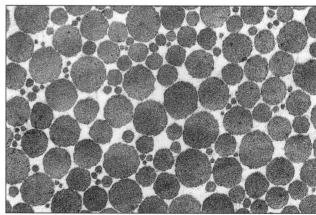

FIGURE 9.5

Photograph taken with transmission electron microscope of a cross-section of an uninjured adult rabbit medial collateral ligament.

frequent mechanism of traumatic ligament injuries is the sudden application of a single load that causes a progressive, sequential failure of fibers until the load is dissipated or the ligament becomes completely disrupted. Clinically, when a ligament is injured in this way, the ligament itself can be damaged at more than one site, and often other structures of the joint can be injured [16]. A second mechanism of traumatic injury is repetitive, subcatastrophic loading that leads to pain and, in some cases, instability. The shoulder and elbow are the joints most frequently injured in this way [17,18]. Immobilization also leads to deterioration in the substance as well as the insertions of an uninjured ligament [19]. Although the deterioration is recoverable, several weeks of immobilization can require several months for recovery; ligament insertions are especially sensitive to immobilization and are slow to recover [19]. Most studies have modeled the complete catastrophic failure and subsequent healing of ligaments because the damage is easier to produce and standardize than for the other causes listed in Table 9.1. Although it is assumed that the healing of all types of ligament damage is similar, this belief remains to be proven. The following discussion focuses on the healing that follows a single traumatic injury.

LIGAMENT HEALING

Descriptions of ligament healing have been defined with animal investigations of knee ligaments, especially the MCL. In general, ligament healing is characterized by a failure to regenerate a normal ligament. In the case of extra-articular ligaments, such as the MCL, these ligaments often heal with a bridging tissue or scar. However, some intra-articular ligaments, such as the ACL, either fail to heal or scar to some other structure (*eg*, posterior cruciate ligament) and no longer function [1]. This section considers ligament healing in the context of joint function, describes general ligament healing using the MCL model, and takes a closer look at what is known about the specific differences between MCL and ACL healing.

General ligament healing

A synovial joint consists of many elements that resist compressive or tensile forces [1]. The joint functions through an equilibrium among these elements (*see* Fig. 9.1). If one particular element (*eg*, a ligament) is damaged, the balance is disturbed and the remaining structures try to establish a new equilibrium to maintain joint function. Three points relevant to ligament function and healing arise from recognizing these mechanisms of joint function. First, a lack of symptoms in a ligament-injured joint does not necessarily mean that an individual ligament has healed, because other structures may simply compensate for it. Second, if other elements or stabilizers are not able to establish a new equilibrium to protect a healing ligament, the load this ligament experiences may be too much, and it may heal poorly or not at all. A lack of healing in this sense is not related to an intrinsic inability of the ligament to heal, but to the excessive load it experiences while healing. Third, one can surmise that certain structures or elements could fail over time if the increased load they carry exceeds their ability to adapt.

A recent study illustrates the equilibrium adjustment and adaptations of a joint where an injury to one ligament causes changes in the other ligaments and soft-tissue structures of the joint [20•]. After an isolated injury to a rabbit MCL, blood flow to the other ligaments and menisci of the same knee was elevated for up to 6 weeks, possibly in response to the increase in loads that are carried by these structures. The blood flow in these structures returns to control levels after this, as loads in these structures decrease as the MCL accepts more load as it heals over time.

Medial collateral ligament healing

Ligament repair follows a process that is qualitatively similar to that described in wound healing. The resultant healing tissue from both processes can be referred to as a scar [3]. There are three main phases of healing that overlap. The inflammatory phase occurs within minutes to days of an injury, with the formation of a blood clot followed by infiltration of polymorphonu-

Table 9.1	**CAUSES OF DAMAGE TO LIGAMENTS**
	Trauma
	Acute (single) event
	Repetitive microtrauma
	Immobilization
	Inflammation
	Intra-articular injections
	High-dose glucocorticoids
	Other causes

clear cells and macrophages to remove damage and attract reparative cells to the area. The proliferative phase begins within days of the injury, lasts several weeks, and is characterized by the formation of granulation tissue. New blood vessels are formed while fibroblasts are recruited from the local environment or circulation to produce and excrete new matrix material. The remodeling phase starts within weeks of the injury and continues for several years. Elements within the tissue reorganize the material produced by the fibroblasts to improve the properties of the healing ligament over time.

Biomechanical tests of healing rabbit MCLs show that although there are substantial improvements in MCL scars over the first 2 to 3 months, over a longer term (up to 1 year) the MCL is larger, with material that is weaker and of inferior quality compared with an uninjured MCL. Whereas the structural properties (stiffness, ultimate load, and energy absorbed to failure) of the healed MCL at 1 year return to about 50% to 70% of uninjured MCL values, the material properties (ultimate tensile strength and modulus) of the healed MCL are worse, ranging from 30% to 50% of control values [21–25]. In contrast, some low-load or viscoelastic properties return toward normal levels considerably sooner (6 to 14 weeks after injury) [3,22].

Biochemically, the amount of collagen returns to normal levels within 12 to 14 weeks of injury, but there are more types III and V collagen (type I collagen is still the most prevalent) and fewer mature collagen cross-links (hydroxypyridinium) in injured ligaments than in normal ligaments [21,26,27•]. The distribution of collagen types I and III returns closer to normal ligament values by 1 year, but the mature collagen cross-links (hydroxypyridinium) remain low, about 45% of normal values. Type V collagen remains elevated (50%) compared with control levels [3,26,27•].

Morphologically, healing MCLs have collagen fibers with smaller cross-sectional diameters, and these fibrils are poorly aligned [3]. Healing MCLs also contain more blood vessels, fat and inflammatory cells, loose or disorganized matrix, and cellular infiltrates (Fig. 9.6). These non–load-bearing components, or "flaws," represent holes in the matrix, potentially serving as stress risers, and are one probable cause of ligament-scar weakness [28•]. Thus, although the MCL heals consistently, it is much weaker, has biochemical abnormalities, and has smaller fibril diameters with more flaws in the healing tissue than in normal MCLs (Table 9.2).

Medial collateral ligament healing versus anterior cruciate ligament healing

Clinically and in the laboratory, different ligaments respond in a tissue-specific manner to various injuries and treatments. This observation is exemplified by comparing the MCL and ACL of the knee [25,29–31]. The reasons for the differences in the functional healing responses of MCLs and ACLs are unknown, but many factors have been suggested. A potential difference between these ligaments is the exposure to a "hostile" synovial environment with injury to the ACL but not the MCL. Some studies, however, have shown positive effects of synovial fluid on ligament healing [32,33]. Another difference between these ligaments is anatomical. Whereas the MCL is surrounded by potential supporting tissues (*eg,* joint capsule) that may keep it in the proper alignment and proximity during healing, the ACL lacks such an anatomic arrangement. Differences in anatomic location may also lead to different load histories for each healing ligament. If one considers the knee joint to function through a balance of compressive and tensile, load-resistant elements, the other tensile stabilizers (*eg,* ligaments) may be able to take

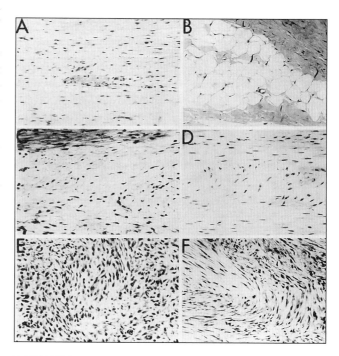

FIGURE 9.6

Photomicrograph of a healing medial collateral ligament showing flaws in the tissue consisting of blood vessels (*panel A*), fat cells (*panel B*), loose collagen (*panel C*), disorganized collagen (*panel D*), cellular infiltrate (*panel E*), and combinations of flaws stained with hematoxylin and eosin (*panel F*).

up the load to allow the MCL to heal following an MCL injury [1]. Conversely, after an ACL injury, the remaining tensile stabilizers may be unable to take up sufficient load to allow ACL healing in a functional sense. Other differences noted between the ACL and MCL include cell morphology, cell adhesion and migration, cellular response to growth factors and hormones, biochemical composition, and biomechanical properties [2,4,34–37,38•]. The role and importance of these differences on the healing potential of these two ligaments remains to be determined.

TREATMENT OF LIGAMENT INJURIES

Several clinical and laboratory studies have been performed to identify methods to improve ligament healing. In vivo studies have looked mostly at knee ligaments, especially the MCL and ACL. This section considers the effects of three clinically relevant treatment variables and also some experimental approaches to improve ligament healing.

Suture repair

Suturing of an MCL has produced only modest improvements in healing in the laboratory, with some differences between models. In a rabbit model comparing 4-mm-gap healing to transection and end-to-end suture repair of an isolated MCL injury, increases in structural and mechanical properties of 10% to 30% occurred with suture repair after 40 weeks of healing [22]. However,

these increases were still significantly less than normal MCL values ($\approx$ 50% to 70% and 40% to 50% for structural and material properties, respectively [22]). Repairing the MCL in a combined MCL and ACL injury where the ACL has been reconstructed has shown that, after 12 weeks of healing, the ultimate load of the femur–MCL–tibia complex (FMTC) was increased 53% in the repair group compared with the nonrepair group, although there were no differences in material properties between these two groups [39]. However, after 52 weeks of MCL healing, there was no longer any improvement in the structural or material properties with suture repair [40].

The issue of repair versus nonrepair for the ACL is more complex. Because of its anatomical location, ruptures of the ACL tend not to heal end to end— the ends either remain unattached or scar to adjacent structures such as the PCL [1]. Repair of the ACL has been disappointing both clinically and in the laboratory. O'Donoghue *et al.* [31,41] reported that suturing together the transected ACL in a dog model resulted in a substantially decreased tensile strength (10% to 60% of controls) at 10 weeks; at longer time periods, resorption of the repair occurred in 14 of 36 repairs. Clinically, repairs of the ACL generally fail with time, and symptoms of instability and signs of increased anterior-tibial laxity return [30,42]. As a result, isolated repair of the ACL is generally not performed. However, if repair is attempted, it is usually augmented with biologic or synthetic grafts [42].

Table 9.2	CHARACTERISTICS OF LONG-TERM HEALING OF THE MEDIAL COLLATERAL LIGAMENT COMPARED WITH THAT OF A NORMAL MEDIAL COLLATERAL LIGAMENT
PROPERTY	**CHARACTERISTICS**
Biomechanics	Larger
	Weaker
	Inferior tissue quality
	Stress-relaxation close to normal
Biochemistry	Total collagen normal
	Increased "minor" collagens
	Decreased mature cross-links
Ultrastructure	Abnormal fibril diameter distribution
	Flaws between fibrils

Motion

Motion in a stable joint after injury affects the healing ligament with improvements in scar stiffness and strength. Immobilization leads to scars that are weaker and not as stiff. A study on rats compared the effects of unrestricted motion versus immobilization on shorter periods of MCL healing (12 days) following an isolated injury [43]. The ultimate load of the FMTCs from animals treated with motion were up to 20% greater than those of the animals treated with immobilization. Using a slightly different study design, the effects of motion on MCL healing up to 48 weeks after injury were investigated [44,45]. Isolated injuries were created in dog MCLs and two treatment regimens were investigated: 1) no repair of the MCL followed by unrestricted motion, and 2) suture repair of the MCL followed by rigid immobilization for 6 weeks. The dogs that were allowed free motion had larger values for ultimate load of the FMTC and ultimate tensile strength of the MCL (15% and 25% more, respectively) compared with those of the immobilized animals. However, even with motion allowed, the structural properties of the FMTCs and the material properties of the MCLs were still significantly less than normal values. The effect of motion on ACL healing is unknown.

Joint instability

The effect of joint instability on ligament healing has been studied using a combined MCL and ACL injury model in rabbits [46]. The healing MCLs in this model are larger, less stiff, regain less strength, and are made of inferior tissue as compared with healing MCLs from an isolated MCL injury. Twelve weeks after injury, the structural properties of the FMTC and the material properties of the MCL from

the combined injury group were around 50% and 35%, respectively, of the corresponding measurements for the isolated MCL injury group. These data imply that too much load can be detrimental to a healing ligament (MCL) in a very unstable joint in which joint motion is allowed.

The negative effects of an MCL and ACL injury on MCL healing can be diminished but not completely eliminated with reconstructions of the ACL, at least for a short-term period [46,47]. On evaluation at 12 weeks, a rabbit model of MCL and ACL injury treated with ACL reconstruction showed that the stiffness and the ultimate load of the FMTCs from the ACL-reconstructed group were 30% and 60% greater, respectively, than those of the ACL-deficient group. There was no difference in the modulus values of the MCLs between the ACL-reconstructed and ACL-deficient groups. However, the structural properties of the FMTCs and the material properties of the MCL from the reconstructed group were approximately 25% and 75% less, respectively, than those from an isolated MCL-injury group [46]. In summary, animal studies indicate that up to 12 weeks after injury, the quality of MCL healing is worse following a MCL and ACL injury compared with an isolated injury, and also that ACL reconstruction improves MCL healing but not to the level of an isolated MCL injury (Fig. 9.7).

Other methods to improve ligament healing

Because all evidence indicates that the tissue quality of healing ligaments is inferior to that of normal ligaments, other methods of treatment require investigation. One such line of investigation examines the use of growth factors to enhance healing. Studies in vitro show that fibroblasts from the MCL and ACL proliferate and increase collagen and total protein

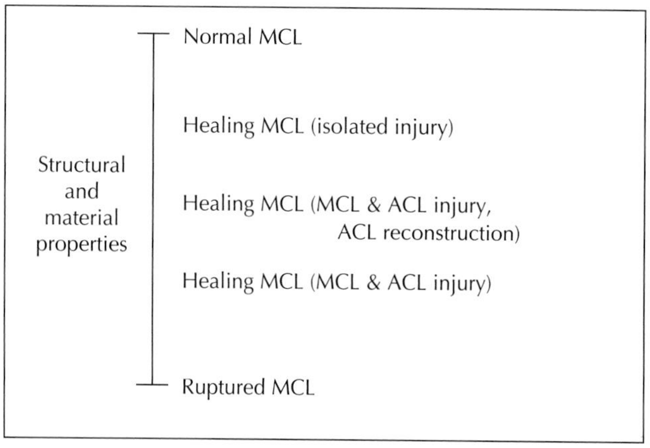

FIGURE 9.7

Relationship of the biomechanical properties of a normal medial collateral ligament (MCL) and the healing MCL 12 weeks after different injuries to the knee.

synthesis in response to selected growth factors. Preliminary in vivo results indicate that early MCL healing can be enhanced with selected growth factors compared with no treatment [38•,48•,49]. Another line of investigation applies gene therapy to ligament healing. Gene therapy offers the potential to deliver genetic information to cells of healing ligaments, which could lead to alterations in the expression of proteins that are known to be important in the healing process. Preliminary studies on gene therapy in musculoskeletal tissues have shown that marker genes can be detected up to 6 weeks after implantation into tendons [50–52].

LIGAMENT RECONSTRUCTION

Following injuries to some ligaments, function does not return to the joint. Some of these ligaments are reconstructed with substitute tissues because predictable results cannot be obtained with suture repair or other treatments. The ACL of the knee is the best example of this, but the same is true of the posterior collateral ligament of the knee and the MCL of the elbow [18]. This section will briefly review the ACL-reconstruction studies as a model for ligament reconstruction; however, the applicability of the ACL model to the posterior collateral ligament and, especially, to the MCL of the elbow (extra-articular structure) is not well characterized.

Substitute tissues for ACL reconstruction include natural tissues (autograft or allograft) and synthetic material (biologic or nonbiologic). Because the synthetic tissues are investigational and not routinely used, this discussion focuses on natural tissue. The natural substitute tissues for ACL reconstruction are mainly tendons, including autografts of the hamstring and patellar tendons and allografts of the Achilles, hamstring, and patellar tendons. Studies have compared the initial (time zero) characteristics of the grafting tissues with those of a normal ACL. The biomechanical properties of the grafting tissues are somewhat variable due to the different sources and sizes of the grafts and also to the different testing methodologies used for evaluation [53,54]. For humans, the patellar tendon (14 mm wide) has the greatest ultimate load and stiffness ($\approx$ 2900 N and $\approx$ 685 N/mm, respectively) of all replacement grafts [55]. The ACL of young human adults fails at lower ultimate loads and is much less stiff ($\approx$ 2160 N and $\approx$ 242 N/mm, respectively) [56]. A single-strand semitendinosus graft has about 55% of the ultimate load of the ACL [55,56]. The sizes of these three structures varied considerably. When compared with a normal ACL, the patellar tendon grafts were 47% larger and the single-strand semitendinosis grafts were 58% smaller in cross-sectional area [55,57]. Large animals such as goats also show differences between the ACL and replacement grafts. Autografts of the central-third patellar tendon had only 33% of the ultimate load and stiffness of control ACLs, even though these structures had very similar cross-sectional areas [58•]. Thus, there exists to date no graft to mimic the biomechanical properties of the normal ACL in humans or animals.

Histologic and biochemical comparisons of the ACL and these grafts have also been reported. Whereas the ACL is composed of rod- or oval-shaped cells, the tendons are composed of spindle-shaped cells. Collagen fibril diameters in the ACL are predominantly small (85% of the area composed of fibrils < 100 nm in diameter). The fibrils in the patellar tendon (45% of area composed of fibrils > 100 nm in diameter) and the semitendinosus tendon (> 70% of the area composed of fibrils > 100 nm in diameter) are larger [59]. The ACL has an overall lower collagen content, but with more type III collagen and more glycosaminoglycans compared with the patellar tendon [4].

Animal studies have been performed on the incorporation and maturation of graft materials used to replace the ACL. ACL grafts undergo histologic modification with necrosis and cell death occurring within the 1st week of healing. Blood vessels and nerve tissue are reestablished in some models within the first 6 to 8 weeks, together with extrinsic cells and matrix production [60–62]. Healing phases similar to those discussed for ligament healing take place in the grafts [59,60]. Biomechanically, a variety of animal models and various autograft and allograft tissues have shown a drop in high-load structural properties that have either not recovered or recovered slowly with time [54,58•,60]. One to 2 years after surgery, tissue grafts have been shown to have stiffness values ranging from 13% to 45% and ultimate load values between 11% to 52% of those for control ACLs [54,58•,60]. Patellar tendon and hamstring autografts studied with an electron microscope appear to be composed of mostly smaller diameter collagen fibrils similar to those in the ACL, but the distribution of these fibers has not revealed normal ACL architectural reconstitution [59]. Biochemical changes include early increases in water content with a return closer to control levels. Total proteoglycan content, collagen-type distribution, and mature collagen cross-links (hydroxypyridinium) approach normal ACL quantities with remodeling for these autograft tendon tissues [60,63•]. In summary, the tendon autografts undergo a substitution and replacement that changes them during the healing process, but the tissue's electron microscopic and biomechanical properties remain different than normal ACL. Thus, whereas many grafts appear to be satisfactory in clinical terms of functional knee stability, they do not become a normal ACL.

CONCLUSIONS

Ligament injury and repair is characterized by an inability to regenerate a normal ligament for reasons that are not clear. In some cases (*eg*, MCL), the healed ligament can lead to the return of joint function, likely because other stabilizing elements in the joint can help compensate for it. However, in other cases (*eg*, ACL), the injured ligament either fails to heal or its healing is of such poor quality that it cannot withstand relevant joint stresses. The other stabilizing structures cannot compensate for the ligament's loss, and, as a result, joint function is diminished.

Much information regarding effects of treatment on ligament healing is available, but many more questions persist. Understanding the roles of all matrix components as well as their functional organization is necessary. Improved definition and characterization of low-load (viscoelastic) and material properties of ligaments would allow more precise correlation of biomechanical, biochemical, and histologic data. Finally, optimization of standard (*eg*, motion and applied stresses) and current investigational treatment methods and the discovery of new treatment strategies are necessary in order to reach the goal of regenerating new ligaments.

ACKNOWLEDGMENTS

The support of the Alberta Heritage Foundation for Medical Research, the Medical Research Council of Canada, and the Canadian Arthritis Society is gratefully acknowledged.

REFERENCES AND RECOMMENDED READING

Recently published papers of particular interest have been highlighted as:
* •   Of special interest
* ••   Of outstanding interest

1.   Frank CB: Ligament healing: current knowledge and clinical applications. *J Am Acad Orthop Surg* 1996, 4:74–83.

2.   Woo SL-Y, Smith BA, Johnson GA: Biomechanics of knee ligaments. In *Knee Surgery*, edn 1. Edited by Fu FH, Harner CD, Vince KG. Baltimore, MD: Williams and Wilkins; 1994:155–172.

3.   Frank CB, Bray RC, Hart DA, *et al.*: Soft tissue healing. In *Knee Surgery*, edn 1. Edited by Fu FH, Harner CD, Vince KG. Baltimore, MD: Williams and Wilkins; 1994:189–229.

4.   Amiel D, Frank C, Harwood F, *et al.*: Tendons and ligaments: a morphological and biochemical comparison. *J Orthop Res* 1984, 1:257–265.

5.   Niyibizi C, Sagarriga Visconte C, *et al.*: Collagens in adult bovine medial collateral ligament: immunofluorescence localization by confocal microscopy reveals that type XIV collagen predominates at the ligament-bone junction. *Matrix Biology* 1995, 14:743–751.

6.   Linsenmayer TF, Gibney E, Igoe F, *et al.*: Type V collagen: molecular structure and fibrillar organization of the chicken a1(V) NH2-terminal domain, a putative regulator of corneal fibrillogenesis. *J Cell Biol* 1993, 121:1181–1189.

7.   Rada JA, Cornuet PK, Hassell JR: Regulation of corneal collagen fibrillogenesis in vitro by corneal proteoglycan (lumican and decorin) core proteins. *Exp Eye Res* 1993, 56:635–648.

8.   Hart RA, Woo SL-Y, Newton PO: Ultrastructural morphometry of anterior cruciate and medial collateral ligaments: an experimental study in rabbits. *J Orthop Res* 1992, 10:96–103.

9.   Parry DAD: The molecular and fibrillar structure of collagen and its relationship to the mechanical properties of connective tissue. *Biophys Chem* 1988, 29:195–209.

10.•   Danielson KG, Baribault H, Holmes DF, *et al.*: Targeted disruption of decorin leads to abnormal collagen fibril morphology and skin fragility. *J Cell Biol* 1997, 136:729–743.
Genetically engineered mice with a deletion of their decorin gene have abnormally large fibrils in their skin and tendons. Biomechanical tests of the skin show increased fragility compared with normal skin, suggesting that proper fibril diameter distribution is important for the mechanical properties of soft tissues.

11.   Frank C, McDonald D, Bray D, *et al.*: Collagen fibril diameters in the healing adult rabbit medial collateral ligament. *Connect Tissue Res* 1992, 27:251–263.

12.   Frank CB, Shrive NG, McDonald DB: Collagen fibril diameters in ligament scars: a long term assessment. *Connect Tissue Res* 1997, in press.

13.   Goldberg VM, Burstein A, Dawson M: The influence of an experimental immune synovitis on the failure mode and

strength of the rabbit anterior cruciate ligament. *J Bone Joint Surg Am* 1982, 64:900–906.

14. Neurath MF: Detection of Luse bodies, spiralled collagen, dysplastic collagen, and intracellular collagen in rheumatoid connective tissues: an electron microscopic study. *Ann Rheum Dis* 1993, 52:278–284.

15. Noyes FR, Grood ES, Nussbaum NS, *et al*.: Effect of intra-articular corticosteroids on ligament properties: a biomechanical and histological study in rhesus knees. *Clin Orthop* 1977, 123:197–209.

16. Garvin GJ, Munk PL, Vellet AD: Tears of the medial collateral ligament: magnetic resonance imaging findings and associated injuries. *Can Assoc Radiol J* 1993, 44:199–204.

17. Neer CS II: *Shoulder Reconstruction*, vol 1, ed 1. Philadelphia: WB Saunders; 1990.

18. Morrey BF: Acute and chronic instability of the elbow. *J Am Acad Orthop Surg* 1996, 4:117–128.

19.• Woo SL-Y, Gomez MA, Sites TJ, *et al*.: The biomechanical and morphological changes in the medial collateral ligament of the rabbit after immobilization and remobilization. *J Bone Joint Surg Am* 1987, 69:1200–1211.

20.• Bray RC, Butterwick DJ, Doschak MR, *et al*.: Coloured microsphere assessment of blood flow to knee ligaments in adult rabbits: effects of injury. *J Orthop Res* 1996, 14:618–625.
Blood flow to a healing rabbit MCL 3 weeks after injury is elevated over 30 times compared with that of normal MCLs and remains elevated (six times greater than controls) at 17 weeks. Blood flow also increases to other ligaments of the same knee after MCL injury and returns to control values by 6 weeks in these other ligaments, illustrating that other ligaments in the same knee adapt to injuries of one of the joint's ligaments.

21. Frank C, Woo SL-Y, Amiel D, *et al*.: Medial collateral ligament healing: a multidisciplinary assessment in rabbits. *Am J Sports Med* 1983, 11:379–389.

22. Chimich D, Frank C, Shrive N, *et al*.: The effects of initial end contact on medial collateral ligament healing: a morphological and biomechanical study in a rabbit model. *J Orthop Res* 1991, 9:37–47.

23. Chimich D, Frank C, Shrive N, *et al*.: No effect of mop-ending on ligament healing: rabbit studies of severed collateral knee ligaments. *Acta Orthop Scand* 1993, 64:587–591.

24. Ohland KJ, Weiss JA, Anderson DR, *et al*.: Long-term healing of the medial collateral ligament (MCL) and its insertion sites. *Trans ORS* 1991, 16:158.

25. Weiss JA, Woo SL-Y, Ohland KJ, *et al*.: Evaluation of a new injury model to study medial collateral ligament healing: Primary repair vs. nonoperative treatment. *J Orthop Res* 1991, 9:516–528.

26. Kavalkovich KW, Yamaji T, Woo SL-Y, *et al*.: Type V collagen levels are elevated following MCL injury and in long term healing. *Trans Orthop Res Soc* 1997, 22:485.

27.• Frank C, McDonald D, Wilson J, *et al*: Rabbit medial collateral ligament scar weakness is associated with decreased collagen pyridinoline crosslink density. *J Orthop Res* 1995, 13:157–165.
Healing ligaments continue to exhibit lower collagen cross-link levels up to 1 year after injury; this is associated with weaker tissue strength. Strategies to increase collagen cross-link levels could potentially lead to greater tissue strength of the healing ligament.

28.• Shrive N, Chimich D, Marchuk L, *et al*.: Soft-tissue "flaws" are associated with the material properties of the healing

rabbit medial collateral ligament. *J Orthop Res* 1995, 13:923–929.
The matrix of healing ligaments contain more "flaws" or holes, which correlates with inferior material properties. These flaws consist of blood vessels, fat and inflammatory cells, disorganized matrix, and cellular infiltrates. Methods to reduce the size and number of flaws could improve ligament healing.

29. Indelicato PA: Isolated medial collateral ligament injuries in the knee. *J Am Acad Orthop Surg* 1995, 3:9–14.

30. Johnson RJ, Beynnon BD, Nichols CE, *et al*.: Current concepts review: the treatment of injuries of the anterior cruciate ligament. *J Bone Joint Surg Am* 1992, 74:140–151.

31. O'Donoghue DH, Frank GR, Jeter GL, *et al*.: Repair and reconstruction of the anterior cruciate ligament in dogs. *J Bone Joint Surg Am* 1971, 53:710–718.

32. Dahlin LB, Hanff G, Myrhage R: Healing of ligaments in synovial fluid: an experimental study in rabbits. *Scand J Plast Reconstr Surg Hand Surg* 1991, 25:97–102.

33. Nickerson DA, Joshi R, Williams S, *et al*.: Synovial fluid stimulates the proliferation of rabbit ligament fibroblasts in-vitro. *Clin Orthop* 1992, 274:294–299.

34. Nagineni CN, Amiel D, Green MH, *et al*. Characterization of the intrinsic properties of the anterior cruciate and medial collateral ligament cells: an in vitro cell culture study. *J Orthop Res* 1992, 10:465–475.

35. Yu WD, Hatch JD, Panossian V, *et al*.: Effects of estrogen on cellular growth and collagen synthesis of the human anterior cruciate ligament: an explanation for female athletic injury. *Trans Orthop Res Soc* 1997, 22:397.

36. Marui T, Niyibizi C, Georgescu HI, *et al*.: The effect of growth factors on matrix synthesis by ligament fibroblasts. *J Orthop Res* 1997, 15:18–23.

37. Schmidt CC, Georgescu HI, Kwoh CK, *et al*.: Effect of growth factors on the proliferation of fibroblasts from the medial collateral and anterior cruciate ligaments. *J Orthop Res* 1995, 13:184–190.

38.• DesRosiers EA, Yahia L, Rivard C-H: Proliferative and matrix synthesis response of canine anterior cruciate ligament fibroblasts submitted to combined growth factors. *J Orthop Res* 1996, 14:200–208.
Growth factors enhance ACL fibroblast proliferation and synthesis of collagen and proteoglycans in vitro. Some combinations of growth factors act synergistically to increase proliferation and synthesis.

39. Ohno K, Pomaybo AS, Schmidt CC, *et al*.: Healing of the medial collateral ligament after a combined medial collateral and anterior cruciate ligament injury and reconstruction of the anterior cruciate ligament: comparison of repair and nonrepair of medial collateral ligament tears in rabbits. *J Orthop Res* 1995, 13:442–449.

40. Yamaji T, Levine RE, Woo SL-Y, *et al*.: Medial collateral ligament healing one year after a concurrent medial collateral ligament and anterior cruciate ligament injury: an interdisciplinary study in rabbits. *J Orthop Res* 1996, 14:223–227.

41. O'Donoghue DH, Rockwood CC Jr, Frank GR: Repair of the anterior cruciate ligament in dogs. *J Bone Joint Surg Am* 1996, 48:503–519.

42. Engebretsen L: The acute repair of anterior cruciate tears. In *The Anterior Cruciate Ligament: Current and Future Concepts*, edn 1. Edited by Jackson DW. New York: Raven Press; 1993:273–279.

43. Hart DP, Dahners LE: Healing of the medial collateral ligament in rats: the effects of repair, motion, and secondary

stabilizing ligaments. *J Bone Joint Surg Am* 1987, 69:1194–1199.

44. Inoue M, Woo SL-Y, Amiel D, *et al.*: Effects of surgical treatment and immobilization on the healing of the medial collateral ligament: a long-term multidisciplinary study. *Connect Tissue Res* 1990, 25:13–26.

45. Woo SL-Y, Gomez MA, Inoue M, *et al*: New experimental procedures to evaluate the biomechanical properties of healing canine medial collateral ligaments. *J Orthop Res* 1987, 5:425–432.

46. Anderson DR, Weiss JA, Takai S, *et al.*: Healing of the medial collateral ligament following a triad injury: a biomechanical and histological study of the knee in rabbits. *J Orthop Res* 1992, 10:485–495.

47. Engle CP, Noguchi M, Ohland KJ, *et al.*: Healing of the rabbit medial collateral ligament following an O'Donoghue triad injury: effects of anterior cruciate ligament reconstruction. *J Orthop Res* 1994, 12:357–364.

48.• Batten ML, Hansen JC, Dahners LE: Influence of dosage and timing of application of platelet-derived growth factor on early healing of the rat medial collateral ligament. *J Orthop Res* 1996, 14:736–741.
The biomechanical properties of the healing rat MCL improve 12 days after injury with the application of PDGF-BB. The greatest effect of growth factors occurs when they are applied immediately after injury of the MCL in this model of ligament healing.

49. Letson AK, Dahners LE: The effect of combinations of growth factors on ligament healing. *Clin Orthop* 1994, 308:207–212.

50. Gerich TG, Kang R, Fu FH, *et al.*: Gene transfer to ligaments and menisci. *Gene Therapy* 1996, 3:1089–1093.

51. Lou J, Manske PR, Aoki M, *et al.*: Adenovirus-mediated gene transfer into tendon and tendon sheath. *J Orthop Res* 1996, 14:513–517.

52. Nakamura N, Horibe S, Matsumoto N, *et al*: Transient introduction of a foreign gene into healing rat patellar ligament. *J Clin Invest* 1996, 97:226–231.

53. Beynnon BD, Johnson RJ, Fleming BC: The mechanics of anterior cruciate ligament reconstruction. In *The Anterior Cruciate Ligament: Current and Future Concepts*, edn 1. Edited by Jackson DW. New York: Raven Press; 1993:259–272.

54. Newton PO, Horibe S, Woo SL-Y: Experimental studies on anterior cruciate ligament autografts and allografts. In

Knee Ligaments: Structure, Function, Injury, and Repair, edn 1. Edited by Daniel DM, Akeson WH, O'Connor JJ. New York: Raven Press; 1990:389–399.

55. Noyes FR, Butler DL, Grood ES, *et al.*: Biomechanical analysis of human ligament grafts used in knee-ligament repairs and reconstructions. *J Bone Joint Surgery Am* 1984, 66:344–352.

56. Woo SL-Y, Hollis JM, Adams DJ, et al: Tensile properties of the human femur-anterior cruciate ligament-tibia complex: the effect of specimen age and orientation. *Am J Sports Med* 1991, 19:217–225.

57. Harner CD, Livesay GA, Kashiwaguchi S, *et al.*: Comparative study of the size and shape of human anterior and posterior cruciate ligaments. *J Orthop Res* 1995, 13:429–434.

58.• Ng GY, Oakes BW, Deacon OW, *et al.*: Biomechanics of patellar tendon autograft for reconstruction of the anterior cruciate ligament in the goat: three year study. *J Orthop Res* 1995, 13:602–608.
Autograft patellar tendon reconstructions in goat ACLs remain weaker than control ACLs up to 3 years after surgery, suggesting problems with remodeling of these grafts. Some osteoarthritis develops in the knees as well.

59. Oakes BW: Collagen ultrastructure in the normal ACL and in ACL graft. In *The Anterior Cruciate Ligament: Current and Future Concepts*, edn 1. Edited by Jackson DW. New York: Raven Press; 1993:209–218.

60. McFarland EG: The biology of anterior cruciate ligament reconstructions. *Orthopedics* 1993, 16:403–410.

61. Aune AK, Hukkanen M, Madsen JE, *et al.*: Nerve regeneration during patellar tendon autograft remodelling after anterior cruciate ligament reconstruction: an experimental and clinical study. *J Orthop Res* 1996, 14:193–199.

62. Spindler KP, Andrish JT, Miller RR, *et al*: Distribution of cellular repopulation and collagen synthesis in a canine anterior cruciate ligament autograft. *J Orthop Res* 1996, 14:384–389.

63.• Ng GYF, Oakes BW, Deacon OW, *et al.*: Long-term study of the biochemistry and biomechanics of anterior cruciate ligament-patellar tendon autografts in goats. *J Orthop Res* 1996, 14:851–856.
A positive correlation between the levels of collagen cross-links and the elastic modulus of patellar tendon autografts exists in this goat model of ACL reconstruction.

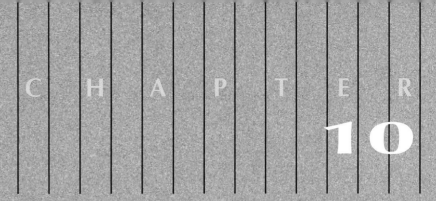

CHAPTER 10

ARTICULAR CARTILAGE BIOLOGY AND HEALING

Joseph A. Buckwalter and E.B. Hunziker

Synovial joints make possible the repetitive, quick, controlled movements necessary for participation in sports. Normal function of these complex structures depends on the unique properties of articular cartilage, which provides a smooth, low-friction gliding surface with stiffness to compression and resilience. It also distributes loads, minimizing peak stresses on subchondral bone, and, perhaps most important, has remarkable durability. Grossly and microscopically, normal adult articular cartilage appears to be a simple inactive tissue with a slick, firm surface that resists deformation. Light microscopic examination shows that it consists primarily of extracellular matrix; has only one type of cell, the chondrocyte; and lacks blood vessels, lymphatic vessels, and nerves (Fig. 10.1) [1,2•,3]. Compared with tissues like muscle or bone, cartilage has a low level of metabolic activity, is less responsive to changes in loading, and cannot repair significant structural damage caused by injury or disease [2–4,5•,6,7]. Yet, detailed study of the morphology and biology of adult articular cartilage reveals not only an elaborate, highly ordered structure but also a variety of complex interactions between the chondrocytes and the matrix that actively maintains the tissue.

In addition, recent work has suggested that it may be possible to facilitate restoration of a damaged articular surface. This article provides an overview of the biology and healing of normal adult articular cartilage. The first two sections summarize the composition and structure of articular cartilage and the interactions between the cells and the matrix that maintain the tissue. The third section discusses the response of articular cartilage to injury. The last section reviews approaches to stimulating articular cartilage repair or regeneration.

ARTICULAR CARTILAGE COMPOSITION

Articular cartilage consists of cells, matrix water, and a matrix macromolecular framework organized to form the bearing surfaces of synovial joints (*see* Fig. 10.1) [2•]. The cells contribute little to the volume of the tissue, about 1% in adult human articular cartilage.

Chondrocytes

Articular cartilage chondrocytes from different cartilage zones differ in size, shape, and probably metabolic activity. All of these cells, however, have a complex relationship with their extracellular matrix and contain the organelles necessary for matrix synthesis, including endoplasmic reticula and Golgi membranes. Nutrients must pass from synovial capillaries through the synovial membrane, the synovial fluid, and then through the cartilage matrix to reach the chondrocytes (*see* Fig. 10.1). These multiple barriers limit the types and concentrations of nutrients available to the cells, leaving chondrocytes with a low oxygen concentration relative to most other tissues; there-

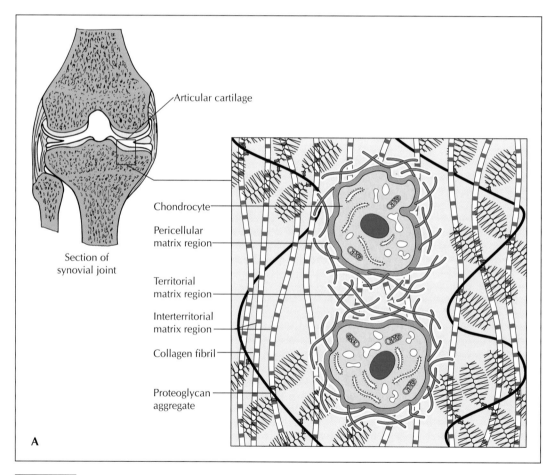

Articular cartilage

Section of synovial joint

Chondrocyte

Pericellular matrix region

Territorial matrix region

Interterritorial matrix region

Collagen fibril

Proteoglycan aggregate

A

FIGURE 10.1

The structure of articular cartilage. This simplified representation shows the lamellar and matrix organization of the tissue. This regional organization is based on chondrocyte proximity and matrix composition. **A,** The three matrix compartments (pericellular, territorial, and interterritorial) of cartilage are shown.

(continued on next page)

fore, they depend primarily on anaerobic metabolism. After completion of skeletal growth, most chondrocytes probably never divide but continue to synthesize collagens, proteoglycans, and noncollagenous proteins. The continuous synthetic activity suggests that maintenance of articular cartilage requires substantial, ongoing internal remodeling of the matrix macromolecular framework [2•]. Enzymes produced by chondrocytes can degrade the matrix macromolecules, and chondrocytes probably respond to the presence of fragmented matrix molecules by increasing their synthetic activity to replace the degraded components of the macromolecular framework. Other mechanisms also influence the balance between syn-

thetic and degradative activity, *eg*, how the frequency and intensity of joint loading influences chondrocyte metabolism. Joint immobilization or marked decreased joint loading alters chondrocyte activity so that degradation exceeds synthesis of at least the proteoglycan component of the matrix [8,9]. Persistent increased joint use may also alter the composition and organization of the matrix, but this has not been clearly demonstrated in skeletally mature individuals [8,9].

Extracellular matrix

The articular cartilage matrix consists of two components: the tissue fluid and the framework of struc-

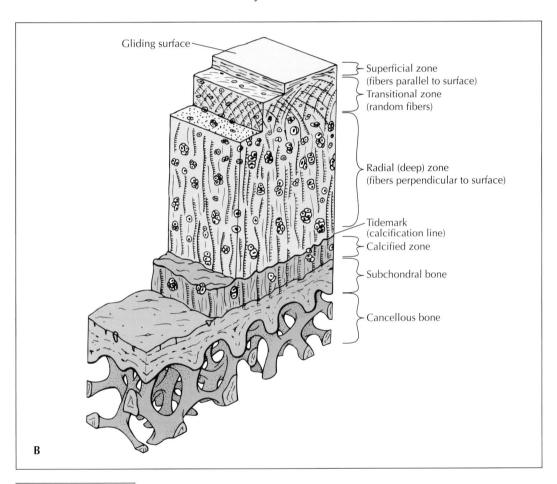

FIGURE 10.1 (continued)

B, The lamellar organization of the tissue (superficial, transition, radial, and calcified zones) is shown. The collagen fibrils form a structural network for the artic-

ular cartilage and provide support for the chondrocytes and proteoglycan aggregates. (*Adapted from* Buckwalter and Martin [42]; with permission.)

tural macromolecules that gives the tissue its form and stability and maintains the tissue fluid within the matrix (*see* Figs. 10.1 and 10.2). The interaction of the tissue fluid and the macromolecular framework makes possible the mechanical properties of stiffness and resilience (*see* Fig. 10.2) [6,10].

Tissue fluid

Water contributes up to 80% of the wet weight of articular cartilage, and the interaction of water with the matrix macromolecules significantly influences the mechanical properties of the tissue (*see* Fig. 10.2) [3,10–13]. This tissue fluid contains gasses, small proteins, metabolites, and a high concentration of cations to balance the negatively charged proteoglycans. At least some of the water can move freely in and out of the tissue. Its volume, concentration, and behavior within the tissue depends primarily on its interaction with the structural macromolecules—in particular, the large aggregated proteoglycans or aggrecans that help maintain the fluid within the matrix and the fluid electrolyte concentrations.

Because these macromolecules are so highly negatively charged, they attract positively charged ions like sodium and repel negatively charged ions like chlorine (*see* Fig. 10.2). The increase in total inorganic ion concentration increases the tissue osmolarity, creating an osmotic or swelling pressure that is resisted by the collagen fibril network [6,10].

Structural macromolecules

The cartilage structural macromolecules—collagens, proteoglycans, and noncollagenous proteins—contribute 20% to 40% of the wet weight of the tissue [3]. Collagens contribute about 60% of the dry weight of cartilage, proteoglycans contribute 25% to 35%, and the noncollagenous proteins and glycoproteins contribute 15% to 20%. The collagen fibrillar meshwork gives cartilage its form and tensile strength [6]. Proteoglycans and noncollagenous proteins bind to the collagenous meshwork or become mechanically entrapped within it, and water fills this molecular framework. Some noncollagenous proteins help organize and stabilize the matrix

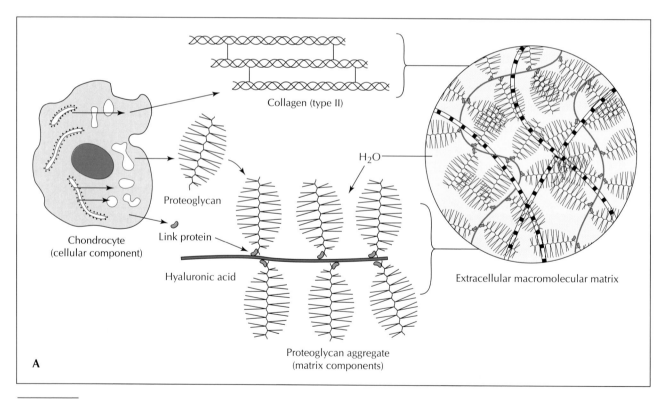

A

Collagen (type II)

H₂O

Chondrocyte (cellular component)

Proteoglycan

Link protein

Hyaluronic acid

Extracellular macromolecular matrix

Proteoglycan aggregate (matrix components)

FIGURE 10.2

The composition of articular cartilage. This simplified representation of articular cartilage composition shows the collagen fibrils and the aggregated proteoglycans, and how the interaction of the proteoglycans and water gives cartilage its stiffness to compression and its resilience. **A,** Chondrocytes synthesize collagen (structural framework) and hydrophilic proteoglycans, which interact with collagen fibrils to form the hydrated macromolecular matrix of articular cartilage.

(continued on next page)

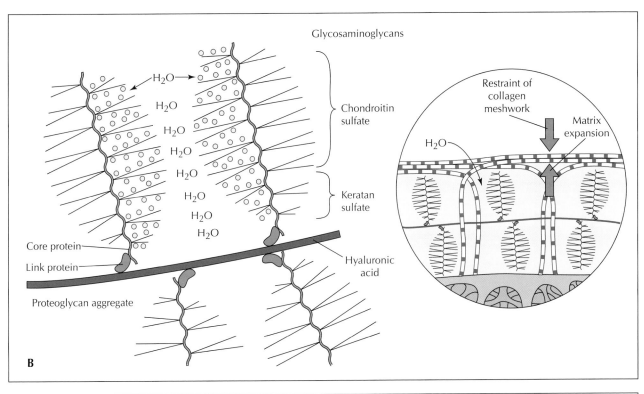

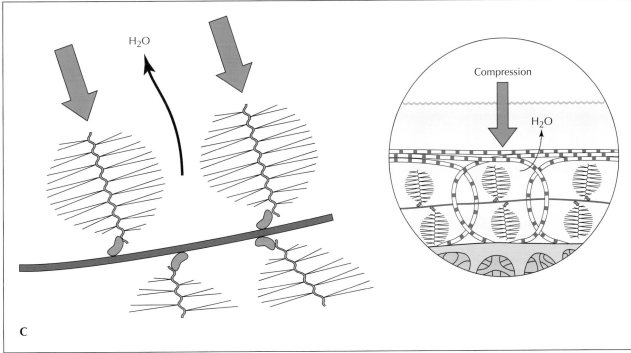

FIGURE 10.2 (continued)

B, Negatively charged glycosaminoglycan side chains repel one another and attract water, increasing matrix volume. Expansion is limited by collagen meshwork. **C,** Compression of matrix pushes glycosaminoglycan side chains together, releasing water and decreasing matrix volume. Decompression allows reexpansion of molecule and matrix volume. (*Adapted from* Buckwalter and Martin [42]; with permission.)

macromolecular framework, whereas others help chondrocytes bind to the matrix macromolecular framework.

Articular cartilage, like most tissues, contains many types of genetically distinct collagen types–specifically, collagen types II, VI, IX, X, and XI. Collagen types II, IX, and XI form the large cross-banded fibrils seen by electron microscopy. A network of finer cross-banded filaments, measuring between 10 and 15 nm in diameter, also exists throughout the matrix (Fig. 10.3). The composition of these structures has not been determined, but their periodicity suggests that they may be a form of collagen. The organization of fibrils and filaments

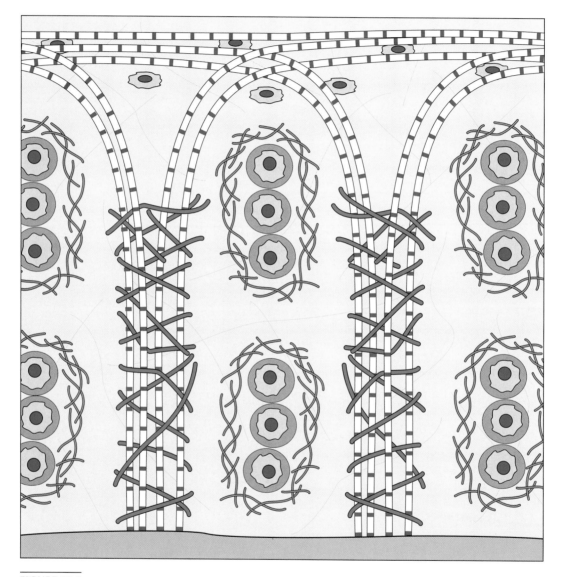

FIGURE 10.3

This representation of articular cartilage shows the relationships of the chondrocytes to the fibrillar components of the matrix and the organization of these components. The pericellular matrix compartment surrounds individual chondrocytes and varies in width; it is free of fibrillar components but contains an abundance of isotropically arranged, cross-banded filaments that extend throughout all matrix compartments. The territori-al matrix contains a basket-like arrangement of collagen fibrils and surrounds the pericellular matrix. The interterritorial matrix forms the bulk of the tissue and contains two populations of fibrils and fibril bundles. The first population consists of fibrils with a highly oriented parallel arrangement that form the arcade-like structures. The second population consists of more randomly oriented fibrils. Aggrecans fill most of the interfibrillar space.

into a tight meshwork that extends throughout the tissue provides the tensile stiffness and strength of articular cartilage and contributes to the cohesiveness of the tissue by mechanically entrapping the large proteoglycans. The principal articular cartilage collagen, type II, accounts for 90% to 95% of the cartilage collagen. Polymerized type II molecules form the primary component of the large cross-banded fibrils. Type XI collagen molecules bind covalently to type II collagen molecules and probably form part of the interior structure of the cross-banded fibrils. Type IX collagen molecules bind covalently to the superficial layers of the cross banded fibrils and project into the matrix where they also can bind covalently to other type IX collagen molecules. The functions of type IX and XI collagens remain uncertain, but, presumably, they help form and stabilize the collagen fibrils assembled primarily from type II collagen. The projecting portions of type IX collagen molecules may also help bind together the collagen fibril meshwork and connect the collagen meshwork with proteoglycans [14]. Type VI collagen appears to form an important part of the matrix immediately surrounding chondrocytes and helps chondrocytes attach to the matrix [15,16]. The presence of Type X collagen found only near the cells of the calcified cartilage zone of articular cartilage and the hypertrophic zone of growth plate (where the longitudinal cartilage septa begin to mineralize) suggests that it has a role in cartilage mineralization.

Proteoglycans consist of a protein core and one or more glycosaminoglycan chains (long, unbranched polysaccharide chains consisting of repeating disaccharides that contain an amino sugar) [14,17,18]. Each disaccharide has at least one negatively charged carboxylate or sulfate group; thus the glycosaminoglycans form long strings of negative charges that repel each other and other negatively charged molecules, and attract cations (*see* Fig. 10.2). Glycosaminoglycans found in cartilage include hyaluronic acid, chondroitin sulfate, keratan sulfate, and dermatan sulfate. Articular cartilage contains two major classes of proteoglycans: large aggregating proteoglycans or aggrecans and small proteoglycans, including decorin, biglycan, and fibromodulin. Aggrecans have large numbers of chondroitin sulfate and keratan sulfate chains attached to a protein core filament (*see* Fig. 10.2). Aggrecan molecules fill most of the interfibrillar space of the cartilage matrix (*see* Figs. 10.1, 10.2, and 10.3). They contribute about 90% of the total cartilage matrix proteoglycan mass, whereas large

nonaggregating proteoglycans contribute 10% or less and small nonaggregating proteoglycans contribute about 3%. Most aggrecans associate noncovalently with hyaluronic acid (hyaluronan) and link proteins, small noncollagenous proteins, to form proteoglycan aggregates (Fig. 10.4) that occupy the space between collagen fibrils. Link proteins stabilize the association between monomers and hyaluronic acid and appear to have a role in directing the assembly of aggregates [19–24]. Aggregate formation helps anchor proteoglycans within the matrix, preventing their displacement during deformation of the tissue, and also helps organize and stabilize the relationship between proteoglycans and the collagen meshwork. The small nonaggregating proteoglycans have shorter protein cores

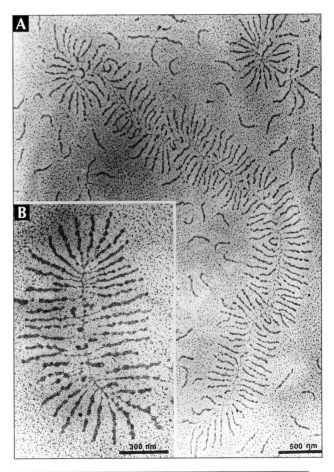

FIGURE 10.4 Electron micrographs of proteoglycan aggregates. **A,** Large aggregate at lower magnification. **B,** Smaller aggregate at higher magnification. The central filament of each aggregate consists of hyaluronan, and the projecting side arms are agrecans. In this preparation, the glycosaminoglycan chains of the aggrecans have collapsed around the aggrecan core proteins.

than aggrecan molecules and, unlike aggrecans, do not fill a large volume of the tissue or contribute directly to the mechanical behavior of the tissue. Instead they bind to other macromolecules and probably influence cell function. Decorin has one dermatan sulfate chain, biglycan has two dermatan sulfate chains, and fibromodulin has several keratan sulfate chains [14]. Decorin and fibromodulin bind with type II collagen and may have a role in organizing and stabilizing the type II collagen meshwork [14]. Biglycan is concentrated in the pericellular matrix and may interact with type VI collagen [14]. The small proteoglycans also can bind transforming growth factor-beta (TGF-beta) and may influence the activity of this cytokine in cartilage [25]. At the articular surface, or on a cut surface of articular cartilage, they may prevent cell adhesion to the matrix.

A wide variety of noncollagenous proteins and glycoproteins exist within articular cartilage, but thus far only a few of them have been studied. In general, they consist primarily of protein and have a few attached monosaccharides and oligosaccharides [26•]. At least some of these molecules appear to help organize and maintain the macromolecular structure of the matrix. Cartilage oligomeric protein, an acidic protein, is concentrated primarily within the chondrocyte territorial matrix, appears to be present only within cartilage, and has the capacity to bind to chondrocytes [27,28]. This molecule may have value as a marker of cartilage turnover and of the progression of cartilage degeneration in patients with osteoarthritis [29,30]. Fibronectin and tenascin, noncollagenous matrix proteins found in a variety of tissues, have also been identified within cartilage. Their functions in articular cartilage remain poorly understood, but they may have roles in matrix organization, cell matrix interactions, and in the responses of the tissue in inflammatory arthritis and osteoarthritis.

ARTICULAR CARTILAGE STRUCTURE

To form articular cartilage, chondrocytes organize the collagens, proteoglycans, and noncollagenous proteins into a unique, highly ordered structure [3]. The composition, organization, and mechanical properties of the matrix, cell morphology, and probably cell function vary with the depth from the articular surface (*see* Fig. 10.1). Matrix composition, organization, and function also vary with the distance from the cell.

Zones

The morphologic changes in chondrocytes and matrix from the articular surface to the subchondral bone make it possible to identify four zones or layers: the superficial zone, the transitional zone, the radial zone, and the zone of calcified cartilage (*see* Figs. 10.1 and 10.3) [1]. The zone matrices differ in concentrations of water, proteoglycan, and collagen and in the size of the aggregates [3]. Cells in different zones not only differ in shape, size, and orientation relative to the articular surface (*see* Fig. 10.3), but they also differ in numerical density and metabolic activity [31,32]. In addition, chondrocytes in different articular cartilage zones may respond differently to mechanical loading, suggesting that development and maintenance of normal articular cartilage depend in part on differentiation of phenotypically distinct populations of chondrocytes.

Superficial zone
The superficial zone consists of two layers: an acellular layer and a deeper cellular layer. The acellular layer consists of a thin covering of amorphous material overlying a deeper sheet of fine fibrils surrounded by a nonfibrillar matrix containing little polysaccharide [1,3]. Underneath the acellular sheet of fine fibrils, flattened ellipsoid-shaped chondrocytes in a collagenous matrix arrange themselves so that their major axes are parallel to the articular surface (*see* Figs. 10.1 and 10.3). They synthesize a matrix that has a high collagen concentration and a low proteoglycan concentration relative to the other cartilage zones. Tissue and cell culture studies show that superficial zone cells degrade proteoglycans more rapidly and synthesize less collagen and proteoglycans than cells from the deeper zones [31,32]. Fibronectin and water concentrations are also highest in this zone.

Transitional zone
As the name "transitional zone" implies, the morphology and matrix composition of the transitional zone is intermediate between the superficial zone and the radial zone. It usually has several times the volume of the superficial zone, and its cells have a higher concentration of synthetic organelles, endoplasmic reticula, and Golgi membranes than do superficial zone cells. Transitional zone cells assume a spheroidal shape and synthesize a matrix that has larger-diameter collagen fibrils and a higher proteoglycan concentration, but lower concentrations of water and collagen than the superficial zone matrix.

Radial (deep) zone

The chondrocytes in the radial zone are spheroidal and tend to align themselves in short columns perpendicular to the joint surface (*see* Fig. 10.1). This zone contains the largest-diameter collagen fibrils, the highest concentration of proteoglycans, and the lowest concentration of water. The collagen fibers of this zone pass into the "tidemark," a thin basophilic line seen on light microscopic sections of decalcified articular cartilage that roughly corresponds to the boundary between calcified and uncalcified cartilage. The nature of the tidemark remains uncertain [33]. It may result from concentration of basophilic calcified material at the interface between calcified and uncalcified matrix, possibly accentuated by the tissue processing, and thus represents a "high water mark" for calcification. Alternatively, one study identified a band of fine fibrils corresponding to the tidemark, suggesting that it represents a well-defined matrix structure [34].

Calcified cartilage zone

A thin zone of calcified cartilage separates the radial zone (uncalcified cartilage) and the subchondral bone. The cells of the calcified cartilage zone have a smaller volume than the cells of the radial zone and contain only small amounts of endoplasmic reticulum and Golgi membranes. Some of these cells are surrounded by calcified cartilage, suggesting an extremely low level of metabolic activity. However, recent work indicates that they may have a role in the development and progression of osteoarthritis [33].

Matrix regions

Variations in the matrix within zones distinguish three regions or compartments: the pericellular region, the territorial region, and the interterritorial region [2•,3] (*see* Figs. 10.1 and 10.3). The pericellular and territorial regions appear to serve the needs of chondrocytes, *ie*, binding the cell membranes to the matrix macromolecules and protecting the cells from damage during loading and deformation of the tissue. They may also help transmit mechanical signals to the chondrocytes when the matrix deforms during joint loading. The primary function of the interterritorial matrix is to provide the mechanical properties of the tissue.

Pericellular matrix

Chondrocyte cell membranes appear to attach to the thin rim of the pericellular matrix that covers the cell surface. This matrix region is rich in proteoglycans and also contains noncollagenous matrix proteins and nonfibrillar collagens, including type VI collagen.

Territorial matrix

An envelope of territorial matrix surrounds the pericellular matrix of individual chondrocytes and, in some locations, pairs or clusters of chondrocytes and their pericellular matrices. In the radial zone, a territorial matrix surrounds each chondrocyte column. The thin collagen fibrils of the territorial matrix nearest to the cell appear to adhere to the pericellular matrix. At a distance from the cell, they decussate and intersect at various angles, forming a fibrillar basket around the cells. This collagenous basket may provide mechanical protection for the chondrocytes during loading and deformation of the tissue.

Interterritorial matrix

The interterritorial matrix makes up most of the volume of mature articular cartilage (*see* Figs. 10.1 and 10.3). It contains the largest-diameter collagen fibrils. Unlike the collagen fibrils of the territorial matrix, these fibrils are not organized to surround the chondrocytes and many of them change their orientation relative to the joint surface 90° from the superficial zone to the deep zone. In the superficial zone, the fibril diameters are relatively small and the fibrils generally lie parallel to the articular surface. In the transition zone, interterritorial matrix collagen fibrils assume more oblique angles relative to the articular surface. In the radial zone, many collagen fibrils form bundles that lie perpendicular (or radial) to the joint surface (*see* Figs. 10.1 and 10.3).

CHONDROCYTE–MATRIX INTERACTIONS

The continuous interactions of chondrocytes and the matrix maintain the tissue throughout life. The mechanisms that control the balance between chondrocyte synthetic and degradative activity remain poorly understood, but cytokines with catabolic and anabolic effects appear to have important roles. For example, interleukin-1 induces expression of enzymes that degrade matrix macromolecules and interfere with synthesis of proteoglycans. Other cytokines such as insulin-like growth factor (IGF)-I and TGF-beta oppose these catabolic activities by stimulating matrix synthesis. In response to a variety of stimuli, chondrocytes synthesize and release these cytokines into the matrix where they may bind to receptors on the cell surfaces (stimulating cell activity either by autocrine or paracrine mechanisms) or become trapped within the matrix. The matrix also protects the chondrocytes from mechanical damage during normal joint use, helps maintain their shape and phenotype, and acts as a signal transducer. The cells bind to the matrix macromolecules through specialized cell-surface receptors, including a variety of integrins. The matrix transmits signals that result from mechanical loading of the articular surface to the chondrocytes, and the chondrocytes respond to these signals by altering the matrix, possibly through expression of cytokines. The details of how mechanical loading of joints influences chondrocyte function remain unknown, but matrix deformation produces mechanical, electrical, and physicochemical signals that may have significant roles in stimulating chondrocytes [35–39]. Loading may also cause persistent changes in matrix molecular organization that alter chondrocyte responses to subsequent loading. Thus, the matrix may not only transduce and transmit signals, it may "record" the loading history of the tissue and alter the response of the cells based on the recorded loading history.

RESPONSE OF ARTICULAR SURFACES TO INJURY

Articular surface injuries can be classified based on the type of tissue damage and the repair response: 1) cartilage matrix and cell injuries (*ie*, damage to the joint surface that does not cause visible mechanical disruption of the articular surface); 2) chondral fissures, flap tears, or chondral defects (*ie*, visible mechanical disruption of articular cartilage limited to articular cartilage); and 3) osteochondral injuries (*ie*, visible mechanical disruption of articular cartilage and bone) [5•,40].

Matrix and cell injuries

Acute or repetitive blunt trauma including excessive impact loading can cause alterations in articular cartilage matrix, including a decrease in proteoglycan concentration and, possibly, disruptions of the collagen fibril framework. The ability of chondrocytes to sense changes in matrix composition and synthesize new molecules makes it possible for them to repair damage to the macromolecular framework. It is not clear at what point this type of injury becomes irreversible and leads to progressive loss of articular cartilage. Presumably, if the fibrillar collagen meshwork remains intact and enough chondrocytes remain viable, the chondrocytes can restore the matrix as long as the loss of matrix proteoglycan does not exceed what the cells can rapidly produce. When these conditions are not met the cells cannot restore the matrix, the chondrocytes will be exposed to excessive loads, and the tissue will degenerate.

Chondral injuries

Acute or repetitive trauma can cause focal mechanical disruption of articular cartilage, including fissures, chondral flaps, or tears and loss of a segment of articular cartilage [40]. The lack of blood vessels and lack of cells that can repair significant tissue defects limits the response of cartilage to injury (Fig. 10.5) [3,6]. Chondrocytes respond to tissue injury by proliferating and increasing the synthesis of matrix macromolecules near the injury. However, the

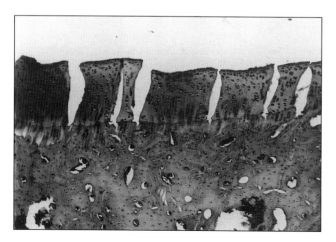

FIGURE 10.5
Light micrograph showing experimentally created defects in rabbit articular cartilage extending from the surface to the subchondral bone. Although the cells may respond to these tissue injuries, they do not migrate into the defects or produce new tissue that fills the defects. (*From* Buckwalter and Mow [6]; with permission.)

newly synthesized matrix and proliferating cells do not fill the tissue defect, and soon after injury the increased proliferative and synthetic activity ceases.

Osteochondral injuries

Unlike injuries limited to cartilage, injuries that extend into subchondral bone cause hemorrhage, fibrin clot formation, and activation the inflammatory response [3,6]. Soon after injury, blood escaping from the damaged bone's blood vessels forms a hematoma that temporarily fills the injury site. Fibrin forms within the hematoma, and platelets bind to fibrillar collagen. A continuous fibrin clot fills the bone defect and extends for a variable distance into the cartilage defect. Platelets within the clot release vasoactive mediators and growth factors or cytokines (small proteins that influence multiple cell functions, including migration, proliferation, differentiation, and matrix synthesis). These cytokines include TGF-beta and platelet-derived growth factor (PDGF). Bone matrix also contains

growth factors, including TGF-beta, IGF-I, PDGF, bone morphogenic protein, IGF-II, and possibly others. Release of these growth factors may have an important role in the repair of osteochondral defects. In particular, they probably stimulate vascular invasion and migration of undifferentiated cells into the clot and influence the proliferative and synthetic activities of the cells. Shortly after entering the tissue defect, the undifferentiated mesenchymal cells proliferate and synthesize a new matrix. Within 2 weeks of injury, some mesenchymal cells assume the rounded form of chondrocytes and begin to synthesize a matrix that contains type II collagen and a relatively high concentration of proteoglycans. These cells produce regions of hyaline-like cartilage in the chondral and bone portions of the defect. Six to 8 weeks following injury, the repair tissue within the chondral region of osteochondral defects contains many chondrocyte-like cells in a matrix consisting of type II collagen, proteoglycans, some type I collagen, and noncollagenous proteins (Fig. 10.6). Unlike the cells in the chondral portion of

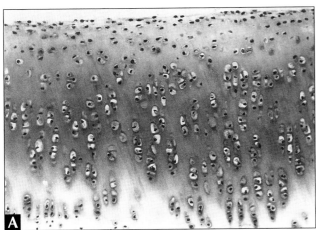

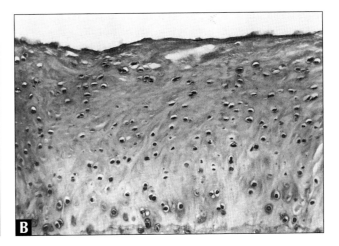

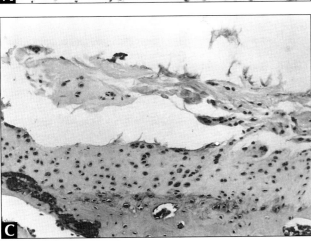

FIGURE 10.6

Light micrographs of rabbit articular surfaces. **A,** Normal articular cartilage; notice the hyaline appearance of the matrix. **B,** Well-formed chondral repair tissue; notice the fibrillar appearance of the matrix. **C,** Fibrillated chondral repair tissue. (*From* Buckwalter and Mow [6]; with permission.)

the defect, the cells in the bone portion of the defect produce immature bone, fibrous tissue, and hyaline-like cartilage.

The chondral repair tissue typically has a composition and structure intermediate between hyaline cartilage and fibrocartilage; and it rarely, if ever, replicates the elaborate structure of normal articular cartilage (*see* Figs. 10.1 and 10.6). Occasionally, the cartilage repair tissue persists unchanged or progressively remodels to form a functional joint surface. In most large osteochondral injuries, however, the chondral repair tissue begins to show evidence of depletion of matrix proteoglycans, fragmentation, and fibrillation. This increases both the collagen content and the loss of chondrocyte-like cells within a year or less (*see* Fig. 10.6). The remaining cells often assume the appearance of fibroblasts as the surrounding matrix comes to consist primarily of densely packed collagen fibrils. This fibrous tissue usually fragments and often disintegrates, leaving areas of exposed bone. The inferior mechanical properties of chondral repair tissue may be responsible for its frequent deterioration [5•,6]. Even repair tissue that successfully fills osteochondral defects is less stiff and more permeable than normal articular cartilage, and the orientation and organization of the collagen fibrils in even the most hyaline-like cartilage repair tissue does not follow the pattern seen in normal articular cartilage. In addition, the repair tissue cells may fail to establish the normal relationships between matrix macromolecules, particularly the relationship between cartilage proteoglycans and the collagen fibril network. The decreased stiffness and increased permeability of repair cartilage matrix may increase loading of the macromolecular framework during joint use, resulting in progressive structural damage to the matrix collagen and proteoglycans. Thus, the repair chondrocytes are exposed to excessive loads, further compromising their ability to restore the matrix.

Clinical experience and experimental studies suggest that the success of chondral repair in osteochondral injuries may depend to some extent on the severity of the injury as measured by the volume of tissue or surface area of cartilage injured and the age of the individual [4]. Smaller osteochondral defects that do not alter joint function heal more predictably than larger defects that may change the loading of the articular surface. Potential age-related differences in healing of chondral and osteochondral injuries have not been thoroughly investigated. However, bone heals more rapidly in children than in adults, and the articular cartilage chondrocytes in skeletally immature animals show a better proliferative response to injury and synthesize larger proteoglycan molecules than those from mature animals. Furthermore, a growing synovial joint has the potential to remodel the articular surface to decrease the mechanical abnormalities created by a chondral or osteochondral defect.

PROMOTING ARTICULAR CARTILAGE REPAIR AND REGENERATION

Better understanding of articular cartilage injuries and recognition of the limitations of the natural repair responses have contributed to the recent interest in cartilage repair and regeneration [3,6,40–42]. Advances in synovial joint imaging and arthroscopic techniques have increased understanding of the frequency and types of chondral defects and made it possible to diagnose and evaluate these lesions with great accuracy. Age-related, nonprogressive superficial cartilage fibrillation and focal lesions of the articular surface must be distinguished from cartilage degeneration due to osteoarthritis [5•,43]. Superficial articular cartilage fibrillation occurs in many joints with increasing age and does not appear to cause symptoms or adversely affect joint function. Focal articular cartilage and osteochondral defects appear to result from trauma that often leaves the majority of the articular surface intact [5•,40,44•]. These commonly occur in adolescents and young adults and in some of these individuals cause joint pain, effusions, and mechanical dysfunction. Although the natural history of isolated chondral and osteochondral defects has not been well defined [45–47], clinical experience suggests that defects involving a significant portion of the articular surface may progress to symptomatic joint degeneration.

In the past three decades, clinical and basic scientific investigations have shown that implantation of artificial matrices, growth factors, perichondria, periostea, and transplanted chondrocytes and mesenchymal stem cells can stimulate formation of cartilaginous tissue in synovial joint osteochondral and chondral defects [5•,41,46,48–50]. Other work has demonstrated that joint loading and motion can influence articular cartilage and joint healing, and that mechanical loading influences the repair process in all of the tissues that form parts of synovial joints [4,8,35,51–53]. The apparent potential of these multiple methods for stimulating formation of cartilaginous articular surfaces has created interest among patients, physicians, and scientists. However, the wide variety of methods and approaches to evaluate results have made it difficult to establish their success in restoring joint function and to define their most appropriate current clinical applications.

Penetration of subchondral bone

Surgeons have developed a variety of methods of penetrating subchondral bone to stimulate formation of a new cartilaginous surface, including drilling, abrasion of the articular surface, and making multiple small-diameter defects or fractures with an awl or similar instrument. Prospective randomized controlled trials of penetrating subchondral bone to stimulate cartilage repair and decrease symptoms have not been reported, but several authors have reviewed series of patients and found that these procedures can decrease the symptoms due to isolated articular cartilage defects and osteoarthritis of the knee [44•,54–58]. Other investigators, however, reported less successful results [59]. Examination of joint surfaces following arthroscopic abrasion has shown that, in some individuals, it results in formation of a fibrocartilaginous articular surface that varies in composition from dense fibrous tissue with little or no type II collagen to hyaline-like cartilage tissue with predominantly type II collagen [56,57]. In some patients with radiographic evidence of cartilage–joint space narrowing, or no radiographically demonstrable joint space, the joint space increased following abrasion [56,57]. Although an increase in radiographic joint space following subchondral abrasion presumably indicates formation of a new articular surface, the development of this new surface does not necessarily result in symptomatic improvement. For example, Bert [60] and Bert and Maschka [61] found that 51% of 59 patients treated with abrasion arthroplasty had evidence of increased radiographic joint space 2 years after treatment, but 31% of these individuals either had no symptomatic improvement or developed more severe symptoms. The lack of predictable clinical benefit from the apparent formation of cartilage repair tissue may result from variability among patients in severity of the degenerative changes, joint alignment, patterns of joint use, age, perception of pain, preoperative expectations, or other factors. It may also result from the inability of the newly formed tissue to replicate the properties of articular cartilage [6].

Periosteal and perichondrial grafts

The potential benefits of periosteal and perichondrial grafts include introduction of a new cell population along with an organic matrix, a decrease in the probability of ankylosis before a new articular surface can form, and some protection of the graft or host cells from excessive loading. Animal experiments and clinical experience show that perichondrial and periosteal grafts placed in articular cartilage defects can produce new cartilage [41,52]. O'Driscoll *et al.* [62,63] described the use of periosteal grafts for the treatment of isolated chondral and osteochondral defects and demonstrated that these grafts can produce a new articular surface. Other investigators have reported encouraging results with perichondrial grafts [64,65]. One study, however, suggests that increasing patient age adversely affects the results of soft tissue grafts. Seradge *et al.* [66] studied the results of rib perichondrial arthroplasties in 16 metacarpophalangeal joints and 20 proximal interphalangeal joints at a minimum of 3 years following surgery. Patient age was directly related to the results. All of the patients in their twenties and 75% of the patients in their thirties had good results following metacarpophalangeal joint arthroplasties. Seventy-five percent of the patients in their teens and 66% of the patients in their twenties had good results following proximal interphalangeal joint arthroplasties. None of the patients over 40 years of age had a good result with either type of arthroplasty. The clinical observation that perichondrial grafts produced the best results in younger patients agrees with the concept that age may adversely affect the ability of undifferentiated cells or chondrocytes to form an articular surface, or that the population of cells that can form an articular surface declines with age [66,67].

Cell transplantation

The limited ability of host cells to restore articular surfaces has led investigators to seek methods of transplanting cells that can form cartilage into chondral and osteochondral defects [3,6]. Experimental work has shown that both chondrocytes and undifferentiated mesenchymal cells placed in articular cartilage defects survive and produce a new cartilage matrix [41]. Recently, Brittberg *et al.* [68,69] compared the results of treating chondral defects in rabbit patellar articular surfaces with periosteal grafts alone; carbon fiber scaffolds and periostea; autologous chondrocytes and periostea; and autologous chondrocytes, carbon fiber scaffolds, and periostea. They found that the addition of autologous chondrocytes improved the histologic quality and amount of repair tissue. Other studies showed that cultured mesenchymal stem cells also can repair large osteochondral defects [70,71•]. In addition to these animal experiments, a group of investigators has reported using autologous chondrocyte transplants for treatment of localized cartilage defects of the femoral condyle or patella in patients [72••]. At 2 or more years following chondrocyte transplantation, 14 of 16 patients with condylar defects and two of seven patients with patellar defects had good or excellent clinical results. Biopsy specimens of the defect sites showed hyaline-like cartilage in 11 of 15 femoral defects and in one of seven patellar defects. More recently, this group of investigators reported the results in a larger group of patients [48]. They found that, at more than 2 years after treatment for chondral defects of the knee, 47 of 66 patients had improved knee function. These results indicate that chondrocyte transplantation combined with a periosteal graft can promote restoration of an articular surface in humans. More work is needed, however, to assess the function and durability of the new tissue and determine if it improves joint function and delays or prevents joint degeneration.

Growth factors

Growth factors influence a variety of cell activities including proliferation, migration, matrix synthesis, and differentiation. Many of these factors, including the fibroblast growth factors, IGFs, and TGF-betas, have been shown to affect chondrocyte metabolism and chondrogenesis [4,41]. Bone matrix contains a variety of these molecules, including IGFs, TGF-betas, bone morphogenic proteins, PDGFs, and others [4,73]. In addition, mesenchymal cells, endothelial cells, and platelets produce many of these factors. Thus, osteochondral injuries and exposure of bone due to loss of articular cartilage may release these agents that affect the formation of cartilage repair tissue, and they probably have an important role in the formation of new articular surfaces after currently used surgical procedures, including penetration of subchondral bone. Local treatment of chondral or osteochondral defects with growth factors has the potential to stimulate restoration of an articular surface. A recent experimental study of the treatment of par-

tial-thickness cartilage defects with enzymatic digestion of proteoglycans (which inhibit adhesion of cells to articular cartilage) followed by implantation of a fibrin matrix and a timed release of TGF-beta showed that this growth factor can stimulate cartilage repair [74•,75]. The cells that filled the chondral defects migrated into the defects from the synovium and formed a fibrous matrix. Despite the promise of this approach, the wide variety of growth factors, their multiple effects, the interactions among them, the possibility that the responsiveness of cells to growth factors may decline with age, and the limited understanding of their effects in osteoarthritic joints make it difficult to develop a simple strategy for using these agents to treat patients with osteoarthritis [67,77,78]. However, development of growth factor–based treatments appears promising for isolated chondral and osteochondral defects and early cartilage degenerative changes in younger people.

Artificial matrices

Treatment of chondral defects with growth factors or cell transplants requires a method of delivering and, in most instances, at least temporarily stabilizing the growth factors or cells in the defect. For these reasons, the success of these approaches often depends on an artificial matrix. In addition, artificial matrices may allow and, in some instances, stimulate ingrowth of host cells, matrix formation, and binding of new cells and matrix to host tissue [78]. Investigators have found that implants formed from a variety of biologic and nonbiologic materials facilitate restoration of an articular surface [5•,41]. These implants included treated cartilage and bone matrices, collagens, collagens and hyaluronan, fibrin, carbon fiber, hydroxylapatite, porous polylactic acid, polytetrafluoroethylene, polyester, and other synthetic polymers. Lack of studies that directly compare different types of artificial matrices makes it difficult to evaluate their relative merits, but the available reports show that this approach may contribute to restoration of an articular surface. Treatment of osteochondral defects of the knee in humans produced a satisfactory result in 77% of 47 patients evaluated clinically and arthroscopically 3 years after surgery [79]. Brittberg *et al.* [80] also studied the use of carbon fiber pads for treatment of articular surface defects. They found good or excellent results in 83% of 36 patients at an average of 4 years after treatment.

CONCLUSIONS

The ability of articular cartilage to provide low-friction joint motion depends on its unique biologic features, including the interactions between chondrocytes and the matrix. Chondrocytes form the tissue matrix macromolecular framework from three classes of molecules: collagens, proteoglycans, and noncollagenous proteins. The matrix protects the cells from injury due to normal joint use, determines the types and concentrations of molecules that reach the cells, and helps maintain the chondrocyte phenotype. Throughout life, the tissue undergoes continuous internal remodeling as the cells replace matrix macromolecules lost through degradation. In addition, the matrix acts as a signal transducer for the cells. Loading of the tissue due to joint use creates mechanical, electrical, and physicochemical signals that help direct chondrocyte synthetic and degradative activity. Prolonged, severely decreased joint use leads to alterations in matrix composition and, eventually, loss of tissue structure and mechanical properties, whereas joint use stimulates chondrocyte synthetic activity and possibly internal tissue remodeling. Recent work shows that the potential for restoration of a damaged articular surface exists. Currently surgeons penetrate subchondral bone with the intent of stimulating formation of a new articular surface

and decreasing symptoms. The results of these procedures vary considerably among patients. Clinical and experimental studies show that chondrocyte and mesenchymal stem cell transplantation, periosteal and perichondrial grafting, synthetic matrices, growth factors, and other methods have the potential to stimulate formation of a new articular surface. Thus far, none of these methods have been shown to predictably restore a durable articular surface in an osteoarthritic joint, and it is unlikely that any one of them will be uniformly successful in the restoration of osteoarthritic articular surfaces.

The available clinical and experimental evidence indicates that future optimal methods of restoring articular surfaces will begin with 1) a detailed analysis of the structural and functional abnormalities of the involved joint, and 2) the patient's expectations for future joint use. Based on this analysis, the surgeon will develop a treatment plan that potentially combines correction of mechanical abnormalities (including malalignment, instability, and intra-articular causes of mechanical dysfunction), debridement (which may nor may not include limited penetration of subchondral bone) and applications of growth factors or implants (which may consist of a synthetic matrix that incorporates cells or growth factors or transplants) followed by a postoperative course of controlled loading and motion.

REFERENCES AND RECOMMENDED READING

Recently published papers of particular interest have been highlighted as:

- • Of special interest
- •• Of outstanding interest

1. Buckwalter JA, Hunziker EB, Rosenberg LC, *et al.*: Articular cartilage: composition and structure. *In* Injury and Repair of the Musculoskeletal Soft Tissues. *Edited by Woo SL, Buckwalter JA. Park Ridge, IL: American Academy of Orthopaedic Surgeons; 1988:405–425.*

2.• Buckwalter JA, Mankin HJ: Articular cartilage I. Tissue design and chondrocyte-matrix interactions. *J Bone Joint Surg Am* 1997, 79:600–611.

This review provides a summary of current understanding of articular cartilage structure, function, and metabolism.

3. Buckwalter JA, Rosenberg LA, Hunziker EB: Articular cartilage: composition, structure, response to injury, and methods of facilitation repair. In *Articular Cartilage and Knee Joint Function: Basic Science and Arthroscopy*. Edited by Ewing JW. New York: Raven Press; 1990:19–56.

4. Buckwalter JA, Einhorn TA, Bolander ME, Cruess RL: Healing of musculoskeletal tissues. In *Fractures*. Edited by Rockwood CA, Green D. Philadelphia: Lippincott-Raven; 1996:261–304.

5.• Buckwalter JA, Mankin HJ: Articular cartilage II. Degeneration and osteoarthrosis, repair, regeneration and transplantation. *J Bone Joint Surg Am* 1997, 79:612–632.

This review provides a summary of current understanding of articular cartilage degeneration and the relationship between cartilage regeneration and osteoarthritis. It also summarizes recent publications concerning basic scientific knowledge and clinical strategies for articular cartilage repair, regeneration, and transplantation.

6. Buckwalter JA, Mow VC: Cartilage repair in osteoarthritis. In *Osteoarthritis: Diagnosis and Management*, edn 2. Edited by Moskowitz RW, Howell DS, Goldberg VM, Mankin HJ. Philadelphia: W.B. Saunders; 1992:71–107.

7. Buckwalter JA, Rosenberg LC, Coutts R, *et al.*: Articular cartilage: injury and repair. In *Injury and Repair of the Musculoskeletal Soft Tissues*. Edited by Woo SL, Buckwalter JA. Park Ridge, IL: American Academy of Orthopaedic Surgeons; 1988:465–482.

8. Buckwalter JA: Activity vs. rest in the treatment of bone, soft tissue and joint injuries. *Iowa Orthop J* 1995, 15:29–42.

9. Buckwalter JA: Osteoarthritis and articular cartilage use, disuse and abuse: experimental studies. *J Rheumatol* 1995, 22(suppl 43):13–15.

10. Mow VC, Rosenwasser MP: Articular cartilage: biomechanics. In *Injury and Repair of the Musculoskeletal Soft Tissues*.

Edited by Woo SL, Buckwalter JA. Park Ridge, IL: American Academy of Orthopaedic Surgeons; 1988:427–463.

11. Lai WM, Mow VC, Roth V: Effects of nonlinear strain-dependent permeability and rate of compression on the stress behavior of articular cartilage. *J Biomech Eng* 1981, 103:61–66.

12. Mankin HJ: The water of articular cartilage. In *The Human Joint in Health and Disease.* Edited by Simon WH. Philadelphia: University of Pennsylvannia Press; 1978:37–42.

13. Maroudas A, Schneiderman R: "Free" and "exchangeable" or "trapped" and "nonexchangeable" water in cartilage. *J Orthop Res* 1987, 5:133–138.

14. Roughley PJ, Lee ER: Cartilage proteoglycans: structure and potential functions. *Micros Res Tech* 1994, 28:385–397.

15. Hagiwara H, Schroter-Kermani C, Merker HJ: Localization of collagen type VI in articular cartilage of young and adult mice. *Cell Tissue Res* 1993, 272:155–160.

17. Hardingham TE, Fosang AJ, Dudhia J: Aggrecan, the chondroitin/keratan sulfate proteoglycan from cartilage. In *Articular Cartilage and Osteoarthritis.* Edited by Kuettner KE, Schleyerbach R, Peyron JG, Hascall VC. New York: Raven Press; 1992:5–20.

16. Marcelino J, McDevitt CA: Attachment of articular cartilage chondrocytes to the tissue form of type VI collagen. *Biochem Biophys Acta* 1995, 1249:180–188.

18. Rosenberg LC: Structure and function of dermatan sulfate proteoglycans in articular cartilage. In *Articular Cartilage and Osteoarthritis.* Edited by Kuettner KE, Schleyerbach R, Peyron JG, Hascall VC. New York: Raven Press; 1992:45–63.

19. Buckwalter JA, Pita JC, Muller FJ, Nessler J: Structural differences between two populations of articular cartilage proteoglycan aggregates. *J Orthop Res* 1993, 12:144–148.

20. Buckwalter JA, Rosenberg LC: Electron microscopic studies of cartilage proteoglycans: direct evidence for the variable length of the chondroitin sulfate rich region of the proteoglycan subunit core protein. *J Biol Chem* 1982, 257:9830–9839.

21. Buckwalter JA, Rosenberg LC: Structural changes during development in bovine fetal epiphyseal cartilage. *Collagen Rel Res* 1983, 3:489–504.

22. Buckwalter JA, Rosenberg LC, Tang LH: The effect of link protein on proteoglycan aggregate structure. *J Biol Chem* 1984, 259:5361–5363.

23. Neame PJ, Barry FP: The link proteins. *Experientia* 1993, 49:393–402.

24. Tang LH, Buckwalter JA, Rosenberg LC: The effect of link protein concentration on articular cartilage proteoglycan aggregation. *J Orthop Res* 1996, 14:334–339.

25. Hildebrand A, Romaris M, Rasmussen LM, *et al.*: Interaction of the small interstitial proteoglycans biglycan, decorin and fibromodulin with transforming growth factor beta. *Biochem J* 1994, 302:527–534.

26.• Heinegard D, Lorenzo P, Sommarin Y: Articular cartilage matrix proteins. In *Osteoarthritic Disorders.* Edited by Kuettner KE, Goldberg VM. Rosemont, IL: American Academy of Orthopaedic Surgeons; 1995:229–237.

This book chapter provides a summary of the current understanding of the wide variety of articular cartilage matrix proteins and their potential importance.

27. DeCesare PE, Morgelin M, Mann K, Paulsson M: Cartilage oligomeric protein and thrombospondin 1: purification from articular cartilage, electron microscopic structure, and chondrocyte binding. *Eur J Biochem* 1994, 223:927–937.

28. Hedbom E, Antonsson P, Hjerpe A, *et al.*: Cartilage matrix proteins: an acidic oligomeric protein (COMP) detected only in cartilage. *J Biol Chem* 1992, 267:6132–6136.

29. Lohmander LS, Saxne T, Heinegard DK: Release of cartilage oligomeric protein (COMP) into joint fluid after knee injury and in osteoarthritis. *Ann Rheum Dis* 1994, 53:8–13.

30. Sharif M, Saxne T, Shepstone L, *et al.*: Relationship between serum cartilage oligomeric matrix protein levels and disease progression in osteoarthritis of the knee joint. *Br J Rheumatol* 1995, 34(4):306–310.

31. Aydelotte MB, Schumacher BL, Kuettner KE: Heterogeneity of articular chondrocytes. In *Articular Cartilage and Osteoarthritis.* Edited by Kuettner KE, Schleyerbach R, Peyron JG, Hascall VC. New York: Raven Press; 1992:237–249.

32. Wong M, Wuethrich P, Eggli P, Hunziker E: Zone-specific cell biosynthetic activity in mature bovine articular cartilage: a new method using confocal microscopic stereology and quantitative autoradiography. *J Orthop Res* 1996, 14:424–432.[KY1]35. Buckwalter JA: Should bone, soft-tissue and joint injuries be treated with rest or activity? *J Orthop Res* 1995, 13:155–156.

33. Oegema TR, Thompson RC: Histopathology and pathobiochemistry of the cartilage-bone interface in osteoarthritis. In *Osteoarthritic Disorders.* Edited by Kuettner KE, Goldberg VM. Rosemont, IL: American Academy of Orthopaedic Surgeons; 1995:205–217.

34. Redler I, Mow VC, Zimny ML, Mansell J: The ultrastructure and biomechanical significance of the tidemark of articular cartilage. *Clin Orthop* 1975, 112:357–362.

36. Buckwalter JA, Lane NE: Aging, sports and osteoarthritis. *Sports Med Arth Rev* 1996, 4:276–287.

37. Buschmann MD, Gluzband YA, Grodzinsky AJ, Hunziker EB: Mechanical compression modulates matrix biosynthesis in chondrocyte/agarose culture. *J Cell Sci* 108:1497–1508, 1995.

38. Gray ML, Pizzanelli AM, Grodzinski AJ, Lee RC: Mechanical and physicochemical determinants of chondrocyte biosynthesis response. *J Orthop Res* 1988, 6:788–792.

39. Grodzinsky AJ: Age-related changes in cartilage: physical properties and cellular response to loading. In *Musculo-skeletal Soft Tissue Aging: Impact on Mobility.* Edited by Buckwalter JA, Goldberg V, Woo S-LY. Rosemont, IL: American Academy of Orthopaedic Surgeons; 1993:137–149.

40. Buckwalter JA: Mechanical injuries of articular cartilage. In *Biology and Biomechanics of the Traumatized Synovial Joint.* Edited by Finerman G. Park Ridge, IL: American Academy of Orthopaedic Surgeons; 1992:83–96.

41. Buckwalter JA, Lohmander S: Operative treatment of osteoarthrosis: current practice and future development. *J Bone Joint Surg Am* 1994, 76:1405–1418.

42. Buckwalter JA, Martin JA: Degenerative joint disease. In *Clinical Symposia.* Summit, NJ: Ciba Geigy; 1995:2–32.

43. Mankin HJ, Buckwalter JA: Restoring the osteoarthritic joint. *J Bone Joint Surg Am* 1996, 78:1–2.

44.• Levy AS, Lohnes J, Sculley S, *et al.*: Chondral delamination of the knee in soccer players. *Am J Sports Med* 1996, 24:634–639.

This clinical series describes the outcome of chondral defects in young, athletic individuals.

45. Maletius W, Messner K: The effect of partial meniscectomy on the long-term prognosis of knees with localized severe

chondral damage: a twelve- to fifteen-year follow-up. *Am J Sports Med* 1996, 24:258–262.

46. Messner K, Gillquist J: Cartilage repair: a critical review. *Acta Orthop Scand* 1996, 67:523–529.

47. Messner K, Maletius W: The long-term prognosis for severe damage to weight-bearing cartilage in the knee: a 14-year clinical and radiographic follow-up in 28 young athletes. *Acta Orthop Scand* 1996, 67:165–168.

48. Buckwalter JA: Cartilage researchers tell progress: technologies hold promise, but caution urged. *Am Acad Orthop Surg Bull* 1996, 44:24–26.

49. Buckwalter JA: Regenerating articular cartilage: why the sudden interest? *Orthopaedics Today* 1996, 16:4–5.

50. Buckwalter JA, Mow VC, Ratliff A: Restoration of injured or degenerated articular surfaces. *J Am Acad Orthop Surg* 1994, 2:192–201.

51. Moran ME, Kim HK, Salter RB: Biological resurfacing of full-thickness defects in patellar articular cartilage of the rabbit: investigation of autogenous periosteal grafts subjected to continuous passive motion. *J Bone Joint Surg Am* 1992, 74:659–667.

52. Salter RB: *Continuous Passive Motion CPM: A Biological Concept for the Healing and Regeneration of Articular Cartilage, Ligaments and Tendons, from Original Research to Clinical Applications.* Baltimore Williams and Wilkins; 1993.

53. Salter RB, Simmons DB, Malcolm BW, *et al.*: The biological effect of continuous passive motion on the healing of full-thickness defects in articular cartilage: an experimental investigation in the rabbit. *J Bone Joint Surg Am* 1980, 62:1232–1251.

54. Ewing JW: Arthroscopic treatment of degenerative meniscal lesions and early degenerative arthritis of the knee. In *Articular Cartilage and Knee Joint Function: Basic Science and Arthroscopy.* Edited by Ewing JW. New York: Raven Press; 1990:137–145.

55. Friedman MJ, Berasi DO, Fox JM, *et al.*: Preliminary results with abrasion arthroplasty in the osteoarthritic knee. *Clin Orthop* 1984, 182:200–205.

56. Johnson LL: Arthroscopic abrasion arthroplasty: historical and pathologic perspective: present status. *Arthroscopy* 1986, 2:54–59.

57. Johnson LL: The sclerotic lesion: pathology and the clinical response to arthroscopic abrasion arthroplasty. In *Articular Cartilage and Knee Joint Function: Basic Science and Arthroscopy.* Edited by Ewing JW. New York: Raven Press; 1990:319–333.

58. Sprague NF: Arthroscopic debridement for degenerative knee joint disease. *Clin Orthop* 1981, 160:118–123.

59. Baumgaertner MR, Cannon WD, *et al.*: Arthroscopic debridement of the arthritic knee. *Clin Orthop* 1990, 253:197–202.

61. Bert JM, Maschka K: The arthroscopic treatment of unicompartmental gonarthoisis. *J Arthroscopy* 1989, 5:25–32.

60. Bert JM: Role of abrasion arthroplasty and debridement in the management of osteoarthritis of the knee. *Rheum Dis Clin North Am*1993, 19(3):725–739.

62. O'Driscoll SW, Keeley FW, Salter RB: Durability of regenerated articular cartilage produced by free autogenous periosteal grafts in major full-thickness defects in joint surfaces under the influence of continuous passive motion. *J Bone Joint Surg Am* 1988, 70:595–606.

63. O'Driscoll SW, Salter RB: The repair of major osteochondral defects in joint surfaces by neochondrogenesis with autogenous osteoperiosteal grafts stimulated by continu-

ous passive motion: an experimental investigation in the rabbit. *Clin Orthop* 1986, 208:131–140.

64. Engkvist O, Johansson SH: Perichondrial arthroplasty: a clinical study in twenty-six patients. *Scand J Plast Reconstr Surg* 1980, 14:71–87.

65. Homminga GN, Bulstra SK, Bouwmeester PM, Linden AJVD: Perichondrial grafting for cartilage lesions of the knee. *J Bone Joint Surg Br* 1990, 72:1003–1007.

66. Seradge H, Kutz JA, Kleinert HE, *et al.*: Perichondrial resurfacing arthroplasty in the hand. *J Hand Surg [Am]* 1984, 9:880–886.

67. Buckwalter JA, Woo SL-Y, Goldberg VM, Hadley EC, Booth F, Oegema TR, Eyre DR: Soft tissue aging and musculoskeletal function. *J Bone Joint Surg Am* 1993, 75:1533–1548.

68. Brittberg M: *Cartilage Repair.* Sweden: Goteborg University; 1996.

69. Brittberg M, Nilsson A, Lindahl A, *et al.*: Rabbit articular cartilage defects treated with autologous cultured chondrocytes. *Clin Orthop* 1996, 326:270–283.

70. Wakitani S, Goto T, Mansour JM, *et al.*: Mesenchymal stem cell-based repair of a large articular cartilage and bone defect. *Trans Orthop Res Soc* 1994, 19:481.

71.• Wakitani S, Goto T, Pineda SJ, *et al.*: Mesenchymal cell-based repair of large, full-thickness defects of articular cartilage. *J Bone Joint Surg Am* 1994, 76:579–592.

This article describes experimental work demonstrating that mesenchymal stem cells may facilitate repair of articular cartilage defects.

72.•• Brittberg M, Lindahl A, Nilsson A, *et al.*: Treatment of deep cartilage defects in the knee with autologous chondrocyte transplantation. *New Engl J Med* 1994, 331:889–895.

This article describes the clinical use of autologous chondrocyte transplantation for patellar and femoral condylar defects in a limited number of patients. The publication of this article stimulated a great increase in the interest of chondrocyte transplantation for clinical use.

73. Buckwalter JA, Glimcher MM, Cooper RR, Recker R: Bone biology II. Formation, form, modeling and remodeling. *J Bone Joint Surg Am* 1995, 77:1276–1289.

74.•• Hunziker EB, Rosenberg LC: Repair of partial-thickness defects in articular cartilage: cell recruitment from the synovial membrane. *J Bone Joint Surg Am* 1996, 78:721–733.

This article describes experimental work demonstrating that growth factors can stimulate repair of partial-thickness articular cartilage defects.

75. Hunziker EB, Rosenberg R: Induction of repair partial thickness articular cartilage lesions by timed release of TGF-Beta. *Trans Orthop Res Soc* 1994, 19:236.

76. Martin JA, Buckwalter JA: Fibronectin and cell shape affect age related decline in chondrocyte synthetic response to IGF-I. *Trans Orthop Res Soc* 1996, 21:306.

77. Pfeilschifter J, Diel I, Brunotte K, *et al.*: Mitogenic responsiveness of human bone cells in vitro to hormones and growth factors decreases with age. *J Bone Miner Res* 1993, 8:707–717.

78. Paletta GA, Arnoczky SP, Warren RG: The repair of osteochondral defects using an exogenous fibrin clot: an experimental study in dogs. *Am J Sports Med* 1992, 20:725–731.

79. Muckle DS, Minns RJ: Biological response to woven carbon fiber pads in the knee: a clinical and experimental study. *J Bone and Joint Surg Br* 1990, 72:60–62.

80. Brittberg M, Faxen E, Peterson L: Carbon fiber scaffolds in the treatment of early knee osteoarthritis. *Clin Orthop* 1994, 307:155–164.

CARDIOPULMONARY PROBLEMS IN ATHLETES

R. Trent Sickles and
Stephen F. Schaal

Cardiopulmonary problems present many interesting challenges to physicians caring for athletes. Recent sudden deaths in several high-profile athletes have increased public interest and awareness of cardiac problems that, although unusual, continue to challenge physicians to diagnose these conditions prior to their potentially catastrophic endpoint. As the population of the United States ages, the number of older athletes also increases. Common cardiovascular conditions that occur in older exercisers, such as hypertension and coronary artery disease, present a different type of challenge. Regular exercise is well accepted as a way of preventing or even treating many cardiovascular risk factors, yet this same group of individuals is at higher risk of myocardial infarction, arrhythmias, and sudden cardiac death from exercise. Respiratory problems are primarily related to obstructive symptoms from either allergies and asthma or from acute vocal cord dysfunction. Acute respiratory illness can also cause impaired performance and cause athletes to seek medical attention. This chapter addresses appropriate screening for cardiopulmonary disease, evaluative methods, and treatment including decisions regarding participation.

CARDIAC PROBLEMS

Screening

Preparticipation evaluation is either required or highly recommended before participation in most school-age athletic programs. The vast majority of sudden death events in this group are due to structural abnormalities of the heart. For this reason, careful attention to a history of syncope, light-headed sensations, dizziness, chest pains, palpitations, or other cardiovascular symptoms is imperative [1••]. A family history of premature cardiac death is also important. Table 11.1 lists important questions to ask as part of cardiopulmonary preparticipation screening. Physical examination is not sensitive enough to detect most cardiovascular abnormalities. The lesions most likely to be detected are aortic stenosis, and coarctation of the aorta with hypertension and decreased femoral pulses. The murmur of hypertrophic cardiomyopathy, if present, begins later in systole, peaks and then diminishes in late systole as outflow decreases. It is exacerbated during the Valsalva maneuver or while standing, in contrast to most other murmurs. Any suspicious murmur or a newly detected or previously undetected murmur that is grade III, VI, or louder should be referred for further evaluation before an athlete is cleared for participation [1••]. Although some authors have advocated the use of echocardiography for mass screening of young athletes [2], the general consensus is that this is not a cost-effective screening tool in the vast majority of environments and that even limited screening echocardiograms are not practical.

In older individuals, the risk of coronary artery disease lurks as the precipitating factor for sudden cardiac death. History of cardiac symptoms remains important. Identification of cardiac risk factors aids in determining whether cardiac stress testing prior to beginning an exercise program is warranted. The American College of Sports Medicine has developed guidelines for recommendation of stress testing [3]. Generally, exercise testing should be considered for men older than 40 and women older than 50 when occult coronary artery disease is suspected based on having two or more risk factors (in addition to age and gender) or a single risk factor that is judged by the clinician to be severe enough to warrant testing.

Once clinical symptoms or cardiovascular risk factors are identified, further diagnostic tests, referral to the athlete's primary care physician, or referral to a cardiologist to make a definitive diagnosis is warranted. Once a definitive diagnosis is made, the consensus panel guidelines of the 26th Bethesda Conference should be used to direct further participation or disqualification from sports [4].

Table 11.1	PREPARTICIPATION EVALUATION CARDIOPULMONARY SCREENING*

Cardiovascular history

Have you ever:
- fainted or passed out during or after exercise?
- had dizziness during or after exercise?
- had racing of your heart (palpitations) or skipped heart beats?
- had high blood pressure?
- had high cholesterol?
- been told that you have (or had) a heart murmur?
- had a physician restrict or not allow your participation in sports because of a heart problem?

Pulmonary history

Do you:
- cough, wheeze, or have trouble breathing before, during, or after exercise?
- have asthma?
- have allergies that require medical treatment?
- take any medication to help your breathing?

Adapted from American Academy of Family Physicians and the Preparticipation Physical Evaluation Task Force [1]; with permission.

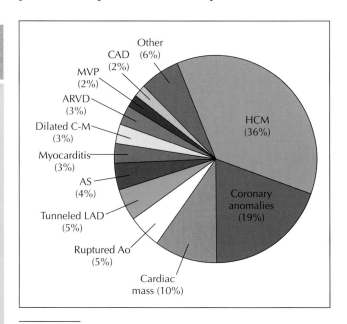

FIGURE 11.1

Causes of sudden cardiac death in young competitive athletes (median age, 17), based on systematic tracking of 158 athletes in the Unites States, primarily from 1985 to 1995. Ao—aorta; ARVD—arrhythmogenic right ventricular dysplasia; AS—aortic stenosis; CAD—coronary artery disease; C-M—cardiomyopathy; HCM—hypertrophic cardiomyopathy; LAD—left anterior descending coronary artery; MVP—mitral valve prolapse. (*Adapted from* Maron *et al.* [7•], with permission.

Normal physiology

Athletic heart syndrome is defined as a series of physiologic adaptations to regular exercise that improves cardiac function and efficiency during exercise. These changes include hypertrophy of the left ventricular musculature, bradycardia, and associated improvement in stroke volume and cardiac output.

Echocardiographic studies have shown an increase in left ventricular mass in both endurance- and strength-trained athletes [5,6]. Left ventricular end-diastolic diameter has also been shown to be increased. In some athletes these normal physiologic changes may be difficult to distinguish from hypertrophic cardiomyopathy on echocardiogram, and other criteria may be needed to aid in differentiating these two diagnoses.

Sinus bradycardia is by far the most common arrhythmia that is seen in conditioned athletes and is present in most collegiate athletes. This is a normal physiologic response to training and can be seen in both strength and endurance athletes. The cause of bradycardia in the athletic heart is increased vagal tone and decreased sympathetic tone.

Sudden death

Sudden death in athletes has received a tremendous amount of attention from the press as well as the general public, primarily because of the unfortunate deaths of several high-profile athletes. Sudden death is generally defined as any cause of death that causes immediate or rapid expiration (within 24 hours) of the athlete and that is associated with exercising. This includes primarily cardiac causes but may include other causes, such as status asthmaticus, anaphylaxis, illicit drug use, heat illness, and others. There are a wide variety of causes of sudden cardiac death in young athletes; hypertrophic cardiomyopathy (36%) and coronary anomalies (19%) are the most common (Fig. 11.1) [7•]. In athletes over 35 years of age, the vast majority of sudden deaths result from complications of atherosclerotic coronary artery disease.

Hypertrophic cardiomyopathy

Hypertrophic cardiomyopathy (HCM) represents the most common cause of sudden cardiac deaths in young athletes. This is a relatively uncommon condition, yet it has garnered much attention in the medical literature. Its overall incidence in the general population is approximately 0.1%–0.2% [8]. It is defined as a hypertrophied, nondilated left ventricle that is present in the absence of any systemic illness that is associated with left ventricular hypertrophy (LVH). Syncope and family history of sudden death prior to age 50 are risk factors for HCM. Their presence warrants careful screening for HCM, including strong consideration of echocardiography prior to clearance for participation in any activity.

A number of recent studies have looked at echocardiographic measurements of athletes' hearts [9–11]. Clearly, a significant number of athletes have higher left ventricular diameter and greater wall thickness. In some cases, left ventricular wall thickness in athletes exceeds the normal range of 12 mm and yet may not be diagnostic of hypertrophic cardiomyopathy. In these circumstances, consultation with a cardiologist who is familiar with athletes and use of other echocardiographic criteria is necessary to distinguish between normal athletes' heart and hypertrophic cardiomyopathy. A recent controversial study by Fananapazir suggested that there may be a subset of patients with HCM who are not at increased risk despite the hypertrophied muscle. Extensive cardiac evaluations in addition to echocardiograms revealed that other than hypertrophied muscle they had otherwise normal hearts; thus it was believed that they could compete safely. Response from other physicians has been extremely cautious and it is generally believed that additional information and studies must be performed before any patients with HCM should be allowed to participate in athletics. The current recommendation from the 26th Bethesda Conference is when there is an unequivocal diagnosis of HCM, athletes should not compete in competitive sports, with the possible exception of low-intensity activities.

Dilated cardiomyopathy

Idiopathic dilated cardiomyopathy is a more unusual cause of death with exercise, accounting for only 3% of sudden death according to Maron *et al.* [7•]. Athletes with dilated cardiomyopathy typically present with dyspnea on exertion or complaints of decreased performance, obviously nonspecific symptoms. Diagnosis is generally confirmed by echocardiography, although cardiac catheterization and cardiac muscle biopsy are often performed to identify a specific cause for the myopathy. Athletes should not participate in any activity until all symptoms have resolved and their test results have completely returned to normal.

Myocarditis

Myocarditis presents with symptoms of fatigue, dyspnea, decreasing performance, palpitations, or syncope. The cause is typically viral in origin, usually Coxsackie B, although others like Coxsackie A, polio, influenza, adeno-, echo-, rubella, and rubeola viruses are known to cause myocarditis. Some cases of apparent idiopathic dilated cardiomyopathy may result from myocarditis. In cases in which there is a question regarding the diagnosis, cardiac muscle biopsy should be considered. Sudden death in acute myocarditis is likely to be related to arrhythmias. As such, withdrawal from all strenuous activity for a minimum of 6 months is recommended. Athletes should be allowed to return to sports only after cardiac structure and function have returned to normal both at rest and with stress, and there is no evidence of arrhythmia either with stress testing or with Holter monitoring [8].

Pericarditis

Acute pericarditis is rarely reported as a cause of sudden cardiac death in athletes. When present in young patients it is usually of viral etiology, similar to myocarditis. Clinical manifestations include fatigue and dyspnea as well as pleuritic-type chest pain. Pericardial friction rub may be present on physical examination. Careful evaluation for evidence of constriction or tamponade should be made. Electrocardiographic changes in acute pericarditis include widespread ST segment elevation. With large pericardial effusions, QRS voltage is reduced. Echocardiography remains critical for evaluation for effusion and constriction. Athletes should not participate in sports until all evidence of disease has resolved. If pericardial constriction results, athletes should not participate in sports. One patient seen by us with pericardial constriction who had a pericardectomy was permitted to return to competitive sports. No guidelines are available with regard to this circumstance.

Anomalous coronary arteries

Anomalous coronary arteries represent the second leading cause of sudden death in young athletes, accounting for 19% of sudden cardiac death according to Maron *et al.* [7•]. The most commonly reported anomaly is the origin of the left main coronary artery from the right sinus of Valsalva. Other anomalies that have been associated with sudden death include origin of the right or left coronary artery from the posterior sinus and hypoplastic coronary arteries. The mechanism of sudden death is probably arrhythmic, resulting from ischemia secondary to compression of the anomalous vessel. Unfortunately, the majority of these patients are asymptomatic until the incident of sudden death. Angina-like symptoms, syncope, or serious arrhythmias in young athletes warrant evaluation with stress testing, echocardiography, or even angiography when no plausible explanation for these symptoms can be found [12].

ARRHYTHMIAS
Sinus arrhythmia

Sinus bradycardia is the most common arrhythmia seen in athletes. Resting heart rates as low as 25 beats per minute have been reported in asymptomatic individuals and sinus pauses of less than

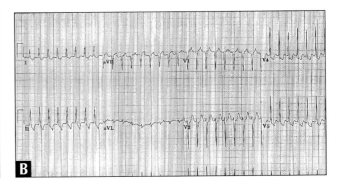

FIGURE 11.2

Normal sinus rhythm (*panel A*) and supraventricular tachycardia (*panel B*) in patients with preexcitation (Wolfe–Parkinson–White) syndrome. Athletes with this condition appear to be at low risk of sudden death but usually will have significant symptoms that may impair performance.

3 seconds in asymptomatic individuals are generally not of concern [13] Wandering atrial pacemaker is a variant of sinus arrhythmia typified by a cyclical change in the RR interval, a gradual shortening of the PR interval, and gradual change in the P wave contour. Atrioventricular junctional escape rhythms are also common in athletes. In asymptomatic individuals, no further evaluation is necessary [13].

Atrioventricular block

First degree atrioventricular block occurs more frequently in athletes than in the general population. Unless the PR interval is prolonged more than 0.3 seconds, further evaluation is not indicated for asymptomatic athletes.

Second degree atrioventricular block of the Wenckebach (Mobitz type 1) variety is also seen more frequently in athletes than in the general population. In addition to a 12-lead electrocardiogram (ECG), these athletes should have an exercise stress test to document improvement or no worsening of the block with exercise and an echocardiogram to exclude structural heart disease. In the absence of these findings athletes should be allowed to compete without restrictions [13].

Type 2 second-degree block and acquired third-degree heart block should be thoroughly evaluated prior to athletic participation. Work-up should include 12-lead ECG, 24-hour ambulatory ECG, echocardiogram, and stress testing. A permanent pacemaker is usually required to permit athletic competition. The Bethesda Conference recommends

that no contact or collision sports be permitted in patients with pacemakers because of the risk of damage to the pacemaker [13].

Supraventricular tachycardia

Athletes with supraventricular tachycardia generally present with symptoms of episodic palpitations. Events may be associated with complaints of dizziness or syncope. Evaluation with a 12-lead ECG and attempts to document the arrhythmia with an ECG event monitor are important. In one of our recent cases, the arrhythmia was documented in a swimmer by having him climb out of the pool and applying electrodes on the pool deck with subsequent documentation of his arrhythmia. In symptomatic athletes electrophysiologic studies may be necessary to fully evaluate the arrhythmia. Ablation therapy is often possible and will generally permit athletes to return to sports without restrictions (Figs. 11.2. and 11.3).

Ventricular pre-excitation

Ventricular pre-excitation (Wolff–Parkinson–White syndrome) is either found surreptitiously on ECG in asymptomatic athletes or in athletes with complaints of intermittent palpitations or tachycardia. Evaluation must include 12-lead ECG, 24-hour ambulatory monitoring, stress testing, and echocardiogram. Electrophysiologic studies have become the gold standard for evaluation and mapping of the pathway in symptomatic patients. Treatment with radiofrequency ablation therapy should be considered, although risk of sudden death in athletes from this condition appears to be small.

Premature ventricular contractions

Premature ventricular contractions (PVCs) are often asymptomatic and are found during preparticipation screening or with evaluation of other cardiac symptoms. Infrequent PVCs are generally believed to be a normal variant, and extensive evaluation is unnecessary. Frequent PVCs warrant stress testing and echocardiography to look for structural abnormalities. If there is an increase in PVCs during stress testing or if complex ventricular arrhythmias (*eg*, multiformed PVCs, nonsustained ventricular tachycardia) occur during stress testing, then further evaluation is needed including imaging studies or catheterization. New onset of PVCs in previously normal athletes should cause thorough investigation

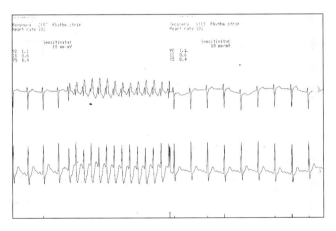

FIGURE 11.3

Electrocardiogram showing the development of supraventricular tachycardia during exercise.

for metabolic causes such as use of diuretics or severe diets with disordered eating. Sudden increases in training intensity have also been known to cause PVCs. A variety of pathologic causes may predispose to PVCs or ventricular tachycardia including cardiomyopathy, myocarditis, congenital coronary anomalies, and occult coronary artery disease. Patients with complex ventricular arrhythmias should not be permitted to participate, particularly when cardiac pathology is identified [13]. Sustained or bursts of monomorphic ventricular tachycardia may be cured with ablation therapy, thereby permitting return to competition (Fig. 11.4).

Bundle branch block

Complete bundle branch block is rare in athletes. When either complete right or left bundle branch block exists complete evaluation including 24-hour ambulatory ECG, echocardiogram, and stress testing should be performed. If no pathology is identified, athletic participation is permitted. Incomplete right bundle branch block occurs in up to 14% of athletes [13], which is believed to be related to hypertrophy of right ventricular muscle mass and is not a contraindication to participation in sports. In asymptomatic individuals, no further evaluation is usually necessary for incomplete right bundle branch block.

VALVULAR HEART DISEASE
Mitral valve prolapse

Mitral valve prolapse (MVP) is a relatively common valvular condition having a prevalence of about 5% in the general population. Whereas the majority of patients with MVP are asymptomatic, some athletes will have symptoms of palpitations, chest pain or pressure, dizziness, or other nonspecific symptoms. The physical examination reveals the characteristic midsystolic click with or without a late systolic murmur. Individuals with significant symptoms of syncope or near syncope, palpitations, a family history of sudden death associated with MVP, or a significant murmur are candidates for echocardiography and event monitoring to attempt to document any arrhythmia. ECG studies are usually normal. In the absence of serious arrhythmias or significant valvular insufficiency, athletes are generally allowed to participate without restrictions. Symptomatic relief of symptoms can usually be obtained with β-blockers, but these drugs may inhibit performance of some athletes and are banned from selected sports (*eg*, rifle, pistol, biathlon).

Mitral valve stenosis

Rheumatic heart disease is the primary cause of acquired mitral stenosis. Although there has been a recent increase in the number of cases of rheumatic fever, the incidence of mitral stenosis remains very low in young athletes. Most patients with significant mitral stenosis are symptomatic such that participation in athletics is not a consideration. The primary symptom is dyspnea as a result of pulmonary hypertension. Left atrial enlargement predisposes to atrial fibrillation. In more severe cases, right heart failure may be present with hepatomegaly and peripheral edema.

Mitral valve regurgitation

The cause of mitral regurgitation is multifactorial. MVP is the number one cause, with rheumatic heart disease, myocarditis, cardiomyopathy, coronary

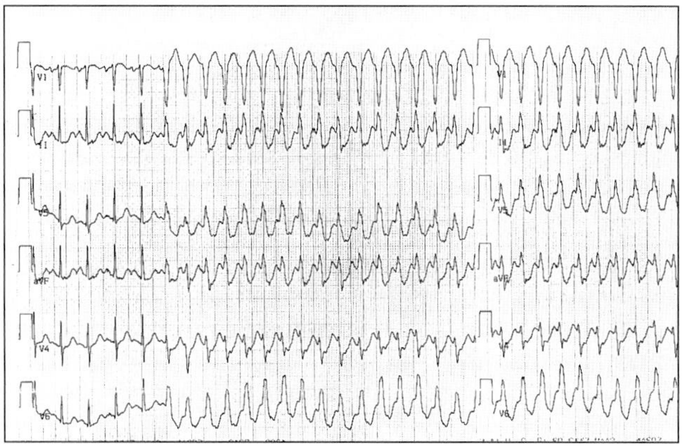

FIGURE 11.4
Electrocardiogram showing exercise-induced ventricular tachycardia. Athletes with this condition should not be allowed to compete until this condition has been thoroughly evaluated and treated successfully.

artery disease (CAD), and connective tissue diseases as some of the other causes. The physical examination will reveal a holosystolic murmur that radiates into the axilla. Evaluation should be directed at identifying the cause of the problem as well as identifying the degree of regurgitation. This can be accomplished noninvasively with Doppler echocardiography. Participation is determined based on clinical symptoms, severity of the regurgitation and the presence or absence of atrial fibrillation (*see* Bethesda Conference Guidelines) [13].

Congenital aortic valve stenosis

Congenital aortic valvular stenosis is readily identified by the systolic ejection murmur at the right second intercostal space with radiation into the carotid arteries. This congenital anomaly is usually identified during well-child examination and is rarely seen as a new finding in athletes. It has been associated with sudden cardiac death, and thus deserves thorough evaluation with echocardiogram and cardiac catheterization before clearance is given to participate in any athletic activities [12].

Marfan syndrome

Marfan syndrome is an autosomal dominant inherited trait characterized primarily by its musculoskeletal findings. Common findings include tall stature, arachnodactyly, increased arm span relative to height, pectus excavatum and joint hypermobility. Diagnosis must include three diagnostic features, which include family history of Marfan syndrome; ocular findings, including dislocated lens, myopia, and retinal detachment; and skeletal findings as discussed previously. Cardiovascular anomalies include an enlarged aortic root with possible aortic root dissection from cystic medial necrosis, MVP, and mitral regurgitation. Aortic rupture accounts for the sudden death risk in athletes with Marfan syndrome. Echocardiographic monitoring of aortic root dimension is recommended at 6-month intervals. Participation in high-intensity or contact/collision sports is not recommended [12].

Coronary artery disease

Coronary artery disease (CAD) remains the number one cause of death in the United States, accounting for nearly 500,000 deaths in 1994 (the last year that the American Heart Association released statistics).

It is clear from innumerable studies that exercise is an extremely beneficial component of any management program for patients just as it is clear that exercise is one of the best preventive measures that can be taken to prevent CAD. For athletes over the age of 35, CAD and myocardial infarction are the highest risk for sudden death.

The American College of Sports Medicine has developed guidelines for exercise stress testing for those individuals who wish to begin a strenuous exercise program (*see* "Screening") [3]. When Patients suspected of having CAD require a careful and thorough evaluation regardless of their physical condition. Patients with multiple risk factors for CAD despite regular exercise may require routine exercise stress testing, even if they are asymptomatic, to monitor for the development of hemodynamically significant coronary artery disease. Although stress ECG is the least sensitive of the stress testing modalities, it remains a cost-effective tool for screening. When suspicion is high or when more sensitivity is needed, stress radionucleotide testing, stress echocardiogram, or even cardiac catheterization may be needed to quantify risk. The 26th Bethesda Conference has developed a risk stratification system based on the presence or absence of specific test findings. Table 11.2 is devel-

Table 11.2 CORONARY ARTERY DISEASE RISK STRATIFICATION*		
	MILDLY INCREASED RISK (ALL OF THE FOLLOWING)	**SUBSTANTIALLY INCREASED RISK (ANY OF THE FOLLOWING)**
Left ventricular ejection fraction	>50%	<50%
Exercise tolerance (age, metabolic equivalents)	<50, >10 mets 50–59, >9 mets 60–69, >8 mets >69, >7 mets	
Exercise-induced ischemia	Negative stress test	Positive stress test
Exercise-induced arrhythmia	No complex ventricular arrhythmia	Complex ventricular arrhythmia
Catheterization (if performed)	No hemodynamically significant lesions (<50% lumen narrowing)	Hemodynamically significant lesions (>50% lumen narrowing)

*Adapted from Thompson *et al.* [4]; with permission.

oped based on the Bethesda Conference recommendations for risk stratification [4].

Identification of CAD should not disqualify an athlete from participation. Appropriate management with adequate control of symptoms or ischemic changes with stress testing should allow return to participation. This is often done through participation in a cardiac rehabilitation program in which exercise can be monitored initially before unrestricted activity resumes. Should angioplasty or open heart surgery be required, return to athletic activity is still possible following cardiac rehabilitation.

Hypertension

About 50,000,000 Americans over 6 years of age have high blood pressure (approximately one in four adults). In 1992, the fifth report of the Joint National Committee on the Detection, Evaluation and Treatment of High Blood Pressure (JNC V) developed a new classification system for hyperten-

sion [14]. The new system has four stages of hypertension in addition to normal and high normal ranges. Hypertension in children is classified based on percentiles by age group. The sixth report of this committee should be available in 1997. Table 11.3 lists classification of hypertension by age as outlined in the 26th Bethesda Conference [15].

Hypertensive athletes are at higher risk for cardiovascular disease, including CAD and its complications (myocardial infarction, congestive heart failure [CHF], atherosclerotic peripheral vascular disease, and stroke). In addition, they have higher risk for renal insufficiency and renal failure. Risk factors for the development of hypertension include male gender (up to the age of 55; from 55 to 74 risk is about equal for men and women; women over the age of 75 have higher risk), African-American descent, increasing age, low socioeconomic status, and family history of high blood pressure.

Elevated blood pressure in athletes is frequently detected during preparticipation screening. Care

Table 11.3	**CLASSIFICATION OF HYPERTENSION BY AGE*†**			
	MILD (STAGE 1), MM HG	MODERATE (STAGE 2), MM HG	SEVERE (STAGE 3), MM HG	VERY SEVERE (STAGE 4), MM HG
Children				
6–9 y				
Systolic	120–124	125–129	130–139	≥140
Diastolic	75–79	80–84	85–89	≥90
10–12 y				
Systolic	125–129	130–134	135–144	≥145
Diastolic	80–84	85–89	90–94	≥95
Adolescents				
13–15 y				
Systolic	135–139	140–149	150–159	≥160
Diastolic	85–89	90–94	95–99	≥100
16–18 y				
Systolic	140–149	150–159	160–179	≥180
Diastolic	90–94	95–99	100–109	≥110
>18 y				
Systolic	140–159	160–179	180–209	≥210
Diastolic	90–99	100–109	110–119	≥120

*Adapted from Maron *et al.* [8]; with permission.
†These criteria apply to patients who are not taking antihypertensive drugs and are not acutely ill. When the systolic and diastolic blood pressures fall into different categories, the higher category classifies the patient's blood pressure status. In adults, isolated systolic hypertension is defined as a systolic blood press ≥140 mm Hg and a diastolic blood pressure ≥90 mm Hg and staged appropriately. Blood pressure values are based on the average of three or more readings taken at two or more visits after the initial screening.

should be taken to appropriately diagnose hypertension by taking serial readings using proper-size cuffs and techniques. Often, normal cuffs are too small for athletes, causing a falsely elevated pressure. When elevated pressures are detected during screening examinations, arrangements must be made for appropriate follow-up with the athlete's primary care physician. Unless stage III or IV hypertension is present at the initial screening, athletes can be cleared to participate while they are undergoing evaluation [15]. When target organ disease is suspected or detected during evaluation, participation should be limited until evaluation is complete and the blood pressure is controlled.

Lifestyle modification remains the cornerstone of initial treatment for hypertension. Many athletes already live healthy lifestyles; however, attempts should be made to obtain or maintain ideal body weight, exercise aerobically at moderate intensity (30 to 45 minutes 3 to 5 times a week), stop smoking (or use smokeless tobacco), limit sodium intake to 6 g of sodium chloride (2.3 g of sodium) per day, and limit alcohol consumption to no more than 2 drinks a day.

When nonpharmacologic methods do not result in blood pressure control, drug therapy must be considered. Treatment of athletes must take into account their activity and the effect that a particular medication might have on their performance. JNC V recommended the use of diuretics and beta-blockers as first-line therapy for hypertension because of their proven reduction in morbidity and mortality in clinical trials [14]. Other first-line agents including calcium channel antagonists, angiotensin converting enzyme (ACE) inhibitors, angiotensin II receptor blockers, alpha-blockers, and alpha-beta blockers are effective in reducing blood pressure, but limited data are available regarding the effects on morbidity and mortality. In athletes the potential adverse effects of diuretics and beta-blockers on performance or even the risk for development of complications such as dehydration and heat illness may limit their effectiveness. Diuretics predispose to electrolyte imbalances and dehydration and must be used with caution in moderate- to high-intensity athletes. In addition, their use is banned in most competitive venues because of the effect that they may have in masking the use of other banned substances through their dilutional effects on the urine. beta-Blockers may have adverse effects on performance by limiting chronotropic response of the heart to exercise. They are banned from most shooting sports.

In our experience, ACE inhibitors and calcium channel antagonists appear to be excellent first-line therapeutic agents for use in physically active patients and athletes. These agents appear to be effective in reducing cardiovascular morbidity and mortality and their side effect profiles are better for use in athletes. Close follow-up with particular attention to questions relating to performance is important.

PULMONARY PROBLEMS
Asthma

Asthma is the most common chronic respiratory problem in competitive athletes, affecting between 10% and 15% of athletes. Although numerous advances in therapy have been made, many athletes remain symptomatic and have significant performance problems from inflammatory or reactive airways.

Asthma is now clearly recognized as a chronic inflammatory disease of the airways. This airway inflammation predisposes to airway bronchoconstriction, increased respiratory secretions, and restricted air flow, all of which cause symptoms of cough, wheezing, tachypnea and dyspnea. Increasing prevalence and increasing morbidity and mortality for asthma led to the publication of the *Global Initiative for Asthma* published by the National Institutes of Health in 1995 [16••]. This publication outlines useful guidelines for diagnostic and management strategies that can easily be used in a primary care office or even in the athletic training room.

Avoidance of triggers is the mainstay of therapy. This obviously creates conflict with athletes when exercise is one of their primary triggers. Modification of training can sometimes decrease symptoms; however, medical therapy is often necessary to achieve optimal control and performance. Classically exercise-induced asthma (EIA) is triggered during periods of intense exercise. Exercise in a cold, dry environment can act as a trigger for some athletes as well. Symptoms usually begin 5 to 10 minutes after the cessation of exercise and last 30 to 60 minutes without intervention. A subset of patients will have a second attack 4 to 6 hours after the initial symptoms (late phase response). Current theory regarding the cause of EIA is that heat and moisture loss from the lungs leads to pH and osmolality changes that trigger the release of histamines from mast cells, which in turn cause bronchoconstriction.

Peak flow meters should be used routinely to monitor the disease process. This allows athletes to see that their disease may be active even when they do not have symptoms, and reinforces the need for compliance with therapy. Peak flow should be measured twice a day both before and after bronchodilator. Patients need to be familiar with proper technique for measuring peak flow and should keep a diary for reference. Treatment and intervention plans should be developed based on zones of performance with peak flow. The zone system is based on traffic light colors to help patients recognize problems early and intervene quickly to maintain optimal control. Green (80%–100% of predicted) represents optimal control. Yellow (50%–80%) represents need for intervention, and red represents emergent need for treatment. A treatment plan should be given to patients that outlines what steps to take, either regarding adjustment of medications or contacting physicians based on their peak flow values [17].

Medical therapy has changed significantly, with the primary focus on use of controller medications to reduce inflammation and prevent exacerbation of symptoms. A stepped approach to diagnosis and treatment has been outlined in the Global Strategy for Asthma Management and Prevention (Table 11.4) With optimal management, athletes should be able to compete successfully at the highest levels without any restrictions. Some medications used for the treatment of asthma are on banned substance lists for various governing bodies. Each list is differ-

Table 11.4	LONG-TERM MANAGEMENT OF ASTHMA: DIAGNOSIS AND CLASSIFICATION OF SEVERITY*†		
	CLINICAL FEATURE BEFORE TREATMENT	**DAILY MEDICATION REQUIRED TO MAINTAIN CONTROL**

Step 4: Severe persistent	Continuous symptoms
	Frequent exacerbations
	Frequent nighttime asthmas symptoms
	Physical activities limited by asthma symptoms
	PEF or FEV_1
	  ≤60% predicted
	  Variability >30%
		Multiple daily controller medications; high doses inhaled corticosteroids, long-acting bronchodilator, and oral corticosteroid (long-term).

Step 3: Moderate persistent	Symptoms daily
	Exacerbations affect activity and sleep
	Nighttime asthma symptoms >1 time/wk
	Daily use of inhaled short-acting beta$_2$-agonist
	PEF or FEV_1
	  >60%–<80% predicted
	  Variability >30%
		Daily controller medications; inhaled corticosteroids and long-acting bronchodilator (especially for nighttime symptoms)

Step 2: Mild persistent	Symptoms >1 time/wk but >1 time/d
	Exacerbations may affect activity and sleep
	Nighttime asthma symptoms >2 times/mo
	PEF or FEV_1
	  ≤80% predicted
	  Variability 20%–30%
		One daily controller medication: possibly add a long-acting bronchodilator to anti-inflammatory medication (especially for nighttime symptoms)

Step 1: Intermittent	Intermittent symptoms <1 time/wk
	Brief exacerbations (from a few hours to a few days)
	Nighttime asthmas symptoms <2 times/mo
	Asymptomatic and normal lung function
	  between exacerbations
	PEF or FEV_1
	  ≤80% predicted
	  Variability >20%
		Intermittent reliever medication taken as needed only; inhaled short-acting beta$_2$-agonist. Intensity of treatment depends on severity of exacerbation; oral corticosteroids may be required.

*Adapted from Global Strategy for Asthma Management and Prevention NHBLI/WHO Workshop Report [16]; with permission.
†The presence of one of the features of severity is sufficient to place a patient in that category.
FEV_1—forced expiratory volume in 1 second; PEF—peak expiratory flow.

ent and athletes need to verify that their medication is not banned prior to competition.

Recent studies are exploring the benefits of new agents for the prevention and treatment of EIA. Heparin has been shown to prevent bronchoconstrictor response in patients with EIA, and in one study inhaled heparin was shown to be more effective than cromolyn in preventing EIA [18]. Zileuton, a 5-lipoxygenase inhibitor also has been shown to attenuate bronchospasm in patients with EIA [19]. Both these agents need further study before they can be routinely used for the management of asthma.

Vocal cord dysfunction

Vocal cord dysfunction (VCD) is recognized as a complex of symptoms that may easily be mistaken for exercise-induced asthma. Symptoms include wheezing with exertion; however, but unlike EIA,

there is typically inconsistency with regard to when symptoms occur. Symptoms usually begin during exercise rather than after exercise, and they generally do not respond to treatment with bronchodilator therapy. Confirmation of the diagnosis is made by directly visualizing the vocal cords during symptoms. Paradoxical narrowing of the vocal cords during the expiratory phase is seen rather than the expected widening of the vocal cords. Treatment with speech and psychotherapy is usually successful in eliminating symptoms [20].

OTHER RECENT REPORTS

The 26th Bethesda Conference yielded a number of reports that should be of interest to the reader. These reports include those of Maron and Mitchell [21], Hutter [22], Maron *et al*. [23], Mitten and Maron [24], Mitchell *et al*. [25], and Cheitlin *et al*. [26].

REFERENCES AND RECOMMENDED READING

Recently published papers of particular interest have been highlighted as:

- •   Of special interest
- •• Of outstanding interest

1.•• American Academy of Family Physicians, Preparticipation Physical Evaluation Task Force (David M. Smith, Chairman): Preparticipation Physical Evaluation [monograph], ed 2. New York: McGraw-Hill.
Comprehensive outline of all aspects of the preparticipation evaluation. Includes suggested forms that can be used for screening examinations.

2. Weidenbener EJ, Krauss MD, Waller BF: Incorporation of screening echocardiography in the preparticipation exam. *Clin J Sport Med* 1995, 5:86–89.

3. American College of Sports Medicine: *Preventive and Rehabilitative Exercise Committee: Guidelines for Exercise Testing and Prescription*, ed 4. Philadelphia: Lea & Febiger; 1991.

4. Thompson PD, Klocke FJ, Levine BD, *et al.*: Task Force 5: coronary artery disease. *J Am Coll Cardiol* 1994, 24:888–892.

5. Fagard RH: Athletes heart: a meta-analysis of the echocardiographic experience. *Int J Sports Med* 1996, suppl 3:S140–S144.

6. Spirito P, Pelliccia A, Proschan MA, *et al.*: Morphology of the athlete's heart assessed by echocardiography in 947 elite athletes representing 27 sports. *Am J Cardiol* 1994, 74:802–806.

7. Maron BJ, Shirani J, Poliac LC, *et al.*: Sudden death in young competitive athletes. clinical, demographic, and pathological profiles. *JAMA* 1996, 276:199–204.

8. Maron BJ, Isner JM, McKenna WJ: The 26th Bethesda Conference: Task Force 3: hypertrophic cardiomyopathy, myocarditis and other myopericardial diseases and mitral valve prolapse. *J Am Coll Cardiol* 1994, 24:880–885.

9. Pelliccia A, Maron BJ, Culasso F, *et al.*: Athlete's heart in women: echocardiographic characterization of highly trained elite female athletes. *JAMA* 1996, 276:211–215.

10. Urhausen A, Monz T, Kindermann W: Sports-specific adaptation of left ventricular muscle mass in athlete's heart. I: An echocardiographic study with combined isometric and dynamic exercise trained athletes (male and female rowers). *Int J Sports Med* 1996 suppl 3:S145–S151.

11. Urhausen A, Monz T, Kindermann W: Sports-specific adaptation of left ventricular muscle mass in athlete's heart. II: An echocardiographic study with 400-m runners and soccer players. *Int. J Sports Med* 1996 suppl 3:S152–S156.

12. Graham TP Jr., Bricker JT, James FW, *et al.*: The 26th Bethesda Conference: Task Force 1: congenital heart disease. *J Am Coll Cardiol* 1994, 24:867–873.

13. Zipes DP, Garson A Jr.: The 26th Bethesda Conference: Task Force 6: arrhythmias. *J Am Coll Cardiol* 1994, 24:892–899.

14. National High Blood Pressure Education Program: *The Fifth Report of the Joint National Committee on Detection, Evaluation and Treatment of High Blood Pressure*. Bethesda: National Heart, Lung and Blood Institute, National Institutes of Health; 1993 [Pub. no. 93–1088.]

15. Kaplan NM, Deveraux RB, Miller HS: The 26th Bethesda Conference: Task Force 4: systemic hypertension. *J Am Coll Cardiol* 1994, 24: 885–888.

16. National Institutes of Health: *Global Initiative for Asthma: Global Strategy for Asthma Management and Prevention. NHLBI Workshop Report*. Bethesda: National Institutes of Health; 1995. [Publication NIH 95–3659.]

17. National Asthma Education Program: Guidelines for the diagnosis and management of asthma (expert panel report). Bethesda: National Heart, Lung, and Blood Institute, National Institutes of Health; 1991. [Publication NIH 91-3042.]

18. Garrigo J, Danta I, Ahmed T: Time course of the protective effect of inhaled heparin on exercise-induced asthma. *Am J Respir Crit Care Med* 1996, 153:1702–1707.

19. Meltzer SS, Hasday JD, Cohn J, Bleecker ER: Inhibition of exercise-induced bronchospasm by zileuton: a 5-lipoxygenase inhibitor. *Am J Respir Crit Care Med* 1996, 153:931–935.

20. McFadden ER Jr., Zawadski DK: Vocal cord dysfunction masquerading as exercise induced asthma. *Am J Respir Crit Care Med* 1996, 153:942–947.

21. Maron BJ, Mitchell JH: The 26th Bethesda Conference: revised eligibility recommendations for competitive athletes with cardiovascular abnormalities. *J Am Coll Cardiol* 1994, 24:848–850.

22. Hutter AM Jr.: The 26th Bethesda Conference: cardiovascular abnormalities in the athlete: role of the physician. *J Am Coll Cardiol* 1994, 24:851–853.

23. Maron BJ, Brown RW, McGrew CA, *et al.*: The 26th Bethesda Conference: ethical, legal and practical considerations affecting medical decision-making in competitive athletes. *J Am Coll Cardiol* 1994, 24:854–860.

24. Mitten MJ, Maron BJ: The 26th Bethesda Conference: legal considerations that affect medical eligibility for competitive athletes with cardiovascular abnormalities and acceptance of bethesda conference recommendations. *JACC* 1994, 24:861–863.

25. Mitchell JH, Haskell WL, Raven PB: The 26th Bethesda Conference: classification of sports. *JACC* 1994, 24:864–866.

26. Cheitlin MD, Douglas PS, Parmley WW: The 26th Bethesda Conference: Task force 2: acquired valvular heart disease. *J Am Coll Cardiol* 1994, 24:874–880.

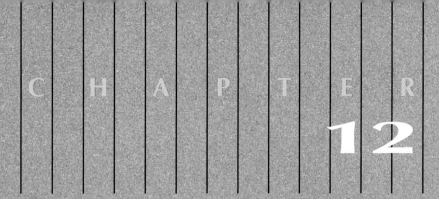

DRUGS IN SPORTS

Robert D. Whitehead

THE WAR AGAINST DRUGS

The association between drugs and sports has become a common household subject. If *Sports Illustrated* magazine is not featuring an article about it, then your local paper probably is. The articles usually feature an athlete who either has tested positive or was arrested for trafficking or possession, or they may tell of some governing body that is going to test a new group of athletes. In the footsteps of our federal government, which has "declared war" on drugs, the various sports governing bodies have declared their own war on drugs. Fines, suspensions, sanctions, banishment from competition, drug tests, and lists of banned substances are all weapons in their arsenal against drugs. A cat-and-mouse game has become commonplace between "tester" and "user," chemist and drug-banning committee. The International Olympic Committee (IOC) will no doubt devise and discuss strategy and weaponry in their 1997 summit to be held in Switzerland.

Who is winning? The IOC says they are, indicating the steadily declining number of positive test results. However, some athletes, authors, and journalists believe the opposite is true.

This chapter discusses many of the commonly used and abused drugs in sports, including performance-enhancing drugs, recreational drugs, and other lesser-used miscellaneous drugs. Current testing is also reviewed.

ERGOGENIC AIDS

Creatine

Creatine is classified as a supplement. However, because of its recent popularity as a performance enhancer, it will be discussed along with the other ergogenic aids. Although the actual incidence of creatine use in athletes is not documented, it is used to gain power during short bouts of strenuous exercise and to increase body mass.

Creatine, a protein first discovered in 1832, has recently become a favorite nutritional supplement of many athletes. A vital energy substrate for muscle contraction, it is synthesized and degraded by the body at a rate of 1 to 2 g/d. Exogenous administration suppresses endogenous production [1].

Creatine is found mainly in skeletal muscle, which contains 95% of the body's total creatine pool. Two thirds of the creatine in muscle is phosphorylated. Type II muscle fibers contain higher levels of phosphorylated creatine then do type I [1–3].

During a muscle contraction, energy is obtained through the high-energy bond of adenosine triphosphate (ATP) as it is hydrolyzed to adenosine diphosphate (ADP). In its phosphorylated state, creatine donates its phosphate to regenerate ADP back into ATP. During the recovery phase of exercise, the "free" nonphosphorylated creatine is rephosphorylated and can then be reused for energy. Creatine may also be used to transport energy from the mitochondria to different adenosine triphosphatase sites in the cytosol. It also modulates glycolysis [1].

The true importance of creatine during exercise has been recently demonstrated. Studies have shown that during high-intensity exercise, the restoration of peak power output is preceded by the resynthesis of creatine to its phosphorylated state [1].

Both dietary sources and endogenous synthesis replenish the muscular stores of creatine. Studies have revealed that significant elevations of creatine in both resting and exercising muscle can be obtained from dietary supplementation [1,4,5]. Doses ranged from 3 to 30 g/d. An average nonvegetarian diet contains 1 g/d of creatine, with fish and meat being the major sources.

Will increasing the body's stores of creatine via supplementation improve exercise performance? It appears so. Multiple studies have revealed that creatine supplementation does enhance performance of dynamic, high-intensity, intermittent exercise of short duration. It may also delay fatigue when adequate recovery time is present [4–10].

Scientists hypothesize that these improvements result from 1) higher preexercise concentrations of muscle creatine and, thus, larger amounts of energy substrate to restore ATP quicker; 2) a buffering effect in the exercising muscle, resulting in a smaller pH drop after lactate accumulation; 3) larger available pools for the rephosphorylation of creatine during recovery periods; and 4) allowing increased work loads during training, resulting in increased lean body weight [1]. These findings, however, have been refuted by some studies [11,12]. Maximal oxygen uptake (VO_2 max) has not been shown to be enhanced by creatine supplementation.

Does creatine supplementation increase body mass? Increases in the total pool of creatine have been accompanied by increased body weight [2]. It is not clear if this is secondary to water retention, increased lean body mass, or a combination of both.

Creatine has few adverse effects. The aforementioned weight gain is one. I have observed both gastrointestinal upset and muscle cramping in athletes. The possible side effects of long-term usage are not known, particularly at the higher doses taken by athletes during supplementation.

Dosage regimens vary among athletes. Studies suggest that 30 g/d for 5 days is adequate to "load" muscle (*ie*, achieve maximal muscle levels of creatine) [1]. A maintenance dose of 3 to 5 g/d can then be used to maintain the loaded creatine levels. If no further supplementation is given after loading, creatine levels will remain elevated for 2 weeks to 3 months.

Creatine is not banned by any governing sports body.

Anabolic steroids

The best known and most widely publicized ergogenic drugs used in athletics are the anabolic steroids (AS). AS are the synthetic derivatives of the hormone testosterone [13]. They are available by injection and in subcutaneous implantable pellets, oral form, scrotal patch, and a newer nonscrotal patch. Since first being isolated in 1935, hundreds of synthetic testosterone derivatives have become available. Modern day use of AS as ergogenic aids began in the 1940s, heightened after the 1950s, and still continues today.

Anecdotal reports and the lay press suggest that current AS use has reached epidemic proportions among professional and amateur athletes. However, self-report surveys and the results of drug testing do not support this proclaimed prevalence. The actual prevalence is not known and is difficult to quantify. Most survey studies suggest high school use to be around 7% and collegiate use to be from 6% to 20% [14–17]. A recent study suggests a decrease in collegiate athletic use [16], and a recent Canadian study found only 0.9% of collegiate athletes admitting to AS use [18]. Tests conducted by the National Football League during 1995 and 1996 found less than 1% of those tested to be positive [19].

The anabolic effects of AS have several proposed mechanisms of action. These include an increase in RNA polymerase and resultant protein synthesis, a decrease in the catabolic effects of cortisol released during high-intensity workouts that result in a positive nitrogen balance, and an increase in aggressive or euphoric behavior [20]. Whatever the physiologic basis, many AS users proclaim that the ability to recover quickly from high-intensity workouts is their most important ergogenic feature.

Few athletes disagree that AS enhance performance. Unfortunately, the scientific literature lacks consensus in data and experimental design, although the efficacy of AS to increase lean body mass and strength is generally accepted by the scientific community. A recent study in humans strongly supports their ergogenic potential [21]. The authors found that supraphysiologic doses of testosterone (600 mg/wk of testosterone enanthate for 10 weeks), especially when combined with weight training, does significantly increase lean body mass (as measured by underwater weighing), muscle size (as measured by MRI) and strength (bench-press and squatting exercises) in normal men. Neither mood nor behavior were altered. Similar findings were also seen in the non–weight-training group but to a lesser degree (Fig. 12.1).

The adverse effects of AS are lengthy and have been generated by the therapeutic literature along with anecdotal reports (Table 12.1). They are reviewed in detail in the previous edition. The actual incidence of these adverse effects in the athletic population is not documented.

Because testosterone receptors exist in the brain, it stands to reason that psychologic and behavioral changes could occur with their use. Investigations and case reports have linked affective and psychotic syndromes with AS use [22]. Psychologic dependence has also been associated with AS use [13,22]. Recent lay press have suggested a link between AS and violence by athletes toward women. The well-controlled study by Bhasin [21] did not support a psychologic effect.

The abuse patterns of AS use have also been studied. AS use is strongly associated with the use of illicit drugs, alcohol, and tobacco. Other high risk-behaviors have also been associated with AS use, including suicidal behavior, driving after drinking alcohol, carrying a weapon, violent behavior, and not using condoms during intercourse. Those with a family history of alcohol or drug abuse are also at an increased risk to use AS [23,24].

Several newer trends in the use of AS as ergogenic aids have occurred. The use of epitestosterone has reportedly increased as an attempt to lower the testosterone-to-epitestosterone (T:E) ratio used in testing for AS use [25••]. Anecdotal reports suggest that another trend is the use of much lower doses than the supraphysiologic doses used in the past. "It's enough to give me that extra edge, but I don't get caught," says one AS user. It is not known whether lower doses reduce or change the adverse effects of AS use or if they have ergogenic effects.

Anabolic steroids are banned by the IOC, the National Collegiate Athletic association (NCAA), and the National Football League (NFL).

Growth hormone

Human growth hormone (hGH), somatotropin, is a polypeptide secreted by the anterior pituitary gland. It is commonly used for replacement in growth hormone–deficient individuals. Currently, large quantities can be produced through recombinant DNA technology. Two types are available: sumatropin, which is identical in amino acid sequence to natural growth hormone, and somatren, which contains one extra amino acid. Multiple complex factors are responsible for hGH release and inhibition. Maintaining linear growth is the major function of hGH [26–28].

The prevalence of using hGH for ergogenic purposes is not known. One study found 5% of high school male athletes reporting its use [27]. Anecdotal reports depict widespread use in professional and amateur sports.

The physiologic effect of hGH is to increase protein synthesis through increased production of messenger RNA and to increase intracellular transportation of amino acids. Promotion of lipolysis and inhibition of glucose uptake by muscle cells also occurs. Collagen synthesis is increased, resulting in axial bone growth when growth plates are open [26].

Human growth hormone promotes growth of skeletal tissue by increasing levels of somatomedin C and insulin-like growth factor. Gigantism occurs when there is hyperproduction of hGH prior to epiphyseal closure. Acromegaly occurs after epiphyseal closure. Nearly every body system is affected by hGH [26,27].

By using hGH, athletes hope to increase body size, strength, and lean body mass while decreasing fat. The various studies conducted in this area have been primarily in laboratory animals and are inconsistent with the true ergogenic effects in normal human muscle tissue. There is a true paucity of scientific data supporting the efficacy of hGH as an ergogenic aid. Anecdotal reports, however, suggest that they do work.

The adverse effects of hGH use include acromegalic appearance, *ie*, a thickening of the bones in the hands, feet, and face. Skin thickening, glucose intolerance, and organomegaly including cardiomyopathy can also occur [26,27]. In athletes, only anecdotal reports of acromegalic facial features exist. Certainly, a common adverse effect is the financial burden on users as the cost can be over $2000 per month of use.

Human growth hormone is banned by the IOC, NFL, and NCAA. However, no test is available to

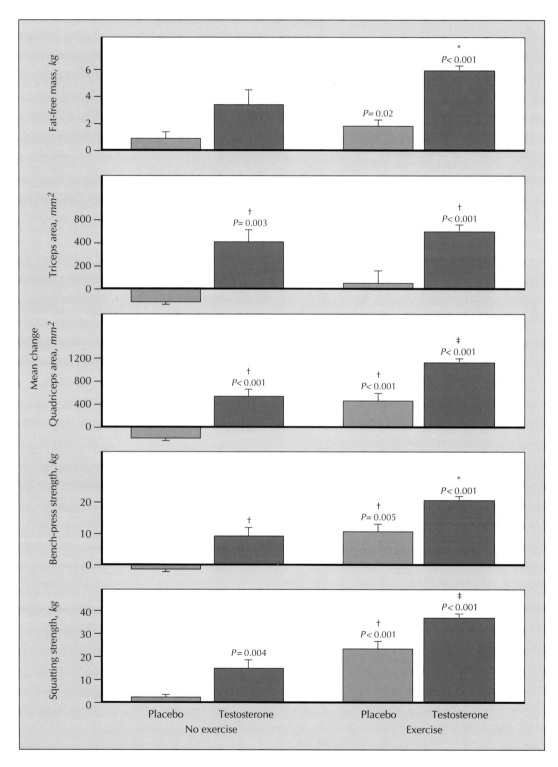

FIGURE 12.1

Changes from base line in mean (±SE) fat-free mass, triceps and quadriceps cross-sectional areas, and muscle strength in the bench-press and squatting exercises over 10 weeks of treatment. The *P* values indicate the comparison between the change indicated and a change of zero. *Asterisks* indicate *P*<0.005 for the comparison between the change indicated and that in either no-exercise group; *daggers* indicate *P*<0.005 for the comparison between the change indicated and that in the group assigned to placebo with no exercise; and *double daggers* indicate *P*<0.005 for the comparison between the change indicated and the changes in all three other groups. (*From* Bhasin *et al.* [21]; with permission.)

detect its presence in the urine, which has prompted some athletes to switch from AS to hGH [28].

Erythropoietin

Erythropoietin is a glycoprotein produced primarily by the kidney to facilitate production of erythrocytes in the bone marrow [29]. Human recombinant erythropoietin (rEPO) became available in Europe and the United States in 1987 and 1989, respectively. Medically, it is used to treat various anemias, including kidney disease. It can be taken intravenously but has a much longer half-life if given subcutaneously. Bone marrow stimulation is unpredictable and can occur from days to weeks after administration [26].

The incidence of rEPO use in sports is unknown. Its use has been reported anecdotally in many endurance events, during which high aerobic metabolism is vital [9,26].

Recombinant erythropoietin stimulates the bone marrow to release reticulocytes and megakaryocytes and increases proliferation and differentiation of stem cells. The resultant elevation in erythrocytes creates an increase in oxygen-carrying capacity, and thus, ultimately, more oxygen reaches the working muscle. Exercise time to exhaustion and VO_2 max have been significantly improved after use of rEPO [30].

The most notable side effect of rEPO is hyperviscosity or "sludging" of the blood, particularly when dehydration occurs. This hyperviscosity syndrome occurs when the hematocrit rises near or above 55%. Headaches, dizziness, vertigo, tinnitus, seizures, elevated blood pressure, visual changes, stroke, angina, claudication (exercise-induced), and thromboembolic events are all symptoms associated with hyperviscosity [26,27] (Dimeff, Unpublished data). The thrombocytosis that occurs may also predispose to thrombotic events.

Multiple deaths (up to 18) have been reported in the European elite cycling community. These "mysterious" deaths began in 1987 and continued through 1990, coinciding with the availability of

Table 12.1 SIDE EFFECTS OF ANABOLIC STEROIDS*			
Endocrine and Reproductive	Altered glucose metabolism(insulin resistance, glucose intolerance)	Alopecia	Hepatoma
Male	Altered thyroid profile (decreased T_3, T_4, TSH, and TBG)	Temporal hair recession	Hepatitis
Decreased reproductive hormones		Skin rash	**Musculoskeletal**
Testicular atrophy	**Cardiovascular and Hematological**	**Subjective**	Increased risk of musculotendinous injury
Oligospermia/azoospermia		Edema	Avascular necrosis of femoral heads
Gynecomastia	Decreased HDL cholesterol	Muscle spasm	Premature epiphyseal closure (in adolescents)
Prostatic hypertrophy	Increased LDL cholesterol	Anxiety	
Prostatic carcinoma	Hypertrophy (sodium and water retention)	Increased urine output	**Psychological**
Priapism	Clotting abnormalities	Headaches	
Altered glucose metabolism (insulin resistance, glucose intolerance)	Myocardial infarction	Dizziness	Aggressive behavior
	Left ventricular hypertrophy	Nausea	Mood swings
Altered thyroid profile (decreased T_3, T_4, TSH, and TBG)	Cerebrovascular accident	Euphoria	Increased or decreased libido
	Renal	Urethritis	Dependency
Female		Scrotal pain	Acute psychosis
Masculinization	Elevated BUN, creatine	Irritability	Manic-depressive episodes
Hirsutism	Wilms' tumor	Suicide ideation and attempts	**Miscellaneous**
Deepening of the voice	**Dermatologic**	**Hepatic**	
Clitoral hypertrophy			AIDS transmission as a result of needle sharing
Menstrual irregularities	Acne	Elevated liver function tests	
Male-pattern alopecia		Cholestatic jaundice	
		Hepatocellular carcinoma († 24 mo of use)	
		Peliosis hepatis († 6 mo of use)	

* *From* Ghaphery [29]; with permission.
BUN—blood urea nitrogen; HDL—high-density lipoprotein; LDL—low-density lipoprotein; T_3—triiodothyronine; T_4—thyroxine; TBG—thyroxine-binding globulin; TSH—thyroid-stimulating hormone.

rEPO in Europe. Speculation has attributed these deaths to rEPO and the hyperviscosity syndrome [28] (Dimeff, Unpublished data).

Recombinant erythropoietin is banned by the IOC and the NCAA, but no test is currently available to detect its presence in urine. Supposed advancements are being made to identify its use [19].

Stimulants

The use of stimulants in the athletic arena dates back to the gladiators of ancient Rome. Today, this class of drugs includes a large number of medications used by athletes. Collectively, their ergogenic effect is rapid in onset and thus can be used on the day of competition.

The common denominator among stimulants is their ability to increase sympathetic nervous system activity through stimulation of both α- and β-receptors. The body's response is multiple, including the classic "fright and flight" response. Some of these responses are listed in Table 12.2.

Common adverse effects of stimulants include tremor, tachycardia, anxiety, palpitation, nausea, lightheadedness, anorexia, dizziness, elevated blood pressure, dependency, and arrhythmias [28,29].

Favorable effects of stimulants that could aid in athletic performance include reduced fatigue, increased concentration, decreased pain sensitivity, improved endurance, increased competitiveness, and bronchodilatation [28,29,31].

The stimulants discussed in this section include clenbuterol, caffeine, amphetamines, and over-the-counter sympathomimetics. They all possess the effects listed above but in varying degrees. For this reason, only the ergogenic activity and side effect that is most distinct to that drug will be discussed. The previously mentioned side-effect profile is applicable in varying degrees to all stimulants.

Clenbuterol

Clenbuterol is a potent oral β_2-adrenergic agonist that has been used by athletes for its ergogenic potential. Some European physicians prescribe it in the treatment of asthma. Clenbuterol took the spotlight during the 1992 Summer Olympic games when two Americans tested positive for its use.

The incidence of use among athletes is unknown. However, for years, veterinarians and livestock breeders have known of the effects of clenbuterol and other β_2-agonists. The drugs have been studied extensively in animals because they were commonly given to increase lean body mass in cattle and other animal food sources for humans. They enhance the deposition of body protein and decrease fat [26,27].

The ergogenic properties of clenbuterol are those common to stimulants listed in Table 12.2. However, unlike other non–β_2-agonist stimulants, clenbuterol has marked anabolic activity. The promotion of muscle growth (10% to 20%) along with large reduc-

Table 12.2	THE BODY'S RESPONSE TO SYMPATHETIC STIMULATION	

Central nervous system	Endocrine
Increased respiration	Increased release of insulin
Increased wakefulness	Increased release of growth hormone
Increased psychomotor activity	Increased release of renin
Decreased appetite	Increased released of various pituitary
Decreased perception of fatigue	hormones
Increased metabolic rate	**Other**
Cardiac	
	Excitation of smooth muscle
Increased contractility	Vasoconstriction of blood vessels to skin
Increased rate	and mucous membranes
Resultant increased cardiac output and	Vasodilatation of blood vessels to skele-
increased blood pressure	tal muscle
Respiratory	Relaxation of smooth muscle of uterus,
	bladder, and gastrointestinal tract
Increased rate	Dilatation of pupils.
Bronchodilatation	

tions in body fat (10% to 20%) makes the β_2-agonist very attractive to athletes looking for an illegal edge [28]. Seemingly, its lipolytic effect is not uniform throughout the body. The intra-abdominal and subcutaneous abdominal fat seem most affected. Likewise, its anabolic effect is not uniform to all skeletal muscle. The type II muscle fibers are most affected [26,27] (Dimeff, Unpublished data).

Attenuation of muscle growth is seen after about 2 weeks of use. This has led athletes to "cycle" on and off clenbuterol for maximal gains. Salbutamol and cimaterol are other β_2-agonists with similar properties to clenbuterol. Side effects are similar to other stimulants.

Clenbuterol is banned by both the IOC, NFL, and NCAA.

Caffeine

Caffeine, a stimulant, is classified as a methylxanthine. It produces the most stimulation of the central nervous system (CNS) when compared with the other xanthines (theophylline and theobromine). This plant derivative is one of the most widely used drugs in America. An estimated 80% of Americans consume coffee or tea daily [26]. Caffeine is also found in soft drinks, chocolate, weight loss and cold preparations, some analgesics, and hundreds of over-the-counter medications (Table 12.3).

Caffeine's pharmacologic effect is caused by blocking the sedative properties of adenosine in the CNS. It spares glycogen and increases lipolysis. Mobilization of intracellular calcium also occurs [28]. These metabolic effects benefit endurance-type activity, although the response to caffeine may be blunted in those who chronically ingest it [27,28]. One notable side effect of caffeine is its diuretic effect. Precaution should always be taken to avoid caffeine products when fluid balance is of concern.

Caffeine was added to the IOC's list of banned drugs in 1984 after being removed from it in 1972. The test is now quantitative in that 12 mg/L of urine or more is the illegal dose (a 500 to 600 mg dose in a 1- to 2-hour period). The NCAA's illegal dose is 15 mg/L. Even so, ergogenic effects have been reported with urinary caffeine levels below the IOC limit [32].

Amphetamines

Ergogenic drug use in the modern era began with the amphetamines. The use of amphetamines was suspected in the 1952 Olympic games and soon after became so widespread that the American Medical Association established a special committee to investigate their effect on performance. Today their prevalence in sports ranges from about 3% to 10% of athletes in self-report studies.

Amphetamines are the prototype stimulant. They act predominantly by releasing sympathetic neurotransmitters, resulting in euphoria, increased alertness, anorexia, heightened confidence, and relief of fatigue. Peripherally, increased lipolysis occurs.

Studies have revealed ergogenic effects in athletes involved in swimming, running, and weight-throwing sports. Strength, power, acceleration, and aerobic and anaerobic capacity have all improved after amphetamine administration [27,29]. More notable adverse effects of amphetamines include confusion, paranoia, and hallucinations. Convulsions and coma can occur with larger doses.

Amphetamines are banned by the IOC, NFL, and NCAA.

Other sympathomimetics

Ephedrine, pseudoephedrine, phenylephrine, and phenylpropanolamine are all widely available as over-the-counter medications. They are commonly present in diet pills, analgesics, and cold remedies.

Table 12.3 COMMON SOURCES OF CAFFEINE*	
BEVERAGES (12 oz)	**CAFFEINE, *mg***
Coffee	
Brewed, drip method	275
Instant	155
Decaffeinated	7
Tea	
Brewed	95–145
Iced	70
Hot cocoa	8
Soft drinks	
Coca-Cola	45
Pepsi	40
Mountain Dew	55
Drugs	
Anacin[†] (2 tablets)	32
Excedrin[‡] (1 tablet)	65
NoDoz[‡] (1 tablet)	100
Dexatrim[§] (1 tablet)	100

*Data from Clark [36].
[†]Whitehall-Robins Healthcare, Madison, NJ.
[‡]Bristol-Meyers Products, New York, NY.
[§]Thompson Medical Co., West Palm Beach, FL.

They are structurally related to amphetamines. Their prevalence as ergogenic aids in sports is poorly documented. However, I have observed excessive use of these agents in several sports.

In high enough doses, these drugs have CNS effects similar to that of amphetamines, and their side-effect profile is also similar. Some athletes use them for their anorexiant and thermogenic effects when weight gain is a concern.

RECREATIONAL DRUGS

Athletes are not immune to the temptations of the general public. Just as recreational or illicit drug use has long been present in the general public, it is and will likely always be present in sports. In fact, professional athletes may be more at risk because of the frequent "down" time or idleness between practices and games. The off season is another example of "free" time. The headlines featuring professional or amateur athletes who have been caught in close association with drugs are always closer to the front page and in larger type—they are often the leading stories. This heightened media attention may falsely raise the perceived prevalence of drug use among athletes. Several national studies suggest that collegiate athletes are not more likely to use alcohol or illicit drugs than their nonathletic peers [15]. In the past several years, however, some high school athletes have been required to undergo illicit drug testing whereas their nonathletic peers have not. The same is true at the collegiate level.

Cocaine

Cocaine is classified as a stimulant and may have ergogenic value. The initiation of its use by athletes is often recreational. Because cocaine has strong addictive potential and is often accompanied with unfavorable social and financial consequences, it has been labeled as the greatest enemy of today's society. Users report that it delivers an unbelievable euphoria.

Cocaine is a potent vasoconstrictor and can cause lethal myocardial infarction, optic neuropathy, arrhythmias, seizures, and stroke [28]. Cocaine-related deaths in athletes have been reported. Any young athlete with chest pain should always be questioned about cocaine or crack use.

Currently, the prevalence of cocaine use in the general population is reported to be on the rise after falling off in the late 1980s and early 1990s. Whether the increase is paralleled in the athletic population is not known. A recent American survey of student-athlete testing policies in universities found that cocaine was the most frequently screened drug [33]. Over half of the universities did not screen for AS.

Cocaine is banned by the IOC, NFL, and NCAA.

Marijuana

Self-report studies have shown marijuana to be the leading illegal recreational drug used by the collegiate population [15]. Its effect on the CNS is touted as having a soothing or relaxing effect on athletes and, therefore, is perceived to have some ergogenic value. Adverse effects include decreased attention span, decreased memory, distortion of time, impaired reaction time, and decreased psychomotor performance.

Marijuana is absorbed by the body and transformed into metabolites that are detectable in the urine 4 to 10 days after smoking a single marijuana cigarette and up to several weeks following use by a chronic abuser. Passive inhalation from a room filled with marijuana smoke is reported to cause detectable levels in the urine [25••].

The IOC does not ban the use of marijuana but tests for it. The United States Olympic Committee (USOC) reserves the right to test for marijuana at competitive events. USOC basketball and boxing, the NCAA, and the NFL have all banned its use.

Alcohol

Ethanol is one of the most commonly abused drugs in today's society. It is the drug of choice on high school and college campuses. Ethanol, particularly beer, is often associated with athletic events and was once promoted by professional athletes. It is often falsely viewed as an excellent source of carbohydrates.

The prevalence of ethanol use among collegiate athletes varies from sport to sport. Use ranges from 80% to 90% of athletes [16]. This is consistent with a more recent Canadian study [33].

Many studies support the fact that ethanol is not ergogenic because it produces psychomotor changes as well as decreased balance, reaction time, motor coordination, visual tracking, and information processing [28]. Studies show no improved performance in sprinters and middle-distance runners after ethanol consumption. Both abuse and dependency may not manifest themselves as poor or decreased performance. Ethanol has also been shown to be acutely cardiotoxic, causing a decrease in contractility, and has been linked to new-onset atrial fibrillation [34].

In some individuals, low doses of ethanol possess anxiolytic properties. It also has the potential to reduce essential tremor and, therefore, has been banned by the IOC and the NCAA in rifle events.

Nicotine

Nicotine is a CNS stimulant present in the tobacco leaf. Professional athletes once heavily promoted the use of smokeless tobacco. Today, "snuff" or "chew" is still very prevalent in the sports world.

Collegiate prevalence is sport- and gender-dependent and ranges from 1% to 10% in female sports and 10% to 60% in male sports. The prevalence in high school is expected to be similar to college because the majority of athletes initiate use at this age [15]. Chronic use is high in baseball. More recently, the use in baseball has dropped off slightly as athletes attempt to find alternatives to chew (*eg*, bubble gum and sunflower seeds). It is also heavily used in collegiate and professional ice hockey, but the actual numbers are poorly documented.

Nicotine is not considered to be a performance enhancer. However, as with any drug, once addiction occurs, performance is perceived to be enhanced with continued use as opposed to enduring withdrawal symptoms during competition.

Nicotine is a vasoconstrictor and elevates the heart rate. It also decreases cardiac stroke volume. Its most ominous adverse effect is its associated risk for oral cancer. My experience is that most users are aware of the cancer risk but choose to continue use.

Nicotine is not banned by the IOC. In 1994, the NCAA banned the use of tobacco by coaches and athletes during practices and competition. A student athlete caught using tobacco could be ruled ineligible for the rest of the practice or game.

MISCELLANEOUS DRUGS
β-Adrenergic blocking agents

β-Blockers are rarely abused antihypertensive medications that, through β-receptor antagonistic activity, exert ergolytic effects on performance when cardiovascular fitness is not of vital importance. Anaerobic capacity, VO_2 max, and endurance are negatively affected by their use [28]. They do possess an anxiolytic property. Because they can reduce tremor and heart rate, they can enhance performance in the shooting events. The β-blockers do not negatively affect strength.

What about athletes with hypertension? Are the β-blockers a good choice for them? In the absence of coronary artery disease, the answer is no. If they are to be used, $β-_1$ selective agents seem to be better tolerated by athletes. Other adverse effects include a decrease in cardiac contractility, bronchospasm in asthma, insomnia, depression, and erectile dysfunction. The angiotensin-converting enzyme inhibitors would be a better selection for the hypertensive athlete.

β-Blockers are banned in shooting events by the NCAA and the IOC. They are also banned in archery, bobsledding, ski jumping, freestyle skiing, sailing, driving, and synchronized swimming.

Ritalin and Cylert

Ritalin (Ciba-Geigy Corporation, Summit, NJ) and Cylert (Abbott Laboratories, Chicago, IL) are amphetamines used successfully in treating both children and adults with attention deficit hyperactive disorder (ADHD). Because the prevalence of ADHD is increasing, it is likely that a collegiate team physician will have athletes being treated for this condition.

The NCAA instituted a ruling in 1993 to allow waivers for these drugs if a letter containing a documented medical history is provided by a physician. The physician's letter should be kept in the student-athlete's campus chart. If the student tests positive, the institution would then apply for a waiver from the NCAA.

Both Ritalin and Cylert are banned by the IOC, NCAA, and NFL.

Diuretics

Athletes use diuretics to lose weight and to dilute urine in hopes of passing drug testing. They possess no true ergogenic qualities. Diuretics are banned by the IOC, NCAA, and NFL.

Probenecid

Taking one drug to prevent the detection of another is the basis for which athletes have used probenecid. It has no ergogenic potential but does have the ability to decrease the urine secretion in users of anabolic steroids. Because of their action, these types of drugs are known as masking or blocking agents. Probenecid is a banned substance. Other masking agents are reportedly used.

DRUG TESTING

Devised as a deterrent for drug use, drug testing has been criticized by many. At present, it remains controversial. The history of drug testing and the necessary characteristics of a successful drug testing program have been thoroughly reviewed [35].

To advocates, the reasons for testing athletes remain constant: to create fair competition by preventing any unfair advantage. In doing so, the beauty of sport is preserved. Also, testing athletes prevents them from suffering the possible adverse effects of banned substances. Critics point out the alleged inefficiencies of testing, infringements on liberties, paternalistic rules, and filtration of advances in technologies.

Current testing is done by the use of urine samples. The sample must not be too diluted or too alkaline or the athlete will be detained at the testing station until satisfactory urine is obtained. Two samples are obtained, labeled, sealed, and sent through the proper chain of command to a laboratory for testing.

Testing for the presence of AS is twofold. With the exception of testosterone, all synthetic AS known to the testing site are easily identified in drug assays. The test result will be positive or negative. However, in the case of testosterone (which can be injected as salts or esters or delivered through skin patches) the extrinsic source is indistinguishable from the body's own testosterone. Because of this, the IOC began using the T:E ratio in 1982.

A ratio of six or above is suspect for a positive test. This number was derived from documenting the T:E ratio in hundreds of male athletes. Although less than 0.8% of specimens in the general population exceed a T:E ratio of six, a mandatory investigation must be performed before the sample is officially declared positive. The positive T:E ratio for women is also six or greater. A T:E ratio of less then six may be obtainable in some athletes using low-dose testosterone.

Newer investigations suggest that ^{13}C technology may be used to distinguish endogenous from exogenous sources of testosterone.

Other dilemmas in drug testing include rEPO and hGH. Distinguishing between extrinsic and intrinsic hGH and rEPO cannot be done with urine testing. Blood testing is controversial in sports. The IOC along with other organizations have launched a $2 million program to implement a valid test for hGH. Because the half-lives of hGH and rEPO are so short, only a small window exists for detecting blood levels. Also, the effect of their use lasts much longer than their detectability [27]. Investigation into improving the testing for AS and other drugs continues.

REFERENCES AND RECOMMENDED READING

Recently published papers of particular interest have been highlighted as:

- • Of special interest
- •• Of outstanding interest

1. Balsom P, Karin S, Ekblom B: Creatine in humans with special reference to creatine supplementation. *Sports Med* 1994; 18:268–280.

2. Greenhaff P, Bodin K, Soderlund K, Hultman E: Effect of oral creatine supplementation on skeletal muscle phosphocreatine resynthesis. *Am J of Physiol* 1994; 266:E725–E730.

3. Greenhaff P: Creatine and its application as an ergogenic aid. *Int J Sports Nutr* 1995, 5(suppl):S100–S110.

4. Harris R, Soderlund K, Hultman E: Elevation of creatine in resting and exercised muscle of normal subjects by creatine supplementation. *Clin Sci* 1992, 83:367–374.

5. Febbrario M, Flanagan T, Snow R, *et al.*: Effect of creatine supplementation on intramuscular tcr, metabolism and performance during intermittent, supramaximal exercise in humans. *Acta Physiol Scand* 1995, 155:387–395.

6. Volek JS, Kraemer WJ, Bush JA, *et al.*: Creative supplementation: effect on muscular performance during high-intensity resistance exercise. *Med Sci Sports Exerc* 1996, 28(suppl):S81.

7. Greenhaff P, Casey A, Short A, *et al.* Influence of oral creatine supplementation during repeated bouts of maximal voluntary exercise in man. *Clin Sci* 1993, 84:565–571.

8. Maughan R: Creatine supplementation and exercise performance. *Int J Sports Nutr* 1995, 5:94–101.

9. Balsom P, Soderlundk B: Skeletal muscle metabolism during short duration high intensity exercise: influence of creatine supplementation. *Acta Physio Scan* 1995, 154:303–310.

10. Ekblom B: Effects of creatine supplementation on performance. *Am J Sports Med* 1996, 24(suppl):S38-S29.

11. Mujika II Chatard J, Lacoste L, *et al.*: Creatine supplementation does not improve sprint performance in competitive swimmers. *Med Sci Sports Exerc* 1996, 11:1435–1441.

12. Odland L, MacDougall J, Tarnpolsky M: Effect of oral creatine supplementation on muscle PCr and short term maximum power. *Med Sci Sports Exerc* 1997, 29:216–219.

13. Bagatelli CJ, Bremmer WJ. Androgens in men: uses and abuses. *N Engl J Med* 1996, 334:707–714.

14. Whitehead RD, Chillag C, Elliot D: Anabolic steroid use among adolescents in a rural state. *J Fam. Pract* 1992, 35:401–405.

15. Anderson WA, Albrecht RR, McKeag D: A national survey of alcohol and drug use by college athletes. *Phys Sports Med* 1991, 19:91–104.

16. Anderson WA, Albrecht RR, McKeag DB: *Second replication of a national study of the substance use and abuse habits of college student-athletes: final report*. Overland Park, KS: National Collegiate Athletic Association; 1993.

17. Buckley WE, Yesalis CE III, Friedl KE: Estimated prevalence of anabolic steroid use among male high school seniors. *JAMA* 1988, 3441–3445.

18. Spence JC, Gauvin L. Drug and alcohol use by canadian university athletes: a national survey. *J Drug Educ* 1996, 26:275–287.

19. Catlin D, Murray T: Performance enhancing drugs, fair competition and Olympic sports. *JAMA* 1996, 276:231–232.

20. Lombardo JA, Hickson RC, Lamb DR: Anabolic/adrogenic steroids and growth hormone. In *Perspective in Exercise Science and Sports Medicine, vol 4: Ergogenics—Enhancement of Performance in Exercise and Sport*. Ann Arbor: Brown & Benchmark; 1991:249.

21. Bhasin S, Storer T, Berman N: The effects of supraphysiologic doses of testosterone on muscle size and strength in normal man. *New Engl J Med* 1996, 335:1–7.

22. Bahrke MS, Yesalis CE, Wright JE: Psychological and behavioral effects of endogenous testosterone and anabolic androgenic steroids. *Sports Med* 1996, 22:367–390.

23. Durant RH, Escobedo L, Heath G: Anabolic steroid use, strength training and multiple drug use among adolescents in the united states *Pediatrics* 1995, 96:23–28.

24. Middleman AB: Anabolic steroid use and associated health risk behaviors. *Sports Med* 1996, 21:251–255.

25.•• Fuentes RJ, Rosenberg JM, Davis A, eds: *Athletic Drug Reference 1996*. Durham, NC: Clean Data Inc.; 1996.
A great resource for banned drug listings.

26. Thein L, Thein J, Landry G: Ergogenic aids. *Phys Ther* 1995, 75:431–439.

27. Wadler G: Drug use update. *Med Clin North Am* 1994; 78:439–455.

28. Wagner J: Enhancement of athletic performance With Drugs. *Sports Med* 1991, 12:250–263.

29. Ghaphery N: Performance enhancing drugs. *Orthop Clin North Am* 1995, 26:433–442.

30. Ekblom B: Blood doping and erythropoietin. *Am J Sports Med* 1992, 24(suppl):S40–S42.

31. Rosenblom D, Sutton J: Drugs and exercise. *Med Clin North Am* 1985, 69:177–186.

32. Spriet LL: Caffeine and performance. *Int J Sports Nutr* 1995, 5(suppl):S84–S99.

33. Fields L, Lange WR, Kreiter NA: A national survey of drug testing policies for college athletes. *Med Sci Sports Exerc* 1994, 26:682–686.

34. Eichner ER. Sports anemia: iron supplements and blood doping. *Med Sci Sports Exerc* 1992, 14:289–303.

35. Lynch JM. Drugs In Sport. In *Current Review Of Sports Medicine*, edn 1. Edited by Johnson RJ, Lombardo JA. Philadelphia: Current Medicine; 1994:191–200.

36. Clark N: What's brewing with caffeine? *Phys Sports Med* 1994, 22:15–16.

PERFORMANCE PSYCHOLOGY AND SPORTS MEDICINE

Chris Carr
and Todd Kays

In today's competitive environment, more performers (whether athletes, musicians, or physicians) are honing their skills with the use of performance psychology skills. The field of sport and exercise psychology explores the relationship between psychological factors and optimal performance. The sports medicine specialist should have some knowledge of the various facets of sport and performance psychology because many of these skills are relevant to the care and management of an athletic population.

The term *performance psychology* is used in this chapter to represent the various environments under which mental skills enhancement can be useful. The term *sport psychology* represents the use of mental skills training within the sport and exercise domain. We have found that many of the techniques used with elite athletes have had comparable successes with elite musicians, actors, and dancers. Therefore, the skills addressed in this chapter, although related in the sport environment, may be helpful for various forms of performance. By absorbing the material presented in this chapter, sports medicine professionals can improve their understanding of the diversity of performance issues and problems that may affect their patients.

Topics addressed in this chapter include 1) a brief history and current status of the field of sport and exercise psychology, 2) a brief review of mental skills training techniques, and 3) specific performance and clinical issues, with specific concerns related to the injured athlete. We review a comprehensive performance psychology model that is coordinated through the sports medicine center at Ohio State University. If a sports medicine professional is to establish a holistic philosophy of care, an understanding of underlying psychological processes is necessary.

HISTORY AND CURRENT ISSUES

The field of sport psychology is relatively young, dating back only to the turn of the 20th century [1]; yet it has a history unrealized by most. The origin of sport psychology is patchy at best, because it has roots in both applied and academic sport psychology. The academic realm of sport psychology is better known than the applied realm because of the researchers' and academicians' law of "publish or perish." Applied sport psychology, although not nearly as visible in the early years, still had more of a role than most realize. Applied sport psychology has been maintained through the use of stories, books, personal anecdotes, presentations, and workshops. The hope for the future of sport psychology would be for these two different areas within the field to recognize and appreciate their uniqueness and how each part can contribute to the development of sport psychology.

The earliest research in sport psychology can be traced to Norman Triplett, who in 1897 conducted one of the first experiment in sport psychology by investigating the performance of cyclists. After finding that young children performed better on a rote motor task in the presence of other children, he concluded that cyclists would usually perform better in the presence of other cyclists. Other studies taking place at about the same time looked at motor behavior by exploring an individual's reaction times as well as how personality development was influenced by sport. None of these experiments and studies, however, were directly applied to athletes or sporting realms.

During the 1920s and 1930s, application of sport psychology began by using principles from the research and academic settings to actual athletic arenas. Coleman Griffith, the father of American sport psychology, had one of the leading roles in the growth of sport psychology during this time. He is credited with developing the first laboratory for studying sport psychology as well as taking sport psychology into "the field." He helped establish the first coaching school in the United States and worked with both the Chicago Cubs baseball team and the Notre Dame football team to improve sport performance. Griffith's vision and insight took applied psychology into the world of sports.

Still, between the 1930s and 1950s, the area of sport psychology remained primarily in the academic realm, with research in the areas of learning and motor acquisition continuing to be strong. At this time, applied sport psychology appeared to be in the hands of physical educators, with much of the scholarly work being done in physical education programs. In fact, through the late 1960s and mid-1970s, physical education had become an established academic discipline and sport psychology a subdiscipline of physical education. Whereas physical education studied the acquisition and improvement of motor skills, sport psychology explored psychological aspects of sport, such as what personality factors influence sport performance and how sport performance influences an individual's personality development.

In the mid-1970s, sport psychology started to grow tremendously, particularly in the applied realm. However, confusion still remained about what was to be the proper focus of sport psychology. Some members in the field argued that sport psychology was primarily educational and should focus on performance issues, whereas other members maintained that sport psychology should focus on the psychological development of the athlete. The advent of the 1984 Olympics began to clear up some of the confusion within the field. For the first time, the idea of sport psychology was presented to a national television audience—a major reason for the strong development of applied sport psychology. Soon after, in 1985, the U.S. Olympic Committee hired its first full-time sport psychologist.

Since 1985, the applied realm of sport psychology has continued to grow tremendously. Journals covering the field began publishing, and Division 47 in the American Psychological Association was established, recognizing for the first time in history the uniqueness offered to the field of psychology in sport. In addition, the 1988 Olympics was the first time teams were accompanied by a sport psychologist to the games. Other advances in the field include the establishment of the Association for the Advancement of Applied Sport Psychology (AAASP) in 1986 and the beginning of the *Journal of Sport Psychology* in 1979. In 1991, as a way to further advance this burgeoning field, the AAASP established criteria designating a "certified consultant" in the field of sport psychology, improving the clarity and understanding of the sport psychologist.

The applied realm of sport psychology has been growing rapidly in use and popularity during the 1990s. This use, however, has not been limited to elite athletes. Applied sport psychology is being applied at the Olympic, professional, college, high school, and youth levels. Many well-known professional athletes in football, baseball, basketball, and golf have been sharing their belief that sport psychology is just as important as physical and technical skills in making a complete athlete. Furthermore, the sport psychology program established by Carr at the collegiate level is setting the standard for sport psychology services in colleges and universities throughout the country (*see* "Performance Psychology Within a Sports Medicine Setting"). Many high school and youth programs are also beginning to use sport psychology more and more. The amount of requests for sport psychology services at high school and elementary school levels and youth camps has grown tremendously in recent years. In fact, we do not have enough time to meet the demands for services within our university let alone an entire city.

Applied sport psychology covers all sports, not just those more visible (football, baseball, and basketball). Sport psychology is being used and sought after in motor sports, mountain biking, rowing, soccer, and rifle and pistol shooting to name just a few. Many physicians, attorneys, and corporate executives are requesting that sport psychology principles be applied to the "performances" in their respective settings. The applied possibilities in performance psychology seem almost endless.

Although the field has come far in the past 10 years, especially in the area of applied sport psychology, it has not been without controversy. Probably the largest debate in the field centers on the definition of and the educational requirements for a sport psychologist. Two primary groups identify themselves as sport psychologists—one from the academic side and the other from the applied side. The academicians and researchers in exercise and sport psychology and physical education are concerned with how an athlete can increase speed, motor control, and other physical capabilities to enhance performance. Sport psychologists in applied settings, on the other hand, typically have been concerned with the mental and emotional well-being of the athlete and the use of psychological theory and concepts in the sport world.

A special note must be made at this point. Individuals do exist who identify themselves as sport psychologists but who have had either very little or no training in psychology, exercise science, or both. Who are these individuals? Some have coached a child's basketball team, or played tennis most of their life, or merely have a subscription to *Sports Illustrated*. Consumers must be wary of people identifying themselves as sport psychologists, but who may have very little or no formal training.

Because of the popularity of sport and the money

and prestige surrounding it, it is quite seductive for people to attach themselves to an area filled with such glamour. As a result, the organizations within sport psychology are currently trying to refine the requirements of a "sport psychologist." (the criteria for identifying oneself as a sport psychologist are discussed later in the chapter). However, in 1991, the AAASP did identify requirements of being a "certified consultant" in the field of sport psychology as a step toward clarifying the training required to be a sport psychologist. Murphy [2••] summarizes those requirements as the following.

1. A doctoral degree
2. Knowledge of scientific and professional ethics and standards
3. Three courses in sport psychology
4. Courses in biomechanics or exercise physiology
5. Courses in the historical, philosophical, social, or motor behavior bases of sport
6. Coursework in pathology and its assessment
7. Training in counseling (*eg*, coursework, supervised practica)
8. Supervised experience with a qualified person in sport psychology
9. Knowledge of skills and techniques in sport or exercise
10. Courses in research design, statistics, and psychological assessment
11. Knowledge of the biological bases of behavior
12. Knowledge of the cognitive–affective bases of behavior
13. Knowledge of the social bases of behavior
14. Knowledge of individual behavior

Although these criteria are a step in the right direction, further work is necessary because they are still somewhat vague and there remains much disagreement in the field. The question is still open as to what constitutes a qualified and competent sport psychologist. Graduate students and individuals looking to enter the field of sport psychology remain somewhat confused. In addition, the opportunities that exist for individuals to gain structured and formal training, especially in applied settings, are minimal. Thus, by having made training very difficult, this lack of clarity within the field will prevent sport psychology from advancing as a discipline.

MENTAL SKILLS IN SPORT

Many coaches and athletes attempt to put in more physical practice to correct mistakes made during competition. However, many times the mistakes are due to *mental* breakdowns as opposed to physical or technical ones. The athletes actually need to practice not only physical skills but mental skills as well. In the same way, physicians working in sports medicine facilities or with athletes sometimes forget or do not realize how mental skills can be used in their work.

Although coaches, athletes, and sports medicine physicians agree that more than 80% of the mistakes made in sport are mental, they still do not attempt to learn or teach mental skills that will assist athletes on the field or during rehabilitation (Carr and Kays, Unpublished data). First, the lack of mental skills knowledge exhibited by sports medicine physicians prevents them from using such skills in their work with athletes. Even though physicians may tell their athletes to "just relax" as they go through rehabilitation of an injury, the athletes are not provided with the knowledge of how to do so.

Second, mental skills in sport are often viewed as part of an individual's personality and something that cannot be taught. Many physicians feel that injured athletes either have the mental toughness to progress through rehabilitation or they simply do not. However, mental skills can be learned! Injured Olympic athletes report practicing mental training on a daily basis. Furthermore, not only can these skills be learned; they also do not require an excessive amount of time, which is another reason why physicians working with athletes have neglected mental training in the past.

The following section briefly discusses some of the mental skills necessary for athletes to improve the chances of optimal performance in their sports, whether on the field or in the training room. These skills are just the basics; space restrictions prohibit a comprehensive description of the power of the mind in sport.

GOAL SETTING

Goal setting is one of the primary mental skills used by athletes. In fact, this skill is helpful and even necessary to develop other mental skills. Csikszentmihalyi [3] discusses goal setting as one of the necessary components of achieving a "flow" experience. He describes flow as an experience in which a person achieves peak performance. Other terms used for this flow experience are "in the zone" and "playing unconscious."

It is not typically a problem to get athletes to identify goals. The difficulty comes in trying to help athletes set the right kind of goals—ones that pro-

vide direction, increase motivation, and guide them to achieving optimal performance. Athletes, and most people for that matter, do not need to be convinced that goals are important. They do, however, need instruction on setting good goals and developing a program that works to achieve them.

Empirical research demonstrates that goal setting can enhance recovery from injury [4]. The research also demonstrates that certain types of goals are most effective in helping athletes achieve these goals. Several goal setting principles that provide a strong base to building a solid goal-setting program have been identified.

1. Set specific goals
2. Set challenging but realistic goals
3. Set long- and short-term goals
4. Set performance goals
5. Write down goals
6. Develop goal-achievement strategies
7. Provide goal support
8. Evaluate goal achievement

Set specific goals

Research illustrates that setting specific goals produces higher levels of performance than planning no goals at all or goals that are too broad [5]. Yet many times physicians tell athletes to "do their best" or "give everything you have" regarding their recovery. Although these goals are admirable, they are not specific and do not help athletes move toward optimal performance. Goal setting needs to be measurable and stated in behavioral terms. Instead of an athlete setting his or her goal to "get better," sport medicine physicians can help these injured athletes set a more appropriate goal like "increasing leg press weight by 25% over the next 2 weeks."

Set realistic but challenging goals

The research indicates that goals should be challenging and difficult, yet attainable [6]. Goals that are too easy to attain do not present a challenge and, therefore, can lead to less than maximal effort. On the other hand, trying to achieve goals that are too difficult often leads to failure, resulting in frustration, which in turn leads to lower morale and motivation. Somewhere between these two extremes are challenging yet realistic goals.

Set both long- and short-term goals

Many times injured athletes discuss a long-term goal of returning to play after a serious injury. This goal is necessary and provides the final destination for the athletes. It is important, however, for physicians to help them focus on short-term goals as a way in which to attain long-term goals. For example, a physician can make certain that an injured athlete sets daily and weekly goals in the rehabilitation process. One way to use this principle is to picture a staircase with the end or long-term goal at the top of the staircase, the present level of performance at the base of the stairs, and the short-term goals as the steps in between.

Set performance goals

It is important for sports medicine physicians to assist athletes in setting goals related to performance rather than outcomes, such as returning to play. Murphy [2] discusses "action goals" versus "result goals" as being extremely important and something that physicians often miss. With action-focused goals, athletes concentrate their energies on the "actions" of a task as opposed to the "outcome." Action goals give focus to the task at hand, are under the athlete's control, and produce confidence and concentration. Result-focused goals, however, are not productive and often lead to slower recovery. These types of goals give focus to irrelevant factors—things outside the control of the athlete—and tend to produce anxiety and tension. For example, if a collegiate tennis player is working back after a serious shoulder injury, physicians can help him or her by setting action goals, such as lifting a certain weight or obtaining a certain degree of flexibility, that will lead to the outcome of full recovery.

Write down goals

Sport psychologists have recommended that goals be written down and placed where they can be easily seen on a daily basis [2,7]. Athletes may choose to write them on index cards and place them in their locker, locker room, or bedroom. Physicians and athletes often spend much time with goal-setting strategies only to see them end up discarded in some drawer. The manner in which goals are recorded varies, but the important fact is that they remain visible and available to athletes on a daily basis.

Develop goal-achievement strategies

This aspect of goal setting is often neglected because goals are set without appropriate strategies to achieve them. An analogy to this faulty process is taking a trip from San Diego to Buffalo without having a map. It will take one much longer to reach the final destination without a map. For example, physicians may encounter an athlete with frequent flu-like symptoms. This athlete needs to employ appropriate strategies that will assist him or her in reducing the frequency of these symptoms, such as working on improving nutrition, sleep hygiene, stress management, and time management.

Provide goal support

Research in the sport psychology literature has demonstrated the vital role that "significant others" play in helping athletes achieve goals [8]. In fact, it has been shown that exercise adherence is strongly affected by spousal support [9]. Sports medicine physicians need to enlist the support of parents, faculty, friends, and others to help athletes focus on the actions required to achieve success (ie, returning to play).

Evaluate goal achievement

Evaluating progress toward goals is one of the most important aspects of goal setting, yet it is frequently overlooked. Injured athletes may spend considerable time in setting goals and devising programs, but it will be for naught if they do not regularly monitor their progress in achieving these goals. To draw an analogy from philosophy: just as an unexamined life is not worth living, unexamined goal setting is not worth doing.

AROUSAL CONTROL
What is arousal control?

Have you ever watched the National Collegiate Athletic Association basketball finals and wondered how a player can make a free throw or last-second shot with thousands of people screaming and millions of people watching on television? It is amazing how athletes are able to remain calm during such times of high pressure and anxiety, but the fact is that these athletes *are* nervous—they *do* have "butterflies" in their stomachs. However, they have developed the ability to use their anxiety as a way to perform their very best—to make the butterflies "fly in formation," so to speak. Similarly, when an athlete becomes injured, he or she typically experiences much anxiety. They experience physical pain, lose their place in the line-up, and are not able to perform something that has been a major part of their life for several years. Sports medicine physicians, however, can help the athletes learn to use the anxiety surrounding their injury as way to help them recover quicker.

The theories of arousal regulation are many—too many for this chapter, in fact—, but some of the more common theories include Yerkes and Dodson's [10] "inverted-U" theory, Hanin's [11] "zone of optimal functioning," the "multidimensional theory of anxiety" developed by Martens *et al.* [12], and the "catastrophe theory" proposed by Thom [13] and mathematically applied by Hardy and Fazey (Paper presented at the annual meetings of the North American Society for the Psychology of Sport and Physical Activity, Vancouver, British Columbia, Canada, 1987). Van Raalte and Brewer [14] reviewed and provided more explicit detail of these theories. The inverted-U theory (Figure 13.1) is most commonly used to describe how performance decrements may occur as a result of physiological arousal levels being either too high or too low. To summarize, an athlete's best performance tends to happen when they are in "the zone," which represents the feeling of controlled and comfortable arousal. Teaching athletes and performers how to control their own levels of arousal is the goal of arousal regulation skills.

Arousal control techniques
Breathing
Perhaps the most simple, yet most important, technique used to regulate anxiety is breathing [15]. It is common for athletes to take short, quick breaths when confronted with a stressful event or situation, such as rehabilitating an injury. With such choppy breaths, the breathing system contracts and does not supply enough oxygen to the body, particularly the muscles. This action results in the muscles becoming tense and fatigued, both of which will prevent optimal performance in recovery. Taking slow, deep breaths allows athletes to supply their bodies with an adequate amount of oxygen that will assist them in better recovery.

Muscle relaxation
One of the most potentially damaging aspects of anxiety for athletes is muscle tension [16]. If an ath-

lete's muscles are tense, he or she will not be able to perform the kinesthetic tasks required by their sport or rehabilitation process in a free-flowing and smooth manner. Therefore, for athletes to perform their best, they must learn to relax their muscles. If their muscles are not relaxed, the athlete's movements will be rigid, short, and tight.

How do athletes learn to relax their muscles? Edmund Jacobson's [17] progressive relaxation technique laid the groundwork for most current relaxation procedures. His technique and other similar ones allow athletes to become aware of different muscle groups, how they hold tension in these areas, and also how to release this tension. It can be extremely helpful for sports medicine physicians to teach these athletes to perform this mental skill, making their rehabilitation less painful and their return to play quicker.

Imagery
What is the mystery in imagery that has helped elite athletes (such as Jack Nicklaus, who has won more major tournaments than anyone in the world) compete so well? There is no mystery at all. Imagery is a human capacity that many people either do not know about or have chosen not to use. It is a skill that very few athletes have developed to its full potential or realized its possible applications.

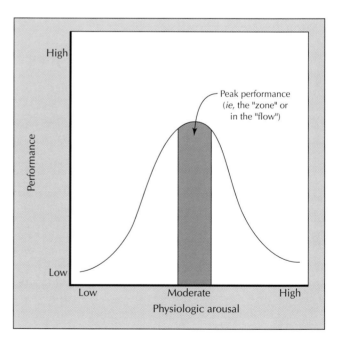

FIGURE 13.1

The inverted-U theory of arousal regulation.

Imagery is a process by which sensory experiences are stored in memory and internally recalled and performed in the absence of external stimuli [2]. Furthermore, imagery is more than visualization, more than just the sense of vision. To maximize its potential, imagery must be a multisensory event and involve as many of the senses as possible, including sound, touch, and movement.

Imagery has many uses for athletes, including regulating arousal level and rehabilitation from injury [4,18]. Imagery is useful for coping with pain and injury by speeding recovery as well as keeping athletic skills from deteriorating. It is difficult for athletes to go through an extended layoff, but instead of feeling sorry for themselves, they can imagine doing practice skills and thereby facilitate recovery.

Cognitive strategies

Self-talk is one of several different cognitive strategies in sport. It occurs whenever an individual thinks, either internally or externally. Sport psychologists are concerned with the self-talk of athletes and how it influences their focus, concentration, arousal level, and performance. The literature in this area is too large to cover in this chapter, but the preponderance of research supports the hypothesis that positive self-talk creates better or "no worse" performance.

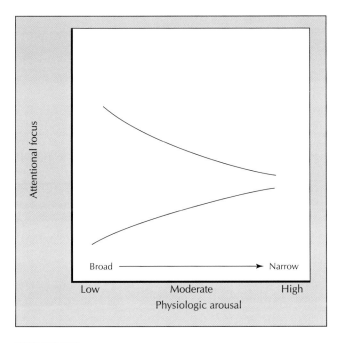

FIGURE 13.2

The narrowing of attentional focus related to anxiety or physiologic arousal.

Self-talk has a direct impact on our emotional experience. If athletes are engaging in negative self-talk, their resulting experience may be one of frustration, anger, or extreme anxiety. These emotional states will challenge breathing, increase muscle tension, and create a loss of concentration and focus that can cause decreased performance. If an athlete's self-talk is positive and relevant, however, the subsequent emotional experience will be one of relaxation, calmness, and centeredness. As a result, the chances of good performance increase dramatically. Sports medicine physicians can assist athletes by teaching and discussing positive self-talk and the differences it can make in recovery.

ATTENTIONAL CONTROL
Concentration

Concentration is the ability to focus all of one's attention on the task at hand. For physicians and their athletes, concentration is being able to direct all attention to the recovery process. When athletes experience anxiety, however, maintaining attention on the task at hand becomes more difficult, and concentration becomes narrow and internally directed toward worry, self-doubt, and other task-irrelevant thoughts [19]. The narrowing of attention related to increases in anxiety or physiological arousal is demonstrated in Figure 13.2.

Part of the definition of concentration involves paying attention to "relevant environmental cues." To give one's full attention to only the relevant parts of a task is sometimes very difficult to do. For example, what cues are relevant to a football player recovering from a serious knee injury? Relevant cues include the rehabilitation process (*eg*, keeping meetings with the physical therapist, good goal setting, and following the physician's recommendations regarding treatment). Irrelevant cues, however, might include the thoughts of friends or the next opponent on the schedule, neither of which have anything to do with rehabilitation. The physical actions required to rehabilitate the knee do not change regardless of the next opponent. Figure 13.3 demonstrates how increases in physiological arousal will elicit a narrowing of attentional focus, so that when the athlete is too aroused, he or she will only be able to focus on one or two task-relevant cues. When the athlete or performer is "in the zone," all of the task-relevant cues have the performer's attention, and the task-irrelevant cues are not attended to by the performer.

Improving concentration skills

It can be extremely beneficial for physicians to help athletes maintain the concentration levels on the task at hand (*eg*, rehabilitating an injury). First, sport physicians can remind the athletes that just as they are skilled to maintain focus in high-pressure situations (*eg*, shooting free throws to win a game), they can do this same thing in the recovery process.

Second, athletes can use cue words to help bring their full attention to the tasks in rehabilitation. For example, a tennis player recovering from an elbow injury might use the term "stay loose" as he or she lifts weights to strengthen the elbow or the word "breathe" to remind him or her that deep breathing will help relaxation during times of intense pain.

Furthermore, much research has demonstrated that routines can focus concentration and be extremely helpful to mental preparation (Moore, Unpublished data) [20,21]. The mind can easily wander during rehabilitation. Injured athletes might worry about losing their position or the reactions of coaches and teammates. These are the times at which routines are ideal. For example, when an athlete is performing rehabilitation exercises, he or she might take a deep breath, imagine what he or she wants to do in the session, and then say one or two cue words to maintain this focus.

Finally, the importance of staying focused in the "here and now" cannot be emphasized enough. Many times athletes get caught up in thinking about past injuries or what might happen to their position on the team after returning, causing them to lose focus on the relevant cues of the rehabilitation process at the present time.

Whether the performance occurs on the playing field, the stage, or in the training room, the use of mental skills for performance enhancement is imperative for optimal growth and potential. The strategies previously discussed all use a cognitive–behavioral orientation in order to assess, intervene, and evaluate behavioral and cognitive change. When the performer (whether an athlete, musician, or physician) uses these mental training skills in the enhancement of his or her own performance, the effects can be wonderful and exciting.

PERFORMANCE PSYCHOLOGY AND CLINICAL ISSUES

In some situations where an athlete or performer seeks individual consultation on a performance problem, additional issues often become the focus of the primary course of treatment. In this brief section, clinical issues that may arise while treating athletes are discussed.

The symptoms associated with many performance issues often parallel diagnostic characteristics of psychological distress. For example, overtraining has been addressed from both the physiological and psychological dimensions with elite athletes [22]. Athletes who suffer from overtraining may meet diagnostic criteria associated with a major depressive disorder as described in the American Psychiatric Association's Diagnostic and Statistical Manual of Mental Disorders [23]. It is imperative that the sports medicine physician be aware of some of these clinical issues rather than assume any emotional or cognitive discomfort reported by an athlete or performer is solely a performance problem. In fact, Carr's clinical experience and review of patient files indicates that 95% of the clients report a "performance-related problem" at the initial intake session, whereas only 30% to 35% of the actual treatment is strictly cognitive–behavioral interventions for performance enhancement. The remaining 65% to 70% of treatment reflects more common psychotherapeutic interventions with various clinical issues. We briefly review some of the more relevant clinical issues that the sports medicine physician may see in his or her practice.

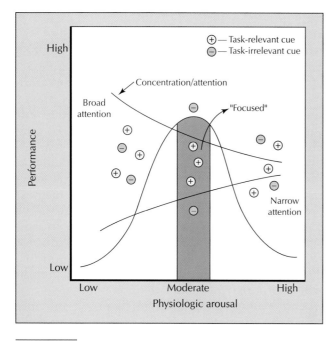

FIGURE 13.3

The impact of physiologic arousal on task-relevant and task-irrelevant cues.

Mood disorders

Disorders that have a disturbance in mood as the predominant feature fall under the category of mood disorders. These disorders can be depressive, bipolar, or based on etiology (*ie*, either substance-induced or due to a general medical condition) [23]. The sports medicine professional should familiarize him or herself with the diagnostic criteria for mood disorders, as they may present either overtly or covertly with an athletic population.

Because athletes and performers are often subjected to environmental stressors that are specific to the performance arena (*eg*, fans, media, coaches), an often normative response to stress is the feeling of a depressed mood. At the Ohio State University Sports Medicine Center, a psychologist on staff can provide consultation with sports medicine physicians when they notice that the mood and affect of a patient is deviating from the previously observed baseline mood. Sports medicine physicians are often privileged to develop close relationships with the athletes for which they provide care, whether on the sideline, while traveling with the team, or at practices. This relationship allows the physician and other sports medicine providers (*eg*, athletic trainers) a unique opportunity to "get to know" the patients. When an athlete presents with a depressed mood, it may be a situational response to an external stressor (*eg*, injury), or it may represent a pattern of depressed cognitive thought and affect that may reflect depression. Early intervention and referral is key to the effective treatment of mood disorders. Consultation with the psychologist—especially when the depression is also being treated psychopharmacologically—is essential to the provision of holistic sports medicine care.

Anxiety disorders

An anxiety disorder may be present when the presenting complaint reflects a change in previous functioning that manifests with increased anxiety, worry, avoidance, cognitive distortion, or experience of a traumatic event. Some anxiety disorders include panic attacks, agoraphobia, specific phobia, social phobia, obsessive–compulsive disorder, posttraumatic stress disorder, acute stress disorder, generalized anxiety disorder, and anxiety disorder due to a general medical condition [23]. The athletic and performance environments are "tailor made" for some anxiety disorders, as injury and performance both represent cognitive interpretations of situational conditions. For example, when an athlete suffers a severe, acute injury, an acute stress disorder may be an appropriate diagnosis after observing diagnostic criteria. Such diagnostic criteria include a subjective sense of emotional numbing or detachment, an absence of emotional response, a reduction in awareness of the patient's surroundings, and depersonalization [23]. The sports medicine physician should be able to refer when the patient begins to describe severe anxiety about competition or when discussing return to play. Some of the athletes seen by a sport psychologist may meet criteria for a generalized anxiety disorder related to their specific performance, especially when the anxiety is interfering with some of their basic functioning and preparation for performance.

Eating disorders

Most sports medicine providers are aware of the female athlete "triad" related to women in athletic environments. The triad identifies amenorrhea, osteoporosis, and disordered eating disorders as being risks specific to female athlete participants [24]. Sports medicine providers should be keenly aware of the "markers" of potential eating disorders, including refusal to maintain body weight over minimal normal weight for age and height; intense fear of gaining weight; distorted body image; absence of at least three consecutive menstrual cycles; recurrent episodes of binge eating, purging (self-induced vomiting), or laxative use; feelings of being "out of control" over eating behavior; and excessive exercise (*eg*, getting on treadmill for 45 minutes after a 3-hour practice). These symptoms, which may represent either anorexia nervosa or bulimia nervosa, may present in preseason physical examinations, during regular season monitoring, or may be assessed when a female athlete is referred for potential stress fracture [23].

Sport psychologists should also be aware of how to assess these symptoms in the context of performance-related issues. For example, some female athletes may attempt to use unhealthy weight-management behaviors (*eg*, disordered eating) to justify increased performance. Additionally, male athletes in some sports may believe that certain behaviors may also increase performance, although the behaviors may be unhealthy or ill-advised (*eg*, wrestlers using laxatives to "make weight"). Readers should review other chapters in this book for more comprehensive dialogue concerning appropriate nutrition and female athlete concerns.

Adjustment disorders

When there is the development of clinically significant emotional or behavioral symptoms in response to identifiable psychosocial stressors, the diagnosis of an adjustment disorder may be appropriate [23]. Because transition is a part of life, many transitions in the athletic realm are often experienced as stressful and overwhelming. When a high school senior who has been an All-State or All-American enters college, the transition can be difficult. With the stressors of leaving home and entering a new social environment and level of athletic competition, the individual may respond with feelings of depression, anxiety, or behavioral problems. The sports medicine professional will acknowledge that these adjustments, although normal, may also manifest emotions and behaviors that interfere with performance and day-to-day functioning. Again, using a referral will allow for further assessment and support.

Athletic injury

A discussion regarding performance issues and barriers to performance would not be complete without discussing the role of athletic injury. The injured athlete experiences a number of stressful and emotionally uncomfortable consequences after the injury. Denial, pain, and cognitive responses (realistic and unrealistic) are normal processes that occur after an athletic injury [25]. A normative response to injury is similar to the grief response of denial, anger, depression, and acceptance. However, there are many individual characteristics that must be taken into consideration when assessing how the athlete responds to an injury. In some situations, the injury is viewed as an external (event) and internal (pain) stressor and may lead to an adjustment disorder with both depressed and anxious moods. The sports medicine physician should be aware of these normal responses, while at the same time attending to potential psychological disturbances in thought, mood, and behavior.

In the authors' experiences, some of the cognitive-behavioral mental skills (*eg*, visualization, imagery, and relaxation training) have been very useful in helping the athlete cope with an injury. Early goal setting, with the assistance of the physician, trainer, and sport psychologist, may lead to better coping and enhanced recovery. Compliance with treatment and rehabilitation protocol may be enhanced with psychological intervention. Often, the mere process of "normalizing" the athlete's response to injury

assists in healthy coping skills. The readers are encouraged to read Heil's *Psychology of Sport Injury* [25••] to further their understanding of the psychological implications of athletic injury.

PERFORMANCE PSYCHOLOGY WITHIN A SPORTS MEDICINE SETTING

Ohio State University Sports Medicine Center

An example of a comprehensive, holistic, performance-oriented sports medicine setting exists at Ohio State University. A brief overview of the model may assist readers in understanding how both sport and performance psychologists can become an integral part of the sports medicine practice and provide a unique component within the athletic and performing community. It should be noted that in this environment the sport psychologist is a licensed psychologist (having earned a PhD in counseling psychology) with specialized graduate training in exercise science and physical education (with an emphasis in sport and health psychology). A postdoctoral fellow with a PhD or PsyD in counseling or clinical psychology and graduate training in the sport sciences is the second integral piece to this model. It is our belief that a wider range of services and revenue generation can be provided by a psychologist with special training in the sport sciences at the graduate level (*eg*, third-party reimbursement is available only to a licensed psychologist but not to a PhD in physical education). Carr also has 1 year (2000 hours) of training experience in the sport science division of the U.S. Olympic Training Center in Colorado Springs, adding to the performance psychology emphasis. Because of the diverse nature of presenting problems at both the individual and system (group or team) level, a licensed professional is recommended in this model.

The sport psychologist works in coordination with primary care (family medicine) physicians trained in sports medicine, orthopedic surgeons, physical therapists, and athletic trainers. At the sports medicine center, the director is the head team physician for the Ohio State University Athletic Department, and the sport psychologist is the head of sport psychology services for athletic department. In this role, team consultation, coaching education, individual athlete counseling and consultation, and support-staff consultation (*eg*, by athletic trainers) is provided by the sport psychologist. As a collaborative member of the sports medicine team, ongoing consultation and referrals are made easily and smoothly, with the patient receiving support throughout the process.

Heil [25] presents four assumptions that guide the comprehensive team-based approach he recommends for sports medicine settings.

1. Sports medicine is a multispecialty discipline amenable to a team approach
2. The interventions of all members of the sports medicine team have a psychological impact
3. Psychological recovery is an essential element in injury rehabilitation
4. Optimal treatment outcomes are based on the careful coordination of care

Within the Ohio State University sports medicine model, the sport psychologist serves an active role in physician consultation, fellow and resident training, and team meetings within athletics to discuss each team's injuries and player status (including recommendations for eating disorder interventions and so on).

In addition to the responsibilities within the athletic department of a large NCAA Division I university, the sport psychologist coordinates private practice counseling and consultation out of his office (in the sports medicine center). The sport psychologist does performance psychology consultation with athletic, performing arts, and business entities, as well as providing community-based educational and performance psychology programming (*eg*, training with the various state coaches' associations and local school districts). Many times, the total sports medicine approach is embraced by these entities, and the goal of optimizing both physical and mental health is reinforced. More information on specific components of this model are available through Carr.

CONCLUSIONS

The role of performance psychology and its impact within a sports medicine setting is increasing in visibility every year. At the same time, the growing pains associated with the development of the field may interfere with the public's knowledge of this dynamic entity. Sports medicine professionals who have a basic understanding of the history, training, "tools," and clinical issues related to the psychology of performance can best benefit their patients' needs. By incorporating some of the mental training skills into practice, a sports medicine professional will be attending to the emotional, cognitive, and behavioral issues that each patient experiences. A more holistic philosophy will embrace the health and optimal functioning of the patients that are served by the sports medicine professional.

REFERENCES AND RECOMMENDED READING

Recently published papers of particular interest have been highlighted as:

- • Of special interest
- •• Of outstanding interest

1. Wiggins DK: The history of sports phsychology in North America. In *Psychological Foundations of Sports*. Edited by Silra JM, Weinberg RS. Champagne, IL: Human Kinetics; 1984:9–23.

2. •• Murphy S: The Achievement Zone. New York: GP Putnam and Sons; 1996.
Easy-to-follow text addressing individual mental skills training for athletes and other performers. Highlights significant findings in the field of sport psycology and applies to individual utilization.

3. Csikszentmihalyi M: *Flow: The Psychology of Optimal Experience*. New York: Harper and Row; 1990.

4. Weinberg RS, Gould D: *Foundations of Sport and Exercise Psychology*. Champaign, IL: Human Kinetics; 1995.

5. Weinberg RS, Weigand D: Goal setting in sport and exercise: a reaction to Locke. *J Sport Exerc Psychol* 19??, 15:88–95.

6. Locke EA, Latham GP: *A Theory of Goal Setting and Task Performance*. Englewood Cliffs, NJ: Prentice Hall; 1990.

7. Botterill C: Goal setting for athletes with examples from hockey. In *Behavior Modification and Coaching: Principles, Procedures, and Research*. Edited by Martin GL, Hrycaik D. Springfield, IL: Charles C. Thomas; 1983.

8. Hardy CV, Richman JM, Rosenfeld LB: The role of social support in the life stress/injury relationship. *Sport Psychol* 1993, 5:128–139.

9. Dishman RK, ed: *Exercise Adherence: Its Impact on Public Health*. Champaign, IL: Human Kinetics; 1988.

10. Yerkes RM, Dodson JD: The relation of strength and stimulus to rapidity of habit formation. *J Comp Neurol Psychol* 1908, 18:459-482.

11. Hanin YL: A study of anxiety in sport. In *Sport Psychology: An Analysis of Athlete Behavior* Edited by Straub WF. Ithaca, NY: Mouvement; 1980.

12. Martins R, Vealy RS, Burton D: *Competitive Anxiety in Sport*. Champaign, IL: Human Kinetics; 1990.

13. Thom R: Structural Stability and Morphogenesis (DH Fowler, translator). New York: Benjamin-Addison Wesley; 1975.

14.• Van Raalte J, Brewer B: *Exploring Sport and Exercise Psychology*. Washington, DC: American Psychological Association; 1996.
Excellent introductory text highlighting psychologic issues in the world of sport and exercise. Chapters provide in-depth exploration of theory, application, and practice issues related to sports psychology.

15. Harris DV: Relaxation and energizing techniques for regulation of arousal. In *Applied Sport Psychology: Personal Growth to Peak Performance*. Edited by Williams JM. Palo Alto, CA: Mayfield; 1986.

16. Landers DM, Boutcher SH: Arousal-performance relationships. In *Applied Sport Psychology: Personal Growth to Peak Performance*. Edited by Williams JM. Palo Alto, CA: Mayfield; 1986.

17. Jacobson E: *Progressive Relaxation*, ed 2. Chicago: University of Chicago Press; 1938.

18. Caudill D, Weinberg R, Jackson A: Psyching-up and track athletes: a preliminary investigation. *J Sport Psychol* 1983 5:231–235.

19. Nideffer RM: Concentration and attentional control training. In *Applied Sport Psychology: Personal Growth to Peak Performance* Edited by Williams JM. Palo Alto, CA: Mayfield; 1993.

20. Cohn PJ, Rotella RJ, Lloyd JW: Effects of a cognitive behavioral intervention on the preshot routine and performance in golf. *Sport Psychol* 1990, 4:33–47.

21. Orlick T: *Psyching for Sport: Mental Training for Athletes*. Champaign, IL: Leisure Press; 1986.

22.• McCann S: Overtraining and burnout. In *Sport Psychology Interventions*. Edited by Murphy SM. Champaign, IL: Human Kinetics; 1995.
Adresses physiologic and psychologic aspects of overtraining in the athletic realm. Required reading for the sports medicine physician who treats athletes in endurance sports.

23. American Psychiatric Association: *Diagnostic and Statistical Manual of Mental Disorders*, ed 4. Washington, DC: American Psychiatric Association; 1994.

24. Yeager KK, Agostini R, Nattiv A, Drinkwater B: The female athlete triad: disordered eating, amenorrhea, osteoporosis. *Med Sci Sports Exerc* 1993, 25:775–777.

25.•• Heil J: *Psychology of Sport Injury*. Champaign, IL: Human Kinetics, 1993.
Excellent overview text for psychologic issues related to athletic injury. Adresses the social, psychologic, and physical demands of the injured athlete and covers special topics in assisting the athlete in total recovery.

OPTIMIZING TRAINING AND CONDITIONING

Jon Divine

DEFINITION OF OPTIMAL TRAINING

What is optimal training? Optimal training should be based on the assessment of individualized goals and physical condition for direction in training. Individualized assessment reduces the potential for musculoskeletal injury and illness associated with inactivity and stresses greater emphasis on the identification of musculoskeletal risk factors for overuse injury. Optimal training outcomes should provide the basic health benefits of regular physical activity, including a general sense of well being (*ie*, "a sound body and a sound mind"). In recreational and competitive athletes, optimal training creates the potential for peak sport performance while avoiding illness and injury associated with overtraining. In order to optimize sport performance, sport-specific training is emphasized.

ASSESSMENT OF INDIVIDUAL TRAINING NEEDS

Planning a program

Beginning an exercise program involves a significant lifestyle change for the majority of people. In fact, based on a 1987 report issued by the Centers for Disease Control and Prevention (CDC), greater than 50% of Americans could be described as sedentary. Many reasons have been discovered for not exercising regularly. These reasons commonly include lack of time, lack of accessible exercise facilities, and lack of energy, or a misconception that in order for exercise to be beneficial, it must be painfully strenuous. Motivation to begin a program of regular exercise requires individual awareness of both the health benefits and the ease with which a program of low to moderate intensity can be followed. In a very good review of exercise prescription with a specific strategy for encouraging primary care patients to begin regular exercise, Will *et al.* [1] makes a strong point that individual motivation to exercise is the key to overcoming the barriers of a sedentary lifestyle. The authors encourage the physician to frequently remind or "plant a seed of knowledge" whenever possible during patient visits—especially those patients for which exercise would improve the complaint. This is done by asking "critical questions" to assess the patient's readiness to begin exercise (Table 14.1). Tools for assessing readiness and suggestions for intervention at different stages of readiness are also included (Fig. 14.1). Assessing individual needs, motivation, and perceptions about exercise training is the first step in establishing an optimal training program for both the competitive athlete and the sedentary individual.

Establishing the goals of training

Numerous reports on the health benefits of regular exercise clearly indicate that regular activity is a crucial component of a healthy lifestyle. Sedentary individuals may want to "tone up" or "lose a few pounds." Recreational athletes—so-called "weekend warriors"—take regular activity one step further by incorporating sports and exercise into an active lifestyle as a form of self-fulfillment and entertainment. Some even enter (or reenter) the arena of competition and regularly train to improve not only their health but their ability to perform. Recreational and competitive athletes may recognize a specific weakness in their "game" and will want to improve on this portion of their training. Input from coaches may identify specific weaknesses in the athlete's aerobic conditioning, strength, or flexibility, and will indicate that the athlete needs to improve in this deficient area. Athletic trainers, team physicians, as well as coaches and other athletes are very interested in injury prevention and would recommend that a portion of one's training focus on areas of conditioning that will reduce the risk of musculoskeletal injuries. For many, improved performance provides increased self-satisfaction and, for others, improves the opportunity to perform well against

Table 14.1	CRITICAL QUESTIONS TO ASSESS PATIENTS' READINESS FOR EXERCISE PROGRAM*

1. What do you know about the benefits of physical activity?
2. Do you think changing your level of physical activity is necessary?
3. Have you ever tried to increase your level of physical activity in the past? If "yes," what happened?
4. Do you think you can increase your level of physical activity now?
5. What are some problems or barriers you may face when changing your level of physical activity?

*From Will *et al.* [1]; with permission.

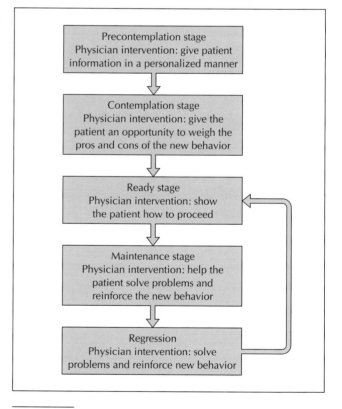

FIGURE 14.1

Stages of patient readiness for behavioral change and suggested physician interventions. (*Adapted from* Will *et al.* [1]; with permission.)

others (winning) in competition. Whether exercising for health, recreation, or improved performance, individual goals must be considered and used as a yardstick for progress to optimize a conditioning program. Asking about these goals prior to forming an exercise program provides the basis for the type of training to be done and has a direct effect on the outcomes of regular training. Understanding an individual's motivation to exercise is an essential portion of designing an optimal training program.

Compliance issues

Factors influencing compliance with training are important for both types of athletes; however, designing a training program that promotes compliance is key in the noncompetitive athlete. Under the best circumstances, compliance is generally 50% after the first year of training, decreasing to around 20% to 30 % after 3 years [2]. Studies of compliance with regular exercise indicate that several factors contribute to a successful adaptation to an active lifestyle. These include positive past experiences with physical activity, appropriate perception of the physical demands of activity, well-adapted time-management skills, feelings of personal responsibility for health, positive environmental influences from family, occupation, access to facilities, weather, and convenience to schedule and location. Immediate cues and regular prompts promoting exercise or increased activity are also helpful [2]. Realistic training goals and expectations of outcomes from training are also important. Unrealistic expectations, such as extreme weight loss or winning an Olympic medal, are unobtainable by most and are met with individual frustration, adversely affecting continued compliance with training.

The role of the professional providing a training program

The role of the individual providing a training program for the athlete is to determine the athlete's purpose, goals, and expectations of a regular training program and to provide expert guidance in obtaining these realistic goals and expectations. After the initial interview and assessment, it is important to reevaluate the individual's physical capabilities and to frequently reexamine their motivation, goals, and expectations and to make the appropriate adjustments. The initial design of a training program should include 1) consideration

for generalized training that can be adapted to multiple locations or environments, 2) frequent reassessment of goals, 3) provision of social support and relevant rewards, 4) appropriate feedback, and 5) the importance of establishing a routine while avoiding boredom. When these factors are considered within the design of an optimal training program, long-term compliance with training will be improved.

The team physician may also take an active role in the design and implementation of the training program. Perhaps what is most important is taking a genuine interest in understanding the basic principles and application of these principles into a training program. Maintaining knowledge of current research of exercise training principles and applications helps to dispel many myths and fads that often are presented to the athlete. The physician's primary medical role is to provide baseline medical information that may influence the initial direction of training. As the athlete is reevaluated throughout the training program, a thorough understanding of the stages of training will help direct the decision as to how to resume training and return (or redirect the path) to the specific training goals and objectives.

Balancing conditioning with skill training

Balancing basic conditioning within a sport-specific skill training program is more difficult for the competitive athlete. Training for many sports lasts the entire year, especially at the collegiate and professional levels. Within a training year, changing levels of aerobic and anaerobic fitness, strength, flexibility, and body composition are influenced most by the type of objectives within each "cycle" of training. These swings in nonspecific fitness-performance variables may be as high as 18% from one portion of the training cycle to the next. For example, the body density and percentage of lean body weight of female gymnasts and elite track athletes are higher during the competitive season than during the noncompetitive season. Elite female swimmers and volleyball players have a peak in body density during the precompetitive season that steadily decreases through the competitive season [3].

Novice athletes are more susceptible to a wider variation in aerobic fitness than elite athletes, due in part to lower relative levels of fitness. Variations of 10% to 22% in VO_2max have been reported between the competitive (more fit) and noncompetitive (less vigorous training) periods [3]. Variation depends on the amount of aerobic energy production specifically required for the sport. For example, athletes with a higher level of aerobic conditioning (such as collegiate wrestlers, swimmers, and track athletes) have less off-season variation in aerobic training parameters. During the competitive season, adverse variation in aerobic conditioning can also be expected in any sport that does not depend on aerobic energy production for sport-specific performance. This adverse variation results from more training time being spent on developing sport-specific skills. For all sports, a minimum level of aerobic conditioning is required in order to reduce fatigue associated with long periods of training or competition. For such sports as football, baseball, and sprinting, the minimum level of aerobic conditioning is not known. Future serial measurements of in-season VO_2max in athletes who have a successful season may shed light on how much aerobic fitness is desirable. Intuitively, in addition to sport-specific training during competitive periods, an unspecified amount of aerobic conditioning should be incorporated into the training program in order to maintain an ideal level of aerobic fitness.

Although less clearly defined in the literature, anaerobic fitness generally refers to an athlete's ability to maintain maximal levels of work output before imminent fatigue. Measurements of anaerobic fitness have included a relative increase in the level of ventilation to the level of oxygen consumption (ventilatory threshold) and increases in circulating lactic acid, generally greater than 4 mmol/L (lactate threshold [LT]). The consensus is that these parameters are not sensitive enough to determine in-season variations

in anaerobic fitness. Studies of runners, cyclists, and swimmers indicate that following a period of intense training, the speed of activity at the LT is increased [4]. The duration of maximal effort beyond the LT is also increased following intense training. It has now become widely accepted that the power output at the LT is one of the major determining factors of endurance performance [5•].

Power athletes (weight lifters, weight throwers, and jumpers) also have seasonal variations in strength and power output. Jumping athletes have a greater variation in jumping ability than nonjumping athletes, with the highest levels reported during the competitive season. Nonjumping athletes have essentially no variation in vertical jump ability throughout the training cycle [6]. Off-season gains in muscular strength and power are difficult to maintain during the competitive season in both nonelite and elite athletes. As expected, during the competitive season, more time and energy is spent on musculoskeletal training for sport-specific skills and less time on pure conditioning or strength training. Fencers, rowers, soccer players, and basketball players all have been reported to lose strength during the competitive season as the majority of time spent training is on sport-specific skills and strategies. On the other hand, wrestlers, weight lifters, and weight throwers, who include weight lifting as a major portion of their training, continue to have increases in strength during the competitive season.

All of these variations in performance parameters emphasize the strong influence of individuality and

| Table 14.2 | AMERICAN COLLEGE OF SPORTS MEDICINE GUIDELINES FOR EXERCISE TESTING AND PARTICIPATION [*] |

Medical exam and graded exercise test needed before beginning a regimen of:

| | APPARENTLY HEALTHY | | HIGHER RISK [†] | | WITH DISEASE [‡] |
	YOUNGER [§]	OLDER	ASYMPTOMATIC	SYMPTOMATIC	
Moderate exercise [¶]	No	No	No	Yes	Yes
Vigorous exercise [**]	No	Yes	Yes	Yes	Yes

[*] *Adapted from ACSM [10••]; with permission.*
[†] Persons with two or more of the following major coronary risk factors: 1) hypertension, treated or untreated; 2) cholesterol ≥ 240 mg/dL; 3) cigarette smoking; 4) diabetes mellitus; and 5) family history of coronary or other atherosclerotic disease in parents or siblings prior to age 55.
[‡] Persons with known cardiac, pulmonary, or metabolic disease.
[§] Men ≤ 40 years of age and women ≤ 50 years of age.
[¶] Exercise intensity of 40% to 60% of maximum oxygen consumption (slow-progression, noncompetitive activity).
[**] Exercise intensity > 60% of maximum oxygen consumption.

the training principle of specificity on sport-specific performance. Performance in nonspecific tasks (*ie,* weight lifting ability in runners) will suffer as training becomes more specific. How much retention of preseason gains in nonspecific performance is needed to carry into the competitive season? As previously mentioned, maintenance of a certain level of aerobic fitness is essential to reduce fatigue and maintain optimal cardiovascular performance and musculoskeletal metabolism. Muscle strength is essential in all sports for optimal performance. As the competitive season progresses, more time is spent on sport-specific training and less on maintenance of basic fitness and strength. The ability to maintain aerobic condition and strength during the competitive season is essential for optimal performance during the current season and for the ability to improve performance in future competitive seasons.

INDIVIDUAL PHYSICAL ASSESSMENT
Medical history and physical assessment

After determining the purposes and goals for the training program, the next step in designing an optimal training program is an individualized physical assessment. To improve the individual specificity of the training program, everyone should receive an individual assessment.

Who requires a medical examination? Although guidelines have varied in the past, more exercise and medical organizations uniformly recognize those guidelines now provided by the American College of Sports Medicine (ACSM) for the necessity of medical evaluation prior to beginning a program of regular exercise (Table 14.2)—especially those with symptoms of cardiovascular disease (Table 14.3). Clearly, because of health status, some indi-

viduals should not exercise (Table 14.4*A*), or should defer beginning an exercise program until their health status is improved (Table 14.4*B*).

With more recent emphasis on the health benefits from low- to moderate-level activities, less emphasis has been placed on the preparticipation or preexercise evaluation. In principle, a medical evaluation of questionable clinical significance is one less obstacle to overcome for most who wish to become more active. However, the opportunity for an individual assessment of health, motivation, and goals may be more beneficial in the long term. If simply becoming more active and reaping the benefits of low- to moderate-level activity is a goal, then initial medical evaluation may not be necessary. If more specific sports performance goals (in addition to the known health benefits of an active lifestyle) are an objective, then a pretraining, individual assessment is necessary.

A basic medical and performance evaluation is recommended prior to beginning any regular training program for all persons who have specific train-

Table 14.4a	DISORDERS THAT EXCLUDE ATHLETES FROM PARTICIPATING IN LOW- TO MODERATE-INTENSITY EXERCISE

Uncompensated heart failure
Uncontrollable arrhythmias
Severe or symptomatic aortic stenosis

Table 14.4b	DISORDERS THAT EXCLUDE ATHLETES FROM EXERCISE UNTIL HEALTH STATUS IMPROVES

Acute or suspected myocardial infarction
Unstable angina
Severe hypertension (systolic > 220, diastolic > 120)
Active or suspected myocarditis or pericarditis
Acute or suspected pulmonary embolus
Thrombophlebitis or intracardiac thrombi
Acute systemic infection or localized infection with constitutional symptoms
Detached retina
Uncontrolled seizures
Complicated pregnancy
Pregnancy-induced hypertension, premature rupture of membranes, persistent bleeding in second and third trimester, incompetent cervix, previous history of preterm labor, or intrauterine growth retardation
Complicated musculoskeletal problems

Table 14.3	MAJOR SYMPTOMS OF CARDIOPULMONARY DISEASE

Chest pain or discomfort consistent with angina (arm, neck, and back pain)
Shortness of breath at rest or low intensity exertion
Dizziness or syncope
Orthopnea or paroxysmal nocturnal dyspnea
Ankle edema
Palpitations or tachycardia
Intermittent claudication
Known cardiac murmur
Unusual fatigue with low-intensity exertion

ing goals. The depth (Table 14.5) and frequency of these evaluations vary. Young athletes have traditionally received a preparticipation physical prior to clearance for sports participation [7•]. The frequency and merit of this traditional type of evaluation has been questioned; however, this is often the only medical contact most adolescents will receive and is required annually in most states prior to sports participation. Initially, a thorough evaluation is warranted. Less in-depth examinations such as reviewing previous injuries and symptoms related to sudden death, cardiovascular disease, or recent infectious illness can be done on an annual basis. In most cases, repetition of the more thorough examination may be required as the athlete enters a higher level of competition, such as from high school to college.

College-age and young adults involved in competitive sports or intensive recreational training also should receive an annual review of cardiovascular and respiratory systems and a cardiovascular and dermatologic screening examination. As at every age and level of competition, a review of significant musculoskeletal injuries occurring in the past year should also be done. A previous injury is a major risk factor for repeat injury. If rehabilitation of an injury is incomplete or residual problems are identified, it is essential to include specific rehabilitation programs within the total training program. In some cases, complete rehabilitation may need to be the main training objective so as to reduce the risk of future problems and time away from training.

An oversight in the traditional preexercise evaluation is the lack of emphasis on the screening of the musculoskeletal system. Clearly, the well-placed emphasis on the evaluation of the cardiovascular health is paramount; however, overuse injuries (often due to correctable muscle imbalances or malalignments) are a more frequent cause for dropping out of a training program than cardiovascular problems. A noncompliant exerciser receives no cardiovascular benefits from exercise training. Certain muscle imbalances in strength and flexibility as well as joint and extremity malalignments have been identified as contributing to the risk of injury, especially overuse injuries (Table 14.6). Time spent in the initial evaluation identifying potential trouble areas will help direct the focus of both the initial and more advanced stages of training.

Table 14.5	EVALUATION DETAILS*

Basic preparticipation, medical history, and physical exam for everyone (if medically warranted)

History-guided, detailed physical and laboratory studies
- Exercise stress testing, nuclear imaging, or both to rule out significant coronary artery disease
- Echocardiogram, gated nuclear studies, or both to rule out significant valvular disease or heart failure
- Baseline pulmonary function testing
- Appropriate imaging and functional testing of previous musculoskeletal injuries

Sport-specific performance-based testing
- Strength measurements
- Power measurements (vertical jump, medicine-ball throw, Cybex testing)
- Flexibility
- Aerobic capacity—VO₂max
- Lactate threshold—sport speed at 4 mmol/L of lactate or percent of VO₂max at blood–lactate concentration 1 mmol/L above extrapolated baseline

Adapted from Kibler [8]; with permission.
VO_2max—maximum oxygen consumption.

Table 14.6	ANATOMIC RISK FACTORS FOR MUSCULOSKELETAL INJURY

Foot pronation $\geq 5°–10°$
Cavus or planus feet
Tibial torsion
Genu varus/valgus of knee
Superior lateral tracking defect of patella
Poor tone vastus medialis obliques muscle
Q-angle $\geq 20°$
Leg length discrepancy
Pelvic obliquity
Hyperlordotic lumbar spine
Inflexibility
   Hamstrings
   Lumbar spine
   Foot plantar and dorsiflexors
   Extensors and flexors of the forearm
Muscle weakness
   Dorsiflexors of foot
   Hamstrings
   Hip rotators
   Spinal intervertebral groups
   Abdominal muscles
   Rotator cuff group
   Cervical flexors and extensors

BASIC CONDITIONING

In order for any training program to provide a successful outcome it should be designed with respect to the five basic principles of exercise training (Table 14.7). Physiologic *adaptation* is the body's ability to adjust to physical stresses. Ideally, by progressively increasing an aerobic or strength-promoting load, the body will respond by gaining endurance or strength. With too much of a load, the body's adaptive response is to breakdown, resulting in poor performance. Frequent reevaluation of performance is important for determining the rate of adaptation. The adaptive process for neuromuscular coordination and metabolic systems are *specific* to the type of training. Runners who specifically run fast during training will adapt and run faster. Lifters who train with heavy weights will adapt and be able to lift heavier weights. Rowers accustomed to training at intensities that require a high amount of lactate production will adapt to higher levels of lactate during competition. Thus, the training principles of *adaptation* and *specificity* are closely related. Appropriate *progression* and *recovery* are also essential principles of training. Because of the adaptive process, the training load must be appropriately increased in order for the adaptive process to continue in a positive direction. The adaptive process takes time, and complete adaptation is dependent on an individual's ability to recover from training loads. The tendency for athletes to overtrain is directly related to incomplete recovery. A training program must by *individualized* to reflect each athlete's unique training goals, sports played, recovery ability, interests, and abilities [9•].

General fitness conditioning

For many years, the foundation for obtaining basic health benefits from exercise conditioning has been based on specific training guidelines established by the ACSM [10•]. Only recently have the ACSM guidelines been significantly modified. Current evidence suggests that the majority of health benefits associated with regular exercise can be gained by less formal exercise training and by adapting a healthy lifestyle. A recently published recommendation coauthored by the CDC and the ACSM emphasizes that every adult should accumulate 30 minutes or more of daily, moderately intense physical activity. Ideally, the increased activity should increase daily caloric expenditure by 840 kJ (1

kJ=0.24 kcal) [10,11]. The 30 minutes of activity may be continuous or intermittent, and can include walking 2 miles, climbing stairs, gardening, housework, and sports activities. Regular resistance and flexibility training should also be a part of regular activity program [11]. Collectively, the goal of the U.S. Department of Health and Human Services' program, *Healthy People 2000*, is to "increase to at least 30% the proportion of people aged 6 and older who engage . . . daily in light to moderate physical activity for at least 30 minutes per day" [12]. Certainly all physicians should strive to meet this goal or better it within their own practice.

Although these guidelines are a major breakthrough in that they will affect the sedentary majority, it is important to remember that the physiologic benefits of exercise follow a dose-dependent response. Based on many years of research, a program of exercise to promote general fitness should include aerobic exercise for 20 to 60 minutes per session, using large muscle groups in a rhythmic fashion at an intensity of 50% to 85% of maximum, repeated three to five times per week. Resistance training should also be included in any general fitness program at least two to three times per week. Regular flexibility training, especially involving the low back, hamstrings, and calves, is beneficial for performance and injury prevention and should be done three to five times per week. Many well-written reviews of aerobic, strength, and flexibility training describe training specifics in greater detail than provided in this review [13•]. Those who design and prescribe an optimal form of exercise training should use and become familiar with the latest edition of the ACSM's *Guidelines for Exercise Testing and Prescription*. This is an invaluable pocket resource for determining the ideal duration, intensity, frequency, and mode of exercise. Additional resources are available on the design of strength training and flexibility programs for general fitness and sport-specific conditioning [14,15].

Table 14.7	BASIC PRINCIPLES OF TRAINING
	Adaptation
	Specificity
	Progression
	Recovery
	Individualization

Sport-specific conditioning

Achieving the specific physiologic benefits that most athletes need to actively pursue sport-specific conditioning and skill development requires more generalized training than simply following an active lifestyle. In a well-described model for sport-specific training, Kibler and Chandler [16•], proposed that optimal athletic performance depends on successful progression from a foundation of general athletic fitness to a program of sport-specific conditioning prior to intensive training that emphasizes the improvement of sport-specific skills (Fig. 14.2). Without an adequate general fitness base, the athlete will have difficulty reaching the high levels of training volume required for sport-specific conditioning and skills training. Beginning with a program of low-intensity, longer-duration exercise provides basic physiologic improvements, such as increased blood volume, cardiac output/stroke volume, and improved metabolic efficiency. Additional training to build basic muscle hypertrophy, capillary density, flexibility, and strength is the foundation on which the more advanced training program will be built.

Following the Kibler and Chandler model, once the competitive athlete has attained the basic benefits of general athletic fitness, the second objective of optimal training is the attainment of sport-specific fitness. The major difference in general fitness training and training for recreational or competitive sports is the emphasis on the specificity of training in the latter. Following the basic principles of training, repetitive demands are placed on the anatomic areas, metabolic systems, muscular force couples, and biomechanical patterns that are essential for a specific sport. The adaptive response to the increased stress determines the level of improvement. In order for the adaptive process to occur, a balance must be maintained between placing too much stress on a system and allowing for complete recovery. An imbalance toward incomplete recovery increases the risks of poor performance, overuse injuries, and the overtraining syndrome. It has been difficult to define an ideal balance that proceeds along the "edge of the envelope" in order to optimize athletic performance.

Periodization

The periodization model for exercise training is an attempt to organize training into specific time periods, each with specific training goals, objectives, and training tasks in order to target and build toward an optimal performance level [17]. By varying the training volume, intensity, and tasks, periodized training attempts not only to optimize performance but also to reduce the risks of training boredom, noncompliance, and overtraining (Fig. 14.3 and Table 14.8). Periodized training schedules, first applied to weight lifters and power athletes, can be applied to sports-specific conditioning and specific skill training for other athletes as well. Periodized training may also be a useful model for a program of general fitness.

Anecdotal evidence suggests that performance is enhanced by following this basic model; however, few peer-reviewed articles provide evidence to support these positive claims. In addition, most periodized training programs are instituted by coaching professionals whose careers depend on the performance of the athletes they coach. For this reason alone, training specifics, especially successful training specifics, are less likely to be shared with others so as not to give away the competitive advantage of their athletes. Periodization training is a good plan because training specifics and progression is individualized. Unfortunately, individuality increases the variability of the training model, thus making powerful statistical conclusions difficult to obtain.

First introduced by Matveyev, a Russian physiologist, the basic principles have been adapted and modified in the United States and have been applied to the training regimens of athletes from several sports [6,14,16•,22]. Training periods or cycles are subdivided based on specific training, performance,

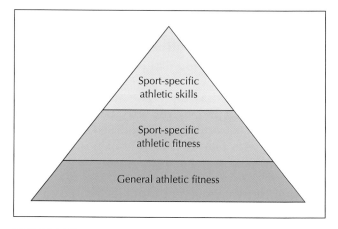

FIGURE 14.2

General athletic fitness as the base on which sport-specific athletic fitness and skills are built.(*Adapted from* Kibler and Chandler [16•]; with permission.)

and competition objectives. The largest time interval, a "macrocycle," generally lasts 1 to 4 years and symbolizes the ultimate training goal (*eg*, optimizing performance at the end of the macrocycle in order to win an Olympic medal). The macrocycle is divided into two or more "mesocycles," each with specific training and competition objectives that complement the macrocycle goal. The training objective of each mesocycle is to build toward an optimal performance at the end of each one. This is accomplished by beginning with high training volume at moderate to heavy training intensity. As the cycle progresses, training volume is decreased, whereas intensity and time spent in sport-specific skill development increase. For example, Figure 14.4 depicts the macrocycle for football. Using a calendar

year as a macrocycle, the period of active rest (transition phase) in which the athlete does no sport-specific activities is the beginning of off-season training. The emphasis during the transition phase is on physical and psychological recovery from the stress of the previous competitive season. The transition phase generally lasts 1 to 4 weeks.

Off-season conditioning begins by establishing a general fitness foundation as a main objective and can be referred to as a general fitness mesocycle. Within this mesocycle, shorter time intervals ("microcycles") focus on aerobic conditioning, muscle hypertrophy, and basic strength improvement. For example, a larger muscle is generally a stronger muscle, so microcycles emphasizing muscle hypertrophy precede microcycles emphasizing strength or power

Table 14.8	PERIODIZATION TRAINING OVERVIEW				
	HYPERTROPHY	**STRENGTH**	**POWER**	**MAINTENANCE (IN-SEASON)**	**ACTIVE REST**
Sets	3–5	3–5	3–5	1–3	Physical activity
Repetitions	8–12	2–6	2–3	1–3	(not necessarily
Volume	High	Moderate to high	Low	Very low	resistance
Intensity	Low	High	High	Very high	training)
	(60%–75% of 1 RM)	(80%–90% of 1 RM)	(90%–95% of 1 RM)	(95%–100% of 1 RM)	
Days per week	3–4	3–5	4–6	1–3	

RM—repetition maximum

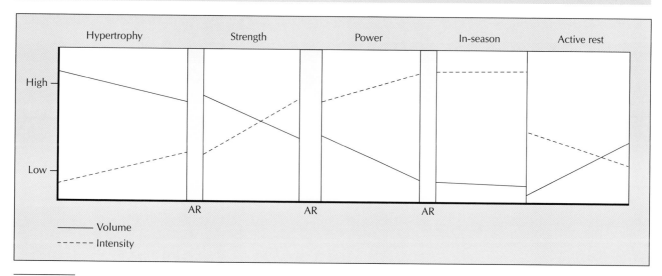

FIGURE 14.3

Periodization program.

development. During hypertrophy cycles, weight training exercises are done at moderate intensities for three to four sets of eight to 12 repetitions. During basic strength cycles, the intensity is increased, the number of repetitions is reduced, and total sets remain the same or increase. Thus, within a mesocycle, the training volume and intensity are manipulated in order to progress the athlete toward an optimal performance at the end of the mesocycle. Training volumes and intensities are adjusted within each microcycle to reflect the training objective and are

based on the results of performance variables (such as strength or 1500-meter time) maintained or improved on during the previous competitive season.

As the preseason approaches, emphasis within the mesocycle shifts away from nonspecific general fitness training towards more sport-specific conditioning. Training time focuses more emphasis on activities that reflect the sport-specific demands on the energy delivery system (aerobic and glycolytic adenosine triphosphate–phosphocreatine cycle), muscle strength, power, and flexibility. Recent infor-

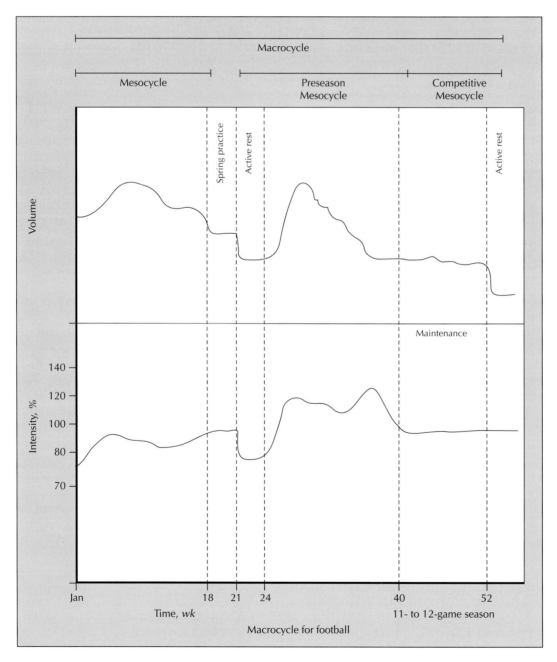

FIGURE 14.4
Macrocycle for football.

mation on performance and injury prevention indicate that training large and small muscles that specifically act as antagonists (rotator cuff and hamstring and calf muscles), should also be emphasized during this portion of the training cycle. Sport-specific conditioning comprises 70% to 80% of the training volume, with work on sports-specific skills taking up the remainder. During the preseason mesocycle, progressively less time is spent conditioning, and more time is spent on skill training.

Once the competitive mesocycle arrives, the vast majority of training time is spent on sport-specific skill training. The obvious objective during this mesocycle is success in competitions. Specific skill training typically involves repetitions of the specific skills required for optimal sport performance. During the competitive season, the objective of training is on sports skill and strategy repetitions; 90% to 95% of training time is spent on specific skill development. Examples for team sports (such as football, soccer, or basketball) include game-simulations; running, cycling, or swimming athletes will perform their sport activities at or above the speed required during competitions. Endurance athletes tend to spend more time on sport-specific conditioning, whereas team-sport athletes usually spend only 5% to 10% of training time on sports-specific conditioning. Microcycles emphasizing these specific training objectives are positioned into the training schedule 1 to 2 weeks before a competitive event or when the athlete desires "peak performance." A brief tapering-off period is desirable a few days before the targeted performance. The length of the competitive season challenges the principles of periodized training; the athlete is required to perform optimally much more frequently than during the off-season. Programs can be designed to prioritize specific games or competitions that are separated by a longer time interval, and training can be adjusted accordingly. However, suboptimal performances can be expected between the priority events.

Opinions on the emphasis of conditioning maintenance during this phase are divided. Some feel that non–sport-specific strength and conditioning gains, although less rapid, can continue through the competitive season. Others feel that nonspecific gains cannot be made during the competitive cycle and that the objective of competitive phase conditioning should be on maintaining levels achieved in the preseason. Regardless of the conditioning outcome, the volume of conditioning training is dramatically reduced to 5% to 10% of total training

time. Intense exercises such as Olympic-style weight lifting, plyometrics, and interval sprints are included within the training program. Adequate rest periods should be taken between intense exercises, intense skill workouts, or competitions. Prolonged, low- to moderate-intensity exercise during the competitive season are only encouraged on active rest days—usually days following competition.

During a competitive season, the demands for peak performances are more frequent. Optimal physical performance is most dependent on the ability of the athlete to skillfully, economically, and strategically maximize power output. It also takes a determined psychological focus and "mental toughness" to maintain and repeat the incredible physical demands placed on the system. In order to improve performance and for the neuromuscular and metabolic systems to adapt, the athlete must repetitively exert maximal or supramaximal effort. Repetitions required to achieve the ideal neuromuscular patterning or coordination to improve skill are numerous. The goal of many athletes and coaches is to physically perform "without thinking"—in other words, to develop a subcortical or reflex level of sport-specific coordination. This also places a metabolic demand on the athlete that is beyond what is required for sport-specific conditioning. Athletes who are able to successfully train at these levels will optimize their individual potential while avoiding injury or illness in the process. Recreational athletes, by genetics, or natural selection, are more susceptible to overuse and overtraining problems than elite-level athletes. Thus, the vast majority of training time for the recreational athlete should be sport-specific conditioning with infrequent, short (5- to 7-day) microcycles. These microcycles should emphasize sport-specific skill training consisting of short bursts or intervals at or above the target performance level for competition.

Sport-specific skills training

Recent training advances have provided valuable information on how specific training principles can be used to improve performance. In order to improve performance and repeat maximal output, the athlete must improve 1) total power output, 2) efficiency of power output, 3) duration of sustained power output, or 4) the time it takes to recover from maximal power outputs. Achieving this requires intense training—training that rides the "edge of the envelope" toward optimal performance. On one side of the edge is too little training in order to improve, and on the other is too much training, which results in breaking down. Because of the intense nature of the training required to optimize performance, athletes must have successfully progressed through a program of general fitness and sport-specific conditioning. Although most research has focused on endurance athletes, the following information can be implemented into a high-level sports-specific conditioning program for team-sport athletes or used during a competitive mesocycle for endurance or power athletes.

Maximal effort places an increased metabolic demand on the athlete resulting in decreased power output over time and early fatigue. Power output at the lactate threshold, the economy of energy generation, and the economy of movement provide the most variation in endurance performance [5•]. Economy of movement will be developed by multiple repetitions of the specific sport skill. The economy of energy generation is partially determined genetically by the relative proportion of Type I muscle fibers, which are metabolically more efficient, and by sport-specific training and conditioning [5•]. Training should focus on exercise that will delay the accumulation of lactate at submaximal exercise loads and improve the tolerance to elevated lactate levels at or near maximal loads. Increasing the volume of high-intensity interval training has been reported to improve submaximal lactate levels; power output at the lactate threshold; and overall performance in elite level runners, cyclists, swimmers and rowers.

Running speed for races longer than 10 km strongly correlates to running speed or velocity at LT [18]. Trained distance runners who added high-intensity (90% to 95% of maximum heart rate) running intervals, decreased lactate levels in the 85% to 90% VO$_2$max range, increased lactate threshold, and improved 10-km times [19]. Trained cyclists who added six to eight repetitions of 5-minute cycling bursts at 80% of peak power, improved 40-kilometer times after 4 weeks of training [20]. Cyclists who had a higher LT (82% of VO$_2$max) were able to continue cycling at a pace corresponding to 88% of VO$_2$max twice as long (60 minutes vs 29 minutes) as those with a lower LT (66% of VO$_2$max) [5•]. Elite rowers also demonstrated a positive correlation between improvement of LT and performance time following periods of intense training [4].

An interesting athletic population are competitive middle- and short-distance runners who exceed both the running speeds associated with LT and VO$_2$max during races. These athletes, either by genetics or

training, are able to tolerate elevated lactate levels during competition for 8 to 11 minutes beyond the LT [21]. In one of few descriptive studies of the training habits of elite runners, Hewson and Hopkins [22] reported a negative correlation between the best short- or middle-distance performance times and the relative training pace during moderate-intensity runs. The study implied that time spent on moderate training had no effect on the ability to run at a higher relative intensity during competitive events. Rowers, like middle-distance runners, tolerate elevated lactate levels; their performance is related to the rate of lactate clearance capabilities [23,24]. Training at supramaximal levels obviously increases blood–lactate levels, which may have a beneficial effect on tolerance to high lactate levels. Successful performance should follow the adaptation to high levels of lactate production, reinforcing the importance of training specificity on the energy generating system.

Cross-training

Cross-training has become vastly more popular in the last 10 years, perhaps due to the popularity and increased participation in triathlons. Activities that use similar muscle groups are effective in maintaining fitness during the competitive season and as an alternative form of conditioning in the off-season. In one of a few studies on well-trained runners, stationary cycling was alternated with running workouts for 5 weeks at the same relative intensity (85% to 90% of VO$_2$max). There were no posttraining differences in 1600-m and 5-km times between the run-trained and cross-trained groups [25]. Cross-training studies combining swimming, stair climbing, and in-line skating with running all indicate that these activities may be substituted for running without affecting run performance [26,27]. Rowers who substituted versiclimber exercise for training with a stationary rowing ergometer had a higher posttraining VO$_2$max than rowers who did only stationary ergometer training or running [28]. Cyclists and swimmers are not able to substitute running without adversely affecting performance time, suggesting greater specificity of the training required for optimal performance of these sports. For performance and aerobic benefit, training with dissimilar modes (different muscle groups) is more beneficial for improving aerobic capacity in persons with lower initial fitness levels and is, thus, ideal for persons in general fitness programs or recreational athletes. Athletes with higher aerobic capacities who cross-train experience less gains from nonspecific training and sport-specific performance and so should not expect sport-specific improvements in performance with regular cross-training [29•].

Intense strength and power training

Intense strength training improves the performance of power athletes such as weight lifters and weight throwers, and is included in the training programs for athletes from many sports. During the preseason phase, these athletes must maximize gains in hypertrophy, strength, and power by appropriately and timely adjusting lifting intensity and total training volume. As the competitive season draws near, training intensities approach maximum and volume is adjusted to optimize high power output. During the competitive season, strength as well as high power output may be maintained up to 6 to 8 weeks by training with four to five weight exercises weekly (*eg*, Olympic-style lifts at intensities from 75% to 90% of maximum for one set of four to eight repetitions).

Endurance athletes generally benefit from including some form of moderate strength training into the off-season and preseason program. During preseason or competitive season, when training emphasis is on intense sport-specific endurance and anaerobic training, there appears to be no benefit from adding nonspecific, intense weight training. Rowers and swimmers had no benefit in performance after periods of intense training that included more then one to two moderate-intensity weight workouts during the competitive season [30,31]. These findings add to the continuing debate over the importance of maintaining non–sport-specific performance during a competitive season.

Jumpers benefit from intense strength training, which also optimizes power output. Heavy weight training, Olympic-style lifting, and plyometric training have traditionally been included in training to improve jumping performance. Recent information from Kramer and Newton [6] suggests that heavy weight training may be detrimental for jumping. During maximal lifts, muscle units are trained to produce high power at a slow velocity. In order to apply the principle of training specificity, squat-lifting exercises done at 30% to 60% of maximum closely corresponds to the maximal mechanical power output (MMPO) during jumping for most athletes. Squat lifts at these intensities performed to mimic jumping (including leaving the ground) have a positive effect on jumping performance [32]. MMPO training can be included into a periodized training schedule for long and high jumpers, basketball players, gymnasts, and all athletes who desire to improve vertical or horizontal jumping abilities. Researchers and coaches may experiment by using similar MMPO-type exercises for the upper body to improve power output in throwers. Due to the high power output required to perform MMPO-type exercises, MMPO training should be done near the end of a mesocycle, appropriately preceded by a sequential program emphasizing muscle hypertrophy, strength, and power development. The use of MMPO during the competitive season may be inappropriate because the load of sport-specific skill development may be adequate to maintain the ability to delivery high power output while jumping.

Volume of training

Increasing the duration or volume of training during the preseason or competitive phases has few reported positive influences on performance. Marathon runners and ultradistance runners have a direct correlation between optimal performance and amount of time spent running at the velocity at the LT [22]. Swimmers who trained twice daily for 6 weeks had no greater improvement in swim performance than those trained at half the training load (once daily). It should be no surprise that the twice-daily swimmers had a comparable *decrease* in swim velocity at the end of the 6-week period during shorter events, suggesting that the extra training was specific for swimming at a slower velocity [33]. Runners, cyclists, rowers, and weight lifters all have less optimal performances when training volume is high. Although it would be difficult to quantify, a performance drop-off in team-sport athletes would be expected when the training volume is high. The increase in training intensity required for competitive success would clearly result in non–peak performance and may lead to unnecessary overuse injuries and symptoms of overtraining. For these reasons, most periodized training schedules have built-in tapering-off periods in both volume and intensity before peak performances are planned.

Conditioning synopsis

Optimal athletic training and conditioning evolves from progressive stages: an active lifestyle, generalized fitness, sport-specific fitness, and sport-specific skill training. The progression between and within these stages is more of an art than a science and presents perhaps the greatest challenge for designing an optimal training program. It is important to keep in perspective the individual goals for training and design the schedule to reflect meeting these goals at an ideal opportunity. By definition of training specificity, optimal performance is reflective of the "appropriate" amount of sport-specific conditioning and skill development. This appropriate amount is totally dependent on the individual and is based on balancing continued improvement in performance with the risk of injury or overtraining. Periodized training, although lacking clear supportive evidence for promoting positive outcomes, appears to be an ideal model for individualized training and providing a "road map" for training progression toward specific performance goals.

OVERUSE INJURIES AND OVERTRAINING

Progressive overload is the basis for exercise training. Excessive overload is the basis for overuse injuries. Athletes of all abilities are susceptible to overuse injuries. The greatest periods of risk are on return from inactivity or injury, when training volume or intensity is increased too rapidly following the addition of a new sport skill. Adequate recovery periods are essential to enable the body's system to positively adapt to training. Incomplete recovery will result in a negative adaptation, *ie*, injury or overtraining. The risk of overtraining is related to the rate of training progression. The progression of training volume should not increase more then 10% per week. Progression greater then 10% per week can result in an overuse injury within 6 to 8 weeks. Progression of 50% per week shortens the time to overuse injury to within 2 to 3 weeks. Increases of 100% per week or more can produce an injury in days [34••].

Risks factors of overuse injuries

Previous injury and amount of exercise (absolute and relative)

In a review of exercise training and injuries confirmed by prospective study data, previous injury and the total exercise exposure time have the most influence on the risks for overuse injuries [35,36•]. In a previous epidemiologic study, male and female runners who run more miles per week have a greater risk of injury [37]. Military recruit studies confirm the increased risks of injuries associated with increased running mileage [35,38].

The risk of overuse injury appears to be greatest in those beginning a program of regular exercise. The previous inactivity of sedentary military recruits is directly related to injury rate, suggesting that novice runners are at greater risk [35,39]. In runners, the relative injury rate (the rate of injury per mile run) is *inversely related* to the amount of total mileage. The relative injury rate tends to level off above 20 miles per week [37]. Studies of military recruits confirm that the relative injury rate *decreases* as the cumulative mileage *increases* [35,38]. These studies suggest that a positive training effect occurs, presumably, as running abilities improve with increased volume. Less epidemiologic data are available for other sports; however, it appears intuitively that beginner or novice athletes should use caution because the relative risk of overuse injury appears to be greatest in the least experienced.

Inexperience

There is perhaps no more clear-cut example of inexperience leading to problems with overuse than studies comparing shoulder overuse problems between experienced and inexperienced baseball pitchers. Inexperienced throwers tend to rely more on arm strength as opposed to total body strength used by experienced throwers. There also appears to be a training effect on the coordination of rapid movements involving the rotator cuff (RTC) muscles during pitching in elite-level pitchers, which is not seen in less experienced pitchers [40]. Too much stress on the shoulder using improper mechanics magnifies problems with coordination, poor endurance, and weakness of the small RTC muscles. These problems lead to several overuse problems including subacromial bursitis, and RTC tendonitis and tears. RTC exercises should be incorporated early in the sport-specific conditioning program and continued into the training program for all overhead athletes.

Effects of small muscle groups

Similar to the RTC muscle groups, loss of relative strength, endurance, or coordination involving active or antagonistic muscle groups can lead to diminished performance and overuse injury. Imbalances in small muscle groups can be found in athletes with chronic low back pain, anterior knee pain, patella tendonitis, and medial tibial stress syndrome (shin splints). Lumbar stabilization exercises help to improve the strength, flexibility, and endurance of the intravertebral muscles in the lumbar region. The use of lumbar stabilization programs early in the training program may reduce down time from training due to low back problems. Inflexibility and weakness to eccentric loads in the dorsiflexors of the foot have recently been found to contribute to anterior knee pain and patella tendonitis (jumper's knee). Theoretically, the inability to handle the eccentric loads associated with running and jumping may also lead to shin splints or stress fractures of the lower leg. Adding eccentric and concentric strengthening exercises for the dorsiflexors of the foot should be incorporated into the training program of jumping athletes [41].

Anatomic factors

Several anatomic factors that have also been identified as presenting an increased risk of overuse injuries are presented in Table 14.6. The anatomic malalignment, rearfoot valgus (pronation), has been reported by many authors to have notable effects on overuse injuries higher up the kinetic chain. Clinically significant pronation is defined as the angle of the Achilles tendon being in excess of 10° (a 4° to 8° pronation is normal). Numerous chronic injuries are associated with excessive pronation, including patella–femoral dysfunction, illiotibial band syndrome, medial tibial stress syndrome, and plantar fasciitis. Most of these clinical problems respond favorably to the addition of orthoses.

In a recent prospective study of 136 European college students followed over a 4-year period of recreational sports activity, Twellaar *et al*. [42•] reported that pelvic obliquity (an imbalance in the heights of the iliac crests) was related to chronic back pain and shin splits. The authors found no other significant relationship to injury between various measurements, including joint flexibility, leg length discrepancy, knee alignment, rearfoot position, cavus/planus foot, or anthropometric measurements. Few other prospective studies of this type have been published. Unfortunately, the amount and type of activity were not quantified in this publication with the same vigor as the body measurements; therefore, a true "overtraining effect" cannot be determined.

Incorporating rehabilitation into the training program

As previously emphasized, it is essential to identify potential anatomic problems that can lead to overuse injury and correct them early to reduce time away from training. However, even in the best circumstances, overuse injuries do occur, and the rehabilitative process becomes the main focus of the training program. Training errors are one of the most common causes of overuse injuries. Therefore, during the rehabilitative process, it is important to reevaluate the training program, both what was planned and what was actually done. In addition to modifying any errors, modification of the training program should reflect a simple rule of thumb: REST or resume exercise below the soreness threshold [34••]. Soreness or pain is an indicator of microtrauma—both will be adversely affected by the repetitive movements and loads that caused the injury in the first place. Using pain as a guide is usually an accurate clinical yardstick as to the state of recovery following an overuse injury. Describing a more detailed rehabilitative program for overuse is beyond the scope of this chapter. For a more indepth presentation, the reader is referred to a very good recent review article by O'Conner *et al*. [43].

Eliminating all painful movements will reduce pain; however, complete elimination of a sport-specific activity is difficult for most competitive athletes and may not need to be the first step in many situations. It is within reason to initially modify training to allow for some sport activity and provide time for adequate recovery. Specific suggestions to modify the training program include reducing the total volume 25% to 50%, the intensity 10% to 20%, and the frequency 25% to 50%. Modification of the program to include cross-training activities that allow the injured area to recover is an option for rehabilitation.

One type of cross-training exercise that deserves mention is water running. Water running has become an alternative to running for injured athletes. Water provides an appropriate low-impact medium to remove the biomechanical stresses associated with running, allowing the healing process to continue. Training benefits are dependent on the running style and previous experience of training, suggesting a learned effect. In a recent study comparing the effects of 6 weeks of water running to "land" running in experienced runners, no differences in VO_2max, LT, or running economy were observed [44]. This finding suggests that water running can be an aid in the maintenance of aerobic fitness and running economy during periods of injury rehabilitation. For exercise prescription purposes, it is important to understand the changes in cardiac output distribution and heart rate that occur during complete water immersion exercise. Depending on the water temperature, cardiac output becomes more cephalic and central blood flow distribution increases. Increases in heart rate are slower and are also directly related to temperature. Until water temperatures approach body temperature (28° to 35°C), near maximal efforts result in a lower heart rate when compared with "land" efforts. This result is due to decreased sympathetic neural output during water exercise. Static lung volumes also decrease during water exercise secondary to increased hydrostatic-induced thoracic pressure. In order to keep up with metabolic demands, breathing frequency must increase to maintain minute ventilation [45].

Inadequate recovery

Too much load without adequate recovery time violates one of the basic training principles and results in several overuse injuries, including an increased risk of tendon injuries. Archanbault *et al.* [46], in a review of tendon overuse injuries, lists training errors (specifically inadequate recovery), inappropriate playing conditions, muscle imbalances, and skeletal malalignments as the biggest contributors to overuse injuries of tendons. From animal studies, tendons adapt well to loads associated with exercise, if allowed time to complete the recovery process. The ideal recovery time varies according to the involved tendon and the relative load placed on the tendon. In humans, 24 hours is considered to be adequate recovery; however, this guideline is based predominantly on information regarding adequate

recovery of metabolic stores (*ie*, glycogen replenishment). The ideal amount of time required to complete the recovery process for muscle and tendons is unknown. Clinical pain is a sign of incomplete recovery and is a late manifestation of the postexercise inflammatory response. The inflammatory response is believed to be the adaptive response to exercise. Persistent pain indicates inadequate tissue recovery and excess inflammation. With early overuse injuries, pain may not be present and will not be a sensitive indicator of inadequate recovery. Additional research is needed to identify the ideal recovery time as well as sensitive markers for incomplete recovery.

Overtraining

Clinical and performance outcomes can benefit from the early identification of chronic incomplete recovery. Chronic incomplete recovery is directly associated with the overtraining syndrome in which performance decreases despite increasing or steady workloads. In addition to overuse injuries, athletes are susceptible to the overtraining syndrome during periods of intense training. Both elite and recreational athletes are equally prone to overtraining, especially those who are multiple-sport or year-round athletes. Well described in several previous publications, overtraining generally refers to a decrease in performance despite increased training [13•,47]. Several physiologic, psychologic, and performance signs and symptoms of overtraining have been recognized (Table 14.9). The most common

Table 14.9	COMMON SIGNS AND SYMPTOMS OF OVERTRAINING*		

Performance aspects
  Failure to improve as season
    progresses
  Inability to complete usual practice
    sessions
  Increased susceptibility to injuries
 	
Psychologic aspects
  Emotional lability
  Decreased motivation and apathy
  Loss of self-confidence
  Depression
	Physiologic aspects
	  Increased resting blood pressure
	  Prolonged recovery time (heart rate
	    and blood pressure)
	  Decreased glycogen stores
	  Decreased appetite
	  Decreased body mass
	  Postural hypertension
	  Excessive thirst
	  Increased serum catecholamines
	  Increased serum cortisol
	  Hypoglycemia with exercise
		Decreased serum testosterone
		Increased muscle enzymes
		Insomnia
		Frequent upper respiratory illness
		Decreased immunoglobulin
		  production
		Increased sedimentation rate
		Decreased serum iron and ferritin
		Subcostal pain
		Muscle soreness without apparent
		  cause	

*From Sevier and Jones [13•]; with permission.

presenting symptom in overtrained athletes is fatigue. It is generally believed that when fatigue or any other clinical findings are present, the athlete has already suffered a decrease in performance and crossed over the "edge of the envelope." Recovery from overtraining may take weeks to months; thus, early recognition and prevention are key.

A well-planned training schedule is one major key to preventing overtraining. By following periods of heavy training with built-in recovery periods, the periodized training design can be beneficial in reducing the risks of overtraining. The basic periodization concept of monitoring and reducing the training volume during cycles of high intensity training also reduces overtraining risks.

It needs to be emphasized that a training plan that is designed to optimize individual performance should be specifically designed for an individual; thus, it defeats the purpose to apply the same training program to all athletes or even athletes on the same team. If a team's abilities are to be more than just the sum of its parts, then each athlete must have a training program individually designed to optimize the potential performance contribution.

Markers for overtraining

Even with the best designs or intentions, overtraining does occur. In addition to reducing training errors, research into identifying early markers of overtraining continue. Research into identifying early biochemical markers remains inconclusive. The serum testosterone/cortisol (T/C) ratio is an index of the catabolic state of the individual—a lower ratio represents a decreased potential for complete recovery. The decrease in the ratio is most often due to prolonged postexercise levels of cortisol, which can remain elevated 24 to 48 hours after strenuous exercise or competition. After prolonged overtraining, testosterone levels will fall, further reducing the T/C ratio. Although adequate testosterone levels are essential for protein synthesis, the clinical relevance of lowered testosterone levels induced by overtraining has yet to be determined. A drop in the T/C ratio of greater than 30% is representative of insufficient recovery and has been associated with a clinical history of fatigue, decreased performance, and heavy training [48,49]. A low T/C ratio, in conjunction with clinical findings, helps to confirm the diagnosis of overtraining. A similar increase in resting norepinephrine

levels in swimmers who had clinical symptoms of overtraining has also been reported [50]. As an early marker for overtraining, the sensitivity of T/C ratio and norepinephrine levels are generally considered to be low.

Recent attention has been given to studies measuring lower resting levels of plasma glutamine (a major energy substrate for the many components of the immune system) in overtrained athletes [51]. Many authors report that glutamine is used at a high rate even when immune cells are quiescent. Speculation that the increased susceptibility to infections in overtrained athletes may be the direct result of depleted glutamine levels following intense, long-duration exercise [52]. Studies examining the effects of glutamine supplementation will inevitably show no systemic effects because nearly all of ingested glutamine is absorbed and used metabolically by intestinal cells. The main source of glutamine is from skeletal muscle. Supplementation with branched-chain amino acids has been shown to prevent postexercise decrease in plasma glutamine concentration [53]. The use of low glutamine levels as a sensitive early marker of overtraining has theoretical promise. The sensitivity of glutamine as an early overtraining marker would probably be enhanced by observing a downward trend in resting levels while simultaneously monitoring performance in clinical findings.

The cytokine interleuken (IL)-6, produced by macrophages in response to infectious and noninfectious agents, induces the liver-cell-mediated acute-phase response that follows infection, stress, and exercise [54]. In the resting state, serum or plasma IL-6 levels are undetectable. Following prolonged strenuous exercise, elevations in serum IL-6 have been reported using the specific 7TD1 immunoassay. Postexercise elevations in cortisol act in a synergistic fashion with IL-6 in stimulating the acute-phase response. Many symptoms of overtraining are less severe symptoms of the acute-phase response initiated by IL-6, including elevated body temperatures, fatigue, cachexia, and elevated resting heart rate. Detectable postexercise or resting elevation in IL-6 may be a potential early marker of overtraining.

CONCLUSIONS

Those pushing the limits of their sport are more likely to be directed by an intuitive art form practiced by gifted coaches than by knowledgeable scientists.

Elite coaches can 1) recognize individual strengths, needs, and level of ability; 2) apply the rate of training volume progression required to obtain optimal performance; and 3) tell when the athlete has strayed from this path—all the while motivating the athlete to consistently follow this regimen.

All would agree that there are few who possess this intuitive ability. What we as scientists (lay coaches?) attempt to do is to analytically tap into the pattern-recognition abilities of the elite coach in order to provide training information for those athletes and coaches lacking in this innate, intuitive sense of ideal training. Elite coaches need not worry, though. We scientists are way behind them.

REFERENCES AND RECOMMENDED READING

Recently published papers of particular interest have been highlighted as:

- Of special interest
- •• Of outstanding interest

1. Will PM, Demko TM, George DL: Prescribing exercise for health: a simple framework for primary care. *Am Family Phys* 1996, 53:579–585.

2. King AC, Martin JE: Adherence to exercise. In *Resource Manual for Guidelines for Exercise Testing and Prescription*, ed 1. Edited by SN Blair, P Painter, RR Pate, *et al.* Philadelphia: Lea & Febigerp; 1988:335–344.

3. Koutedakis Y: Seasonal variation in fitness parameters in competitive athletes. *Sports Med* 1995, 19:373–392.

4. Billat LV: Use of blood lactate measurements for prediction of exercise performance and for control of training: recommendations for long distance runners. *Sports Med* 1996, 22:157–175.

5.• Coyle E: Integration of the physiologic factors determining endurance performance ability. *Exer Sport Sci Rev* 1995,23:25–63.
This article is helpful to understand the latest theory and basic principles of optimal endurance performance.

6. Kraemer WJ, Newton RU: Training for improved vertical jump. *Sports Science Exchange* 1994, 7:1–5

7.• *Preparticipation Physical Evaluation*, ed 2. Edited by The Preparticipation Physical Evaluation Task of the AFP, AMSSM, AOSSM, AOASM. Minneapolis: McGraw-Hill; 1997.
A prerequisite for performing preparticipation exams; well-diagramed with excellent tables.

8. Kibler WB: *The Sport Preparticipation Fitness Examination.* Champaign, IL: Human Kinetics Books; 1990.

9.• Wilmore JH, Costill DL: *Physiology of Sport and Exercise.* Champaign, IL: Human Kinetics Books; 1994.
Overall, an excellent reference text on exercise science.

10.•• *ACSM's Guidelines for Exercise Testing and Prescription*, ed 5. Baltimore: Williams and Wilkins; 1995.
Essential, easy-to-use, pocket-book reference for those who want to accurately design an exercise program; the "gold standard" used by exercise physiologists.

11. Pate RR, Pratt M, Blair SN, *et al.*: Physical activity and public health: a recommendation from the Centers for Disease Control and the American College of Sports Medicine. *JAMA* 1995, 273:402–407.

12. US Department of Health and Human Services: *Healthy People 2000: National Health Promotion and Disease Prevention Objectives.* Washington D.C.: US Department of Health and Human Services; 1991. [DHHS Publication no. (PHS) 91-50212.]

13.• Sevier TL, Jones JW: Optimizing training and conditioning. In *Current Reviews of Sports Medicine*, ed 1. Edited by Johnson RJ, Lombardo J. Philadelphia: Current Medicine; 1994:248–265.
Excellent explanation of energy systems and a basis for flexibility and strength training.

14. Fleck S, Kraemer W: *Designing Strength and Conditioning Programs.* Champaign, IL: Human Kinetics Books; 1987.

15. Anderson B: *Stretching* Bolinas, CA: Shelter Publications; 1980.

16.• Kibler WB, Chandler J: Sport specific conditioning. *Am J Sports Med* 1994,22: 424–432.
Well-written description of the general and specific application of periodization. Specific training programs for football and tennis are included.

17. Baechle, T: *Strength and Conditioning.* Champaigne, IL: Human Kinetics Books; 1994.

18. Allen WK, Seals DR, Hurley BF, *et al.*: Lactate threshold and distance running performance in young and older endurance athletes. *J Appl Physiol* 1985, 58:1281–1284

19. Acevedo EO, Goldfarb AH: Increased training intensity effects on plasma lactate, ventilatory threshold, and endurance. *Med Sci Sports Exerc* 1989, 21:563–568.

20. Lindsay FH, Hawley JA, Myburgh KH, Schomer HH, Noakes TD, Dennis SC. Improved athletic performance in highly trained cyclists after interval training. *Med Sci Sports Exerc.* 1996,28:1427–1434.

21. Brandon LJ: Physiological factors associated with middle distance running performance. *Sports Med* 1995, 19:268–277.

22. Hewson DJ, Hopkins WG: Specificity of training and its relation to the performance of distance runners. *Int J Sports Med* 1996, 17:199–204

23. Bangsbo J, Mchalsik L, Peterson A: Accumulated O_2 deficit during intense exercise and muscle characteristics of elite athletes. *Int J Sports Med* 1993, 14:207–213.

24. Messonnier L, Freund H, Bourdin M, *et al.*: Lactate exchange and removal abilities in rowing performance. *Med Sci Sports Exerc* 1997, 29:396–401

25. Mutton DL, Loy SF, Rogers DM, *et al.*: Effect of run vs. combined cycle/run training on VO_2max and running performance. *Med Sci Sports Exerc* 1993, 25:1393–1397.

26. Snyder AC, O'Hagen KP, Clifford PS, *et al.*: Exercise responses to in-line skating: comparisons to running and cycling. *Int J Sports Med* 1993, 14:38–42.

27. Melanson EL, Freedson PS, Jungbluth S: Changes in VO$_2$max and maximal treadmill time after 9 weeks of running or in-line skating. *Med Sci Sports Exerc* 1996, 28:1422–1426.

28. Brahler CJ, Blank SE. VersaClimbing elicits higher VO$_2$max than does treadmill running or rowing ergometry. *Med Sci Sports Exerc* 1995, 27:249–254.

29.• Loy SF, Hoffinan JJ, Holland GJ: Benefits and practical use of cross training in sports. *Sports Med* 1995, 19:1–8.
A good, broad, and simplified explanation of cross-training principles and techniques

30. Bell GJ, Syrotuik DG, Atwood K, *et al.*: Maintenance of strength gains while performing endurance training in oarswomen. *Can J Appl Phys* 1993, 18:104–115.

31. Tanaka H, Costill DL, Thomas R, *et al.*: Dry-land resistance training for competitive swimming. *Med Sci Sports Exerc* 1993, 25:952–959.

32. Wilson GJ, Newton RU, Murphy AJ, Humphries BJ: The optimal training load for the development of dynamic athletic performance. *Med Sci Sports Exerc* 1993, 25:1279–1286.

33. Costill DL, Thomas R, Robergs RA, *et al.*: Adaptations to swimming training: influence of training volume. *Med Sci Sports Exerc* 1991, 23:371–377.

34.•• Scott WA: Overuse injuries. In *ACSM's Essentials of Sports Medicine*. Edited by Sailis RE, Massimino F. St. Louis: Mosby; 1996:517–527.
Easy-to-follow outline form with excellent tables.

35. Jones BH, Cowan DN, Knapik JJ: Exercise, training and injuries. *Sports Med* 1994, 18:202–214.

36.• Van Mechelen W, Twisk J, Molendijk A, *et al.*: Subject-related risk factors for sports injuries: a I year prospective study in young adults. *Med Sci Sports Exerc* 1996, 28:1171–1179.
One of a few prospective studies on injury risk factors that includes psychological factors.

37. Koplan JP, Powell KE, Sikes RK, *et al.*: An epidemiologic study of the benefits and risks of running. *JAMA* 1982, 248:3118–3121.

38. Jones BH, Cowan DN, Tomlinson JP, *et al.*: Epidemiology of injuries associated with physical training among young men in the army. *Med Sci Sports Exerc* 1993, 25:197–203.

39. Jones BH, Bovee MW, Haffis JM, Cowan DN: Intrinsic risk factors for exerciserelated injuries among male and female army trainees. *Am J Sports Med* 1993, 21:705–710.

40. Kvitne RS, Jobe FW, Jobe CM: Shoulder instability in the overhead or throwing athlete. *Clin Sports Med* 1995, 14:917–935.

41. WalshWM: Patellofemoral joint. In *Orthopaedic Sports Medicine: Principles and Practice*. Edited by DeLee JC, Drez D. Philadelphia: WB Saunders Co.; 1994:1163–1248.

42.• Twellaar M, Verstappen FTJ, Hudson A, Van Mechelan W: Physical characteristics as risk factors for sports injuries: a four year prospective study. *Int J Sports Med* 1997, 18:66–71.
Essentially from the same data pool as Van Mechelen *et al.* (*Med Sci Sports Exercs E*996, 28:1171–1179).

43. O'Conner FG, Howard TM, Fieseler CM, Nirschl RP: Managing overuse injuries: a systemic approach. *Phys Sports Med* 1997, 25:88–113.

44. Wilber RL, Moffatt RJ, Scott BE, *et al.*: Influence of water run training on the maintenance of aerobic performance. *Med Sci Sports Exerc* 1996, 28:1056–1062..

45. Frangolias DD, Rhodes EC: Metabolic responses and mechanisms during water immersion running and exercise. *Sports Med* 1996, 22:38–53.

46. Archanbault JM, Wiley JP, Bray RC: Exercise loading of tendons and the development of overuse injuries: a review of current literature. *Sports Med* 1995, 20:77–89.

47. Lehmann M, Foster C, Keul J: Overtraining in endurance athletes: a brief review. *Med Sci Sports Exerc* 1993, 25:854–862.

48. Adlercreutz H, Harkonen M, Kuoppasalm *et al.*: Effect of training on plasma anabolic and catabolic steroid hormones and their response during physical exercise. *Int J Sports Med* 1986, 7:27–28.

49. Urhausen A, Kullmer T, Kindermann W: A 7-week follow-up study of the behavior of testosterone and cortisol during the competition period in rowers. *Eur J Appl Physiol* 1987, 56:528–533.

50. Hooper SL, MacKinnon LT, Gordon RD, Bachmann AW: Hormonal responses of elite swimmers to overtraining. *Med Sci Sports Exerc* 1993, 25:741–747.

51. Rowbottom DG, Keast D, Goodman C, Morton AR: The haematological, biochemical and immunological profile of athletes suffering from the overtraining syndrome. *Eur J Appl Physiol* 1995, 70:502–509.

52. Newsholme EA: Biochemical mechanisms to explain immunosuppression in welltrained and overtrained athletes. *Int J Sports Med* 1994, 15(suppl):S142–S147.

53. Newsholme EA, Parry-Billings M, McAndrews N, Budget R: A Biochemical mechanism to explain some characteristics of overtraining. *Med Sci Sports Exerc* 1991, 32:79–93.

54. Northoff H, Berg A: Immunologic mediators as parameters of the reaction to strenuous exercise. *Int J Sports Med* 1991, 12(suppl):S9–S15.

15

WOMEN IN
SPORTS

Margot Putukian

The opportunities for girls and women to participate in sports have increased dramatically and, with the support of title IX legislation, continue to demonstrate remarkable growth. Although there are many similarities in the way female and male athletes respond to training and recover from injuries, there are differences that underscore the need to be familiar with entities specific to the female athlete. Obviously, menstrual dysfunction and pregnancy are medical issues that only relate to the female athlete. However, other entities, such as patellofemoral dysfunction, anterior cruciate ligament (ACL) injuries, and nutrition issues, are different in the female athlete compared with their male counterparts. The literature relating to the female athlete is slowly increasing, and the purpose of this chapter is to discuss some of these issues, with the intent to spark additional interest and improve the medical care given to the female athlete.

The benefits of exercise and competitive sport are numerous, with beneficial effects on hypertension, coronary artery disease, diabetes, osteoporosis, and obesity, and improvement in overall health and quality of life [1–3]. These benefits are incurred by both male and female subjects, yet only recently has exercise been promoted for the female population. In young girls, the positive effects of exercise include important health behaviors such as lower teen pregnancy, decreased substance use, and higher graduation rates. Psychologic effects include an increase in self-esteem, more positive body image, better feeling of well-being, and a lower incidence of depression [4,5]. Finally, the skills of teamwork, cooperation, acceptance of weaknesses in others, and goal-setting are all tools often learned during participation in sports, and are important for overall success in all facets of life.

Some early myths regarding women and exercise include the beliefs that women were unable to participate in sports because they were inherently weak, and that the stress of exercise was dangerous and would further weaken their ability to function and have children. Pregnancy, as well as the time of menstrual bleeding, was believed to be a time when women needed to be bedridden. Only recently have girls and women been allowed to fully reap the benefits of exercise. With the passage of Title IX legislation in 1972, women were finally given the opportunity to participate equally in intercollegiate sports. Recently, professional leagues have formed for women's basketball, and a professional league for women's soccer will soon be a reality as well. With the increased opportunities, not only have women shown that they can benefit from participation but also that they can excel.

The literature in sports medicine as it applies to the female athlete is limited, with much work in progress. There are certain issues that have been assessed rather well, including exercise and pregnancy and exercise and the menstrual cycle. There are other entities, such as the female athlete triad (menstrual dysfunction, disordered eating, premature osteoporosis), that have recently been elucidated; however, much research is still necessary to answer all of the questions. The nutritional needs of the female athlete, as well as strength and conditioning issues and specific injury patterns are all being more closely assessed, with insights that are helpful for all those taking care of the female athlete.

PHYSICAL VARIABLES FOR WOMEN IN SPORTS

It is important to recognize differences in physiologic variables between male and female athletes. Much of the information in the exercise medicine literature is based on studies performed in men. The cardiovascular system, skeletal system, and hematopoietic system are different in men versus women, and other factors such as body composition and overall strength and fitness parameters are also different. It is important to be familiar with the gender-specific psychologic variables and to understand how these differences may relate to some of the differences in performance between male and female athletes.

The skeleton

From birth until adulthood, increased growth in terms of height and weight follow a double sigmoid pattern [6]: the first dramatic increase occurs in infancy and early childhood, and the second occurs during adolescence and continues until completion of growth during the second decade. For boys, the peak height velocity ranges from 12.5 to 15 years, whereas in girls it ranges from 10.5 to 13 years, and peak weight velocity occurs approximately 6 months after peak height is attained [7]. Menarche normally occurs approximately 1 year after peak height velocity is attained. The age at which closure of the primary and secondary ossification centers, termed *skeletal maturity*, is different for girls and boys. Girls are generally skeletally mature at age 18 versus age 21 to 22 for boys. When growth is complete, men are approximately 10% taller than women.

Other skeletal differences include the pelvis, which in women is shallower and wider. The bones in women are thinner and lighter than in their male counterparts, which puts them at risk for osteoporosis. In addition, at menopause, the withdrawal of estrogen can also lead to an increase in the loss of bone from the skeleton. These topics will be discussed in further detail in a later section. Women are more likely to demonstrate femoral neck anteversion, with varus at the hip and valgus at the knee. To compensate, the tibial tubercle externally rotates with pronation at the hindfoot. This may lead to an increased Q angle, which is the angle formed by the intersection of a line drawn down the femoral shaft and a line drawn from the center of the patella to the tibial tubercle [8]. An increased Q angle is one of many risk factors for the development of patellofemoral dysfunction, which will be described later. The musculoskeletal evaluation of the female athlete is important and should be performed with an understanding of these special physical demands [9].

Body composition

Women have a higher body fat than men, by approximately 8% to 10% [10]. The absolute amount of storage fat is essentially the same in men and women, and the difference is found in the amount of essential fat, which in women is 9% to 12% versus 3% in men. The average body fat for average college-aged women and men is 23% to 27% and 15% to18%, respectively [10]. The percent body fat is different for each individual and varies among sports. A very great risk for the development of eating disorders can be seen when athletes strive for a "number" instead of allowing for individual differences in skeletal structure and energy needs.

Strengthening and conditioning

There does not appear to be major differences between men and women in terms of the response to strengthening and conditioning exercise. Strength of girls compared with boys changes as growth continues, with girls having 90% of the strength of boys at ages 11 to 12, but only 75% of their strength by the ages 15 to 16 [11]. The types of muscle fibers used, the ability to metabolize fat, and the physiologic responses to exercise in male and female subjects are similar [12–14]. Although there is an absolute difference in some of these physiologic variables, many of these differences disappear when related to lean body weight [10,15].

Women do not tend to develop the same muscle hypertrophy in response to strength training as men do, mostly because hypertrophy is primarily testosterone-regulated. In fact, strength in women can increase by 44% without an increase in muscle mass [16]. Strength training is useful for increasing strength, especially if used in a sport-specific manner. It may protect the skeletal system from injury by strengthening the musculature of the trunk and around joints. When used in a sport-specific manner, it may also improve performance by increasing the force with which a ball can be struck or by increasing muscular endurance in repetitive activities. Young girls and women should be encouraged to participate in an individualized sport-specific strength-training program as part of their training.

Cardiovascular system

The volume of the heart, systolic and diastolic blood pressure, lung volumes, and thoracic cavities are smaller in women compared with men. In prepubescent girls and boys, VO_{2max} is the same, and peaks between the ages of 16 and 20 years. The smaller heart size and volume in women means a smaller stroke volume (SV) and thus a higher heart rate (HR) to achieve the same cardiac output (CO) (CO = HR × SV) [8]. Finally, because women have 6% fewer erythrocytes and 10% to 15% less hemoglobin than men; their oxygen-carrying capacity is also less [17,18]. Absolute VO_2 (L/min) differences at adulthood differ by 52%, but this difference decreases to 20% to 30% if given in relation to body weight (L/kg/min) and to 15% when expressed in relation to fat-free weight (FFW) (L/kg FFW/min). Overall, with increases in VO_{2max}, there is a decrease in mortality risk [19], thus exemplifying the benefits of an aerobic exercise program.

MENSTRUAL CYCLE FUNCTION

Normal menstrual cycle function depends on an intact reproductive tract and normal hypothalamic-pituitary-ovarian function. This delicate balance of functions involves several hormones and mediators. Some of the alterations in menstrual function occur as a result of a normal exercise stimulus and have no significant health effects. However, when menstrul dysfunction occurs, it should be closely assessed; it can be associated with significant health concerns, including eating disorders, altered bone health and lipid profiles, and infertility. It is not "ok" for an athlete to miss menstrual cycles because she is "in season," as is still often told. This is especially important because more and more athletes are now involved in year-round training. In addition, other medical problems can present as mentrual dysfuntion and should not be missed just because a woman is involved in competive sport.

It is important to understand the use of oral contraceptives as well as other regimens for the overall health and well-being of the female athlete, as well as the effects of the menstrual cycle and oral contraceptives on performance. Much additional research is needed in this area, with important implications for management decisions for the female athlete with normal menstrual function as well as those female athletes with menstrual dysfunction.

The mechanisms by which exercise affects menstrual cycle function and the hormones that regulate it remain unclear. How the reproductive hormones affect exercise and performance is a question that has been looked at by various researchers. Menstrual dysfunction occurs more commonly in athletes than the general population, and the mechanisms involved are becoming clearer. The health care provider taking care of female athletes needs to understand how the normal cycle affects performance and the risks and benefits of exogenous hormonal medications. It is important to address menstrual function and dysfunction during the preparticipation physical examination so that young athletes understand that there are risks, both acute and long term, associated with menstrual dysfunction, and that it is not "ok" to have abnormal menstrual cycles just because they are "in season." Finally, menstrual dysfunction, although often due to exercise, can also be caused by other more serious medical problems, thus warranting a complete and thorough work-up.

The normal menstrual cycle

The normal menstrual cycle requires an intact female genital system and is regulated by hormones secreted from the hypothalamus, posterior pituitary, and ovary. Assuming normal anatomy, proper function depends on the interaction of hormonal signals and feedback systems. The median eminence of the hypothalamus releases gonadotropin hormone-releasing hormone (GnRH), which acts on the anterior pituitary to produce follicle-stimulating hormone (FSH) and luteinizing hormone (LH). The menstrual cycle is divided into a follicular phase and a luteal phase (Fig. 15.1).

In the follicular phase, FSH stimulates the granulosa cells to produce estradiol, which in turn stimulates further growth of the follicle. A negative feedback eventually occurs at the level of the pituitary, and FSH production diminishes. The dominant folli-cle is able to continue growing despite this, and a positive feedback system at the pituitary increases LH release during the mid to late follicular phase. Just before ovulation, in the late follicular phase, the progesterone levels increase slightly; this increase in combination with estrogen causes an increase in the release of LH and FSH. Estradiol levels reach their peak (about 300 pg/mL), the LH surge occurs approximately 14 to 24 hours later, and ovulation occurs approximately 34 to 36 hours later [20]. During the luteal phase, progesterone levels increase and act on the granulosa cells producing the corpus luteum, which has a life span of approximately 14 days. The uterus prepares for potential implantation of a fertilized ovum, and if this does not occur, then endometrial sloughing occurs, causing menstrual blood flow.

The normal cycle is 23 to 35 days, with 10 to 13 cycles per year. Women with this menstrual pattern

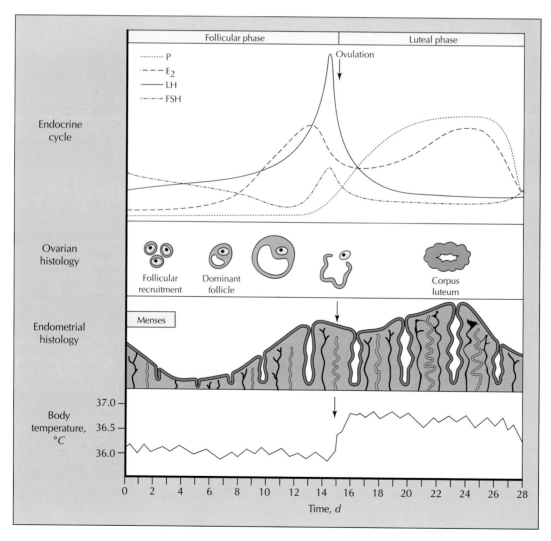

FIGURE 15.1

The hormonal, ovarian, endometrial, and basal body temperature changes and relationships throughout the normal menstrual cycle. E_2—estrogen; LH—luteinizing hormone; FSH—follicle-stimulating hormone; P—progesterone (*Adapted from* Carr and Wilson [149]; with permission.)

are called "regular" or "eumenorrheic." Three to six cycles per year at intervals generally greater than 35 days is called *oligomenorrhea*. *Amenorrhea* is defined as the absence or cessation of menstrual flow and is the clinical manifestation of a variety of disorders [20]. *Primary amenorrhea* is the absence of menarche by the age of 16. *Secondary amenorrhea* is the absence of 3 to 12 consecutive menstrual periods after normal menarche has occurred.

Menopause occurs when the number of ovarian follicles has diminished, and is accompanied with a decrease in ovarian hormone production. As this process starts occurring, the length of cycles will often shorten and some are anovulatory, which leads to missed menstrual cycles or irregular cycles. The average age of natural menopause is 51, and diagnosis is often made by levels of FSH, which have increased, along with a typical history that often includes vasomotor symptoms and other symptoms associated with estrogen deficiency [21].

Vasomotor symptoms include hot flashes, which occur in approximately 75% of women and are variable in severity. Estrogen deficiency is associated with genitourinary atrophy, which can cause dyspareunia and vulvovaginal pruritus as well as urinary tract infections and urinary incontinence. Estrogen is a cardioprotective hormone, and thus the benefits women derive from estrogen are lost once estrogen production diminishes. This explains the increase in cardiovascular risk that occurs after menopause. Finally, estrogen is also a permissive hormone for calcium accumulation, and estrogen deficiency is associated with an increased risk for the development of osteoporosis. This last effect of estrogen deficiency may well be one of the most important, given the major effect osteoporosis and resultant fractures have in terms of morbidity and mortality in women.

Hormonal replacement therapy has been used to treat menopausal women and can prevent many of the previously described consequences of estrogen deficiency. This is an exciting area of research that has significant implications. As will be discussed later, menstrual dysfunction can also be associated with diminished or unopposed estrogen, and the risks and benefits of hormonal replacement therapy are also applicable to this younger population of women. It is therefore important to be familiar with these risks as well as benefits in taking care of active women.

THE MENSTRUAL CYCLE AND ORAL CONTRACEPTIVES: EFFECT ON EXERCISE AND PERFORMANCE

The effects of the menstrual cycle as well as oral contraceptives on performance have recently been reviewed. Conflicting results have been found when assessing individual physiologic responses and the effects of oral contraceptives during different phases of the cycle. There is some subjectivity, which makes these effects difficult to assess, and many studies do not properly document cycle phase by measuring basal body temperatures or direct hormone levels. Nonetheless, a review of some of the literature is useful.

Cardiovascular system

How the cardiovascular system is effected by the menstrual cycle has been addressed by following several variables, including hemoglobin, heart rate, free fatty acids, oxygen uptake (VO_2), ventilation, and respiratory exchange ratio. When the stage of the cycle has been documented, there are conflicting results for some of these variables.

An increase in plasma volume with a concomitant but lesser increase in erythrocyte volume is a well-known response to endurance training. This increase in volume results in a "pseudoanemia" based on dilution, and may represent an adaptation that occurs to make the blood flow more easily through the vasculature. In some studies, both hemoglobin and hematocrit levels were lower during the luteal phase [22,23], whereas in another, no significant difference was noted [24].

Some authors have noted an increase in heart rate during the luteal phase [25], whereas others have again noted no significant difference [24,26,27]. There is no significant difference in rating of perceived exertion and oxygen uptake during different phases of the menstrual cycle [22,27], and there is no significant difference in ventilation [22,24,26,27]. Although some of the specific variables differ regarding the cardiovascular response during the menstrual phase, there does not appear to be much effect on performance. Only one study [26] demonstrated an increase in the VO_2 during the luteal phase of the cycle at rest, but this difference disappeared with exercise.

The data regarding the effects of menstrual function on cardiovascular response with oral contraceptive medications have been similarly equivocal. In one study, although cardiac index, pulmonary distendability, heart rate, and blood pressure did not vary in women taking a estrogenprogestin–combined pill compared with a progestin-only pill or placebo, cardiac output was greater in the combined pill compared with the progestin-only pill and in both pill formulations compared with placebo [28]. In another study, a higher blood volume, stroke volume, and cardiac output were demonstrated in women taking lynestrenol- and mestranol-containing contraceptives [29].

Theoretically, if an increase in cardiac output occurs along with an increase in blood volume, then one might expect to see an improvement in performance. In addition, oral contraceptive use is often associated with a decrease in menstrual flow and, therefore, a decrease in the amount of iron loss. In combination with an increased cardiac output, one might expect to see a potential increase in performance. Contrary to this finding, Lebrun [30] demonstrated a small though insignificant decrease in VO_{2max} with oral contraceptive use. More research is needed to better delineate the effects of oral contraceptives on performance variables.

Ventilatory response

The changes that occur in ventilatory response during the menstrual cycle and with oral contraceptive administration appear to be related to progesterone, although estrogen may have an enhancing effect. Progesterone appears to increase the ventilatory response seen during the luteal phase in women and has been seen in studies in which medroxyprogesterone is given to men [31–33]. During the luteal phase, an increased sensitivity to both hypoxia and hypercarbia has been demonstrated [32,33]. Changes in ventilation do not appear to have any effect on performance variables.

Strength changes

There do not appear to be any strength gains during different parts of the menstrual cycle [34,35]. Earlier studies have shown a decrease in strength during the luteal phase of the cycle [36], but a recent prospective study [30] did not show any difference in isokinetic knee extension and flexion strength during luteal and follicular phases. Although the data are limited, oral contraceptives do not seem to alter strength either.

Thermoregulatory changes

The relationship of thermoregulation and the menstrual cycle has been addressed by several studies, and again the results are conflicting. Some studies have not shown any change in the heat–stress response during different parts of the cycle [37,38]. Others have demonstrated core temperature increases before and after exercise during the luteal phase, as well as a decrease in exercise performance related to altered thermoregulation [39,40]. Sparse data exist assessing the effect of oral contraceptives on heat–stress responses.

Metabolic changes

Estradiol alters resting metabolism by increasing triglyceride synthesis and high-density lipoprotein-2 levels, increasing lipolysis in fat and muscle tissue and inhibiting gluconeogenesis and glycogenolysis [41]. Estrogen spares glycogen during exercise to favor lipid metabolism [42]. In the luteal phase, glycogen sparing occurs secondary to a lower lactate production [43]. Progesterone also acts to increase the uptake of glucose into both liver and muscle [44]. Oral contraceptives may have a negative effect on the blood lipid profile, but may have a positive effect on the utilization of glucose during high-intensity endurance exercise [45].

Performance and the menstrual cycle

Many female athletes subjectively report poor performance during menses [46], whereas others have felt no effect on performance [47]. Some studies have demonstrated a subtle increase in performance, measured by time to exhaustion [43,48], or increased VO_{2max} [49], whereas others have found no significant difference in performance variables [50,51].

It is difficult to assess the effects of oral contraceptive pills on performance, because different preparations are used and the caliber of athletes assessed differ. Oral contraceptives have been reported to have no effect on performance in some studies [52,53], whereas more recent data suggest that low-dose oral contraceptives may be associated with a 5% to 8% decline in VO_{2max} [54]. Premenstrual symptoms such as cramps, bloating, nausea, vomiting, breast tenderness, and emotional lability are often lessened when women are active compared with when they are inactive. In a prospective study of soccer players, those on oral contraceptives had fewer injuries than those not on oral contraceptives [55]. This difference in injury rate was believed to be secondary to the decreased incidence of molimenal symptoms that oral contraceptives had on these women. More well-controlled studies are needed to address whether performance varies throughout the menstrual cycle, and what effect, if any, oral contraceptives have on performance.

MENSTRUAL DYSFUNCTION

Menstrual dysfunction is common in the female athlete and is manifested by a spectrum of clinical presentations, ranging from amenorrhea to oligomenorrhea to menometrorrhagia. Menstrual dysfunction is often associated with abnormalities in estrogen production, progesterone production, or both. Estrogen plays an important role in many different systems, including the endocrinologic, hematologic, reproductive, and skeletal systems. Without estrogen, there may be an increased risk for coronary artery disease, diabetes mellitus, hypertension, embolic disease, stroke, and cancer along with the increased risk for stress fractures and osteoporosis. Amenorrheic runners have higher low-density lipoprotein (LDL) cholesterol levels than regularly menstruating runners and regularly menstruating sedentary control subjects [56]; thus the absence of normal menstrual function may negate the positive effects of exercise on the lipid profile.

Delayed puberty has been demonstrated in athletic compared with inactive girls [57]. Variables that may lead to menstrual dysfunction include exercise-related changes in the sex and stress hormones, nutritional factors, and "energy drain," as well as changes in body composition.

Chronic exercise can result in changes in mentsrual function. Variables that have been identified that may lead to menstrual dysfunction include exercise-related changes in the sex and stress hormones, nutritional factors, body composition, and "energy drain" [58–62]. Athletes have a reduction in the frequency and amplitude of the LH surge [63], and this may be the first abnormality of menstrual function that occurs. Additionally, naloxone, an opiate antagonist, has been shown to restore the normal LH surge and amplitude in some amenorrheic athletes [64].

Frisch [65], as early as 1974, proposed that a minimum body fat of 17% was necessary in order to initiate menarche, and that menarche could not be maintained with a body fat below 22%. Although body fat is a factor, it has since been shown that it is not the only factor. Normal menstrual flow has been seen in athletes with body fats as low as 4% [66]. Diet and nutrition are also important in maintaining normal menstrual function. Diets low in protein, fat, or calories carry a higher risk for amenorrhea [67,68]. Marcus *et al.* [66] found that in elite runners, 50% of amenorrheic versus 40% of normally cycling runners were getting less than two thirds of the recommended daily allowance for calcium. Iron and protein consumption was also lower in the amenorrheic versus eumenorrheic runners.

The incidence of menstrual irregularity appears to be higher in athletes than in the general population. The incidence of amenorrhea has been reported as 3.4% to 66% in athletic women [69,70] compared with 2% to 5% in the general population [71]. Three main subsets of menstrual dysfunction are seen in response to training: luteal phase deficiency, anovulation [72], and exercise-associated amenorrhea (EAA).

Luteal phase deficiency is a shortening of the luteal phase, which is associated with decreased levels of progesterone. Abnormal FSH:LH ratios consistent with luteal phase shortening and progesterone deficiency have been documented in studies in swimmers and runners [73,74]. The menstrual cycle length and pattern is unchanged, and therefore these abnormalities in function may go undetected. Luteal phase deficiency has important clinical significance because it has been related to decreased bone density [75] and infertility [76].

In anovulation, estrogen is present without progesterone, and cycles are irregular, with cycle lengths as short as 21 days or as many as 35 to 150 days between bleeding [75]. In this situation, the main concern is unopposed estrogen, which is associated with an increased risk for endometrial hyperplasia, adenocarcinoma, and breast cancer [77,78]. Anovulation has many causes, and prompts further evaluation and treatment.

Exercise-associated amenorrhea

Exercise-associated amenorrhea is the most frequent cause of amenorrhea in athletes, yet it is essential to understand it as a diagnosis of exclusion. Its cause is multifactorial, with the common final pathway to menstrual dysfunction being an alteration at the hypothalamic-pituitary level. Factors that seem to play a role in the development of EAA include nutrition, changes in body composition, exercise-induced changes in hormones, stress, amount of training and training intensity, and reproductive immaturity (nulliparity, delayed menarche, and oligomenorrhea) [79].

The low to absent levels of estrogen present in amenorrheic athletes is associated with lower bone mineral density than that seen in their eumenorrheic counterparts [80, 81, 82]. Low bone mineral density is a risk factor for osteoporosis and stress fractures, and therefore has significant clinical importance. Amenorrheic runners lose the improvements in lipid profiles seen with exercise compared with runners with normal menstrual cycles [83] and also face an increased risk for infertility [76].

Bone formation is enhanced by exercise [84–86], and weight-bearing exercise increases bone mass more than non–weight-bearing exercise [75]. If, however, exercise leads to amenorrhea, these beneficial results may be lost. A study in 1984 demonstrated that amenorrheic women had a 22% to 29% decrease in bone mineral density at the spine compared with age-matched eumenorrheic control subjects, and uniformly low estrogen levels [82]. In individuals amenorrheic for longer than 2 years, the bone loss was greater than those amenorrheic for less than 1 year.

These findings were later confirmed in athletes in whom the vertebral bone mineral density as well as the estradiol levels and peak progesterone levels in amenorrheic runners were significantly lower than those seen in eumenorrheic runners [81]. If these athletes spontaneously regain their menses, the bone mineral density increases, though never to a level equivalent to that seen in athletes with normal menstrual function [87], causing concern that the bone loss seen in menstrual dysfunction may not be reversible.

In a later study by Drinkwater *et al.* [88], menstrual patterns were compared with bone density. A linear relationship was found, with the highest bone mineral density being present in those individuals with currently normal and historically normal cycles, and the lowest bone mineral density seen in those with a history of amenorrhea who were currently amenorrheic. Athletes who had occasional irregularities in their menstrual cycle had a bone density 6% less than those with normal cycles (1.18 g/cm^2), and runners who were always irregular had

a bone density 17% lower (1.05 g/cm^2). Thus, both the current menstrual status and the past history of menstrual abnormalities are important in terms of decreased bone mineral density.

Individuals with menstrual dysfunction have an increased incidence of stress fractures compared with those with normal menstrual function. In a retrospective study, individuals with stress fractures had more menstrual irregularity, as well as lower bone density, lower calcium intake, and lower oral contraceptive use [89]. Similar findings were found in other studies [90–92]. The lower bone mineral density seen in individuals with menstrual dysfunction improves when normal menses returns. In Drinkwater *et al.*'s study [87], in which amenorrheic runners spontaneously regained their menses, an initial 6.2% increase in bone density occurred. However, the following year the increase in bone density was only 3%, and over the following 2 years, remained unchanged. Four years later, the bone mineral density of these individuals remained significantly lower than those runners who had never been amenorrheic.

These data demonstrate that menstrual dysfunction, especially amenorrhea, is associated with low bone mineral density and that decreased bone mineral density is associated with an increased risk for stress fractures and premature osteoporosis. The data also seem to question whether the effects of menstrual dysfunction on bone health are reversible. This concern underscores the need to detect and treat menstrual dysfunction as early as possible.

Evaluation and treatment of menstrual dysfunction

The evaluation of menstrual dysfunction should be thorough and include a complete physical examination, including pelvic examination as well as laboratory information. This includes a pregnancy test (the most common cause of amenorrhea) as well as FSH, LH, prolactin, and thyroid function tests. Additional tests may be indicated if prompted by the history or physical examination. An algorithm for evaluation is presented in Figure 15.2. It is important to individualize evaluation and treatment based on the history and physical examination.

The next step in the evaluation of amenorrhea is administering a "progesterone challenge," which consists of 5 to 10 mg of medroxyprogesterone acetate per day for 7 to 10 days. If the uterus is "estrogen-primed" and simply lacks progesterone, administering progesterone will cause menstrual bleeding to occur within 3 to 4 days. If no bleeding occurs, then the body lacks both estrogen and progesterone. It is important to perform this step, as the risks and treatment regimen for hypoestrogenism and unopposed estrogen are different.

If the progesterone challenge test produces bleeding, then unopposed estrogen is the concern. Treatment can be cyclical oral progesterone for 10 days at the end of the cycle (or 10 days out of a month if they are amenorrheic) or oral contraceptives. If the progesterone challenge test is negative, then hypoestrogenism is present and one can either use cyclical estrogen and progesterone (as in postmenopausal estrogen therapy) or oral contraceptive pills. The most common postmenopausal regimen is 0.3 to 0.6 mg estrogen each day for 25 days, along with 5 to 10 mg medroxyprogesterone for

days 14 to 25. The treatment options must be individualized and should consider whether contraception is an issue, whether pregnancy is desired, and whether risk factors for hormonal treatment are present.

The administration of estrogen is based on research in postmenopausal women in whom estrogen along with supplemental calcium administration reduced the frequency of arm and hip fractures by 50% to 60% and reduced the frequency of vertebral fractures by 80% [93]. The optimal regimen in regard to effect on bone mineral density [94] remains unclear, and more information specific to exercise-associated amenorrhea is needed. An advantage to using oral contraceptives is the additional protection against pregnancy that they provide, which is an important consideration in the sexually active woman. Additionally, the side-effect profile of oral contraceptives is good, and the ease of administration often makes this regimen the one most easily and successfully adhered to by athletes.

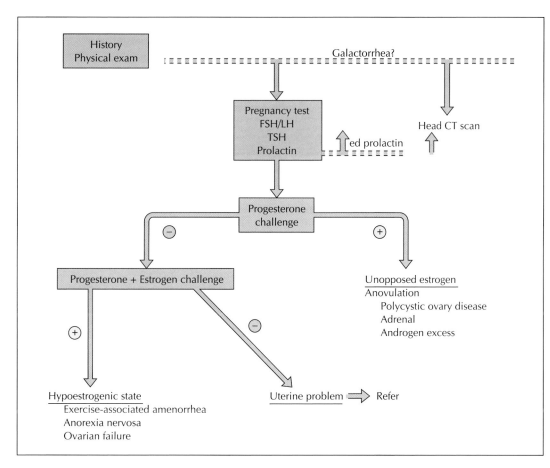

FIGURE 15.2

Algorithm for amenorrhea work-up. FSH/LH—follicle-stimulating hormone and luteinizing hormone; TSH—thyroid-stimulating hormone. (*Adapted from* Putukian [153]; with permission.)

The absolute contraindications to systemic estrogen therapy are given in Table 15.1.

The treatment of menstrual dysfunction should also include an assessment of training patterns and body composition as well as an assessment for the presence of disordered eating. Treatment therefore may include decreasing training intensity by 10%, increasing body weight or body fat percentage if too low, and ensuring adequate caloric intake, including a qualitative assessment of specific needs such as calcium, iron, and protein intake. Estrogen, progesterone, or both should be considered individually as discussed previously.

It is often difficult for young athletes to adhere to a regimen in which they must lessen their training duration or intensity, or gain weight. Few athletes want to comply with these types of demands and often see amenorrhea as evidence that they are training adequately, and they certainly do not mind missing the monthly inconvenience and expense of maintaining a normal menses. It is important to educate trainers, coaches, parents, and athletes themselves about the risks associated with menstrual dysfunction and the need for early detection and treatment. Even if the long-term risks of osteoporosis may not concern the athlete, many are aware of the consequences of stress fracture.

MENSTRUAL DYSFUNCTION, DISORDERED EATING, AND THE FEMALE ATHLETE TRIAD

Menstrual dysfunction is common in athletes, and is often caused by an interaction of multiple factors, all of which appear to result in a disruption of the hypothalamic-pituitary-ovarian axis. Disordered eating includes a spectrum of abnormalities; in its mildest form, the condition presents as abnormal eating behaviors, and at its most extreme, it presents as classic anorexia nervosa. Eating disorders and menstrual dysfunction have both been associated with low estrogen and low bone mineral density, with a resultant increased risk for stress fractures and premature osteoporosis. Eating disorders, menstrual dysfunction, and osteoporosis have become known as the "female athlete triad" [95, 96], which represents a significant concern for the health care providers of female athletes. Eating disorders are difficult to treat successfully and may be associated with significant morbidity and mortality. The detection, treatment, and most importantly prevention

through education is paramount for the future of healthy participation by girls and women in sports [97, 98].

Osteoporosis

Bone is constantly forming and undergoing remodeling. It serves as a reservoir for both calcium and phosphorus, and is essential in calcium homeostasis. Bone is composed of both trabecular and cortical components, with varying amounts of each found in different sites throughout the body. Trabecular bone is found in the spine, pelvis, ends of long bones and the flat bones, and is more metabolically active than cortical bone. Cortical bone is found in the shafts of long bones and comprises two thirds of the skeleton. The various methods for measuring bone density are demonstrated in Table 15.2.

Osteoporosis is a decrease in bone mass and tensile strength that leads to microarchitectural deterioration, which results in an increased risk of skeletal fragility and fracture. The condition has been defined as a bone mineral density more than 2.5 SD below the mean value, with osteopenia being present if the bone mineral density is between 1.0 and 2.5 SD below the mean. The clinical diagnosis of osteoporosis depends on several factors [99], with bone mineral density representing only one of these criteria.

Osteoporosis causes more than 1,300,000 fractures per year and an annual cost of $6 billion in the United States. In many individuals it represents the "final straw" of independent life, and 20% of those with a hip fracture die within a year [100]. Of menopausal women, 44% will sustain at least one osteoporotic fracture, thus increasing the impor-

Table 15.1 CONTRAINDICATIONS TO SYSTEMIC ESTROGEN THERAPY*
Vaginal bleeding, unexplained
Pervious history of cerebrovascular accident
Deep vein thrombosis
Cardiac disease with right to left shunting
Breast cancer
Uterine cancer
Cervical cancer
Active hepatic disease
Pregnancy

*Data from White and Hergenroeder [77].

tance of identifying risk factors [101]. Identifiable risk factors are listed in Table 15.3.

Normal estrogen levels and establishing an adequate calcium intake, especially in childhood and young adulthood when peak bone mass is forming, is essential. Calcium intake of 1200 to 1500 mg/d as well as adequate vitamin D intake has been recommended by the National Institutes of Health (NIH) Consensus Conference [102]. Exercise and estrogen therapy have both been shown to prevent bone loss in postmenopausal women [103–105]. Snow [106] demonstrated in premenopausal women that the bone mineral density of the femoral neck and lumbar spine and radius were independently predicted by hip abductor and grip strength. The primary prevention of osteoporosis is maximizing the attainment of peak bone mass, whereas the mainstay of treatment for established osteoporosis is estrogen therapy [107]. Other treatment protocols, including calcium, calcitonin, and fluoride, are currently under investigation.

Disordered eating

Eating disorders make up the third component of the female triad, and because 90% of eating disorders occur in women (and the incidence is higher in active women compared with their sedentary counterparts), they remain a significant concern for the female athlete. Eating disorders are associated with a high morbidity and mortality rate, and health care providers for the active female population need to be familiar with eating disorders. In addition, trainers, coaches, parents, and athletes themselves should be familiar with the signs of disordered eating, methods to help identify and treat athletes, and the short- and long-term health consequences of these disorders.

There are three subsets of eating disorders: anorexia nervosa, bulimia nervosa, and eating disorders not otherwise specified (EDNOS). The definitions for anorexia and bulimia are given in Table 15.4, and EDNOS is often used for individuals who have disordered eating patterns yet do note fall into

Table 15.2 COMPARISON OF BONE DENSITY MEASUREMENT METHODS*			
TECHNIQUE	**SITE**	**RAD. EXP.**	**COST**
Single-photon absorptiometry	Radius (integral bone)	10	$60–100
Dual-photon absorptiometry	Spine/hip (trabecular)	100	$125–150
Quantitative computed tomography scanning	Spine/hip (integral and trabecular)	1000	$250–350
Dual-energy x-ray absorptiometry	Spine/hip/total bone mineral density (integral)	3	$75–100

*Adapted from Pearl [150]; with permission.

Table 15.3 RISK FACTORS FOR OSTEOPOROSIS
Female gender
Asian or white race
Age
Sedentary lifestyle
Thinness
Tobacco use
Decreased bone mineral density
Prolonged corticosteroid use
Decreased calcium level
Estrogen deficiency

either of the other two categories. Anorexia nervosa and bulimia nervosa may be very different in their presentation, health risks, and in terms of the individual's willingness to receive treatment; yet they also have certain similarities.

Anorexia nervosa is a psychiatric syndrome of severe weight loss by self-starvation due to an extreme desire to be thin, along with a distorted body image. It is seen most commonly in the adolescent and young adult age group. Anorexic individuals are often very difficult to identify because of their denial and secretive behavior.

Bulimia nervosa shares a similar desire for thinness, but in these individuals, body weight is often at or above normal. Bulimia nervosa is characterized by recurrent bingeing episodes usually followed by purging behavior. This can include self-induced vomiting, laxative use, or diuretic use. Weight fluctuations are very common, as is an awareness that the eating behavior is abnormal.

Often, individuals will be fearful of their inability to control their eating behaviors. EDNOS are characterized by individuals that are usually of average weight. There is a preoccupation with body image and weight, and guilt surrounding eating. Individuals with EDNOS can be thought of as anorexic patients who are not amenorrheic and as bulimic patients who do not binge.

The statistics for eating disorders are of concern, especially in athletes, although the numbers reported in the general population may be underestimates. Anorexia occurs in 0.5% to 1.0%, bulimia occurs in 2% to 5% [71], and EDNOS occur in 3% to 5% of women aged 15 to 30. The numbers in athletes are higher, ranging anywhere from 15% to 62% depending on the study.

Athletes are at an increased risk for eating disorders, mainly because many of the characteristics that describe our best athletes also describe those individuals at risk for eating disorders. These

Table 15.4 DIAGNOSTIC AND STATISTICAL MANUAL OF MENTAL DISORDERS-IV DIAGNOSTIC CRITERIA FOR ANOREXIA AND BULIMIA*	
ANOREXIA NERVOSA	**BULIMIA NERVOSA**
Refusal to maintain normal body weight at or above a minimally normal weight for age and height (*eg*, weight loss leading to maintenance of body weight < 85% of that expected; or failure to make expected weight gain during period of growth, leading to body weight < 85% of that expected).	Recurrent episodes of binge eating. An episode of binge eating is characterized by both of the following: Eating, in a discrete period of time (*eg*, within any 2-hour period) an amount of food that is definitely larger than most people would eat during a similar period of time and under similar circumstances.
Intense fear of gaining weight or becoming fat, even though underweight.	A sense of lack of control over eating during the episode (*eg*, a feeling that one cannot stop eating or control what or how much one is eating).
Disturbance in the way in which one's body weight or shape is experienced; undue influence of body weight or shape on self-evaluation; denial of the seriousness of the current low body weight.	Recurrent inappropriate compensatory behavior in order to prevent weight gain, such as: self-induced vomiting; misuse of laxatives, diuretics or other medications; fasting; or excessive exercise.
In postmenarchal females, amenorrhea (the absence of at least three consecutive menstrual cycles). A woman is considered to have amenorrhea if her periods occur only following hormone, *eg*, estrogen, administration.	The binge eating and inappropriate compensatory behaviors both occur, on average, at least twice a week for 3 months.
Restricting type: During the episode of anorexia nervosa, the person does not regularly engage in binge eating or purging behavior (*ie*, self-induced vomiting or the misuse of laxatives or diuretics).	Self-evaluation in unduly influenced by body shape and weight.
Binge eating/purging type: During the episode of anorexia nervosa, the person regularly engages in binge eating or purging behavior (*ie*, self-induced vomiting or the misuse of laxatives or diuretics).	The disturbance does not occur exclusively during periods of anorexia nervosa.
	Purging type: The person regularly engages in self-induced vomiting or the misuse of laxative or diuretics.
	Nonpurging type: The person uses other inappropriate compensatory behaviors, such as fasting or excessive exercise, but does not regularly engage in self-induced vomiting or the misuse of laxatives or diuretics.

Adapted from Task Force on the Diagnostic and Statistical Manual of Mental Disorders-IV [151]; with permission.

include a heightened body awareness, perfectionism, compulsivity, and high achievement expectations. Additionally, athletes are always trying to gain the extra edge in competition and will often go through extraordinary measures to reach the weights they feel will give them the performance advantage. Unfortunately, subtle messages given by parents, teammates, or even the coach can reinforce disordered eating behaviors.

Etiology of disordered eating

The origin of eating disorders is multifactorial and includes social climate, family issues, biologic issues, response to victimization, identity issues, low self-esteem, and role conflicts. There are certainly societal issues that contribute to the development of disordered eating behaviors, by normalizing many of these pathogenic behaviors that prize thinness. Persons with disordered eating are often from families where coping skills have not been learned and in whom self-worth has been related to and centered on appearance. Biologic changes can occur as the result of severe dieting, and these may affect the psychologic and physiologic cues for satiety. Of persons with eating disorders, 20% to 35% report a history of sexual abuse, and 67% of bulimics report sexual and/or physical abuse. Unfortunately, many individuals with eating disorders do not have high self-esteem, and controlling their eating is one of few areas in their life that they feel they are able to feel good about. They may not be able to control how they are treated, how well they do in school, or whether they start on the team, but they *can* control what they eat, and therefore for many, eating disorders are a desperate result of trying to gain control over some part of their lives.

Risks of disordered eating

The risks of eating disorders are numerous, and nutritional deficiencies are by far the rule. This impairs wound healing and the ability to fight infections. Long-term sequelae include infertility, electrolyte disturbances, gastrointestinal disease, psychiatric problems, decreased immune function, malnutrition, and decreased bone density. Approximately 6% to 12% of anorexic individuals will die from starvation, sepsis, cardiac arrhythmias, or suicide, with the latter accounting for most of the mortality [71].

Identification

Identifying individuals with eating disorders can often be very difficult and yet remains crucial to successful treatment. The morbidity and mortality is significant, and the earlier these individuals can be recognized, the more likely they are to recover. It is often difficult to detect individuals with eating disorders and differentiate them from healthy athletes. There are often common features that make this important task quite difficult. Some of the features that athletes share with those with eating disorders, and some of the features that can be used to help distinguish athletes from those with eating disorders, are shown in Table 15.5.

Table 15.5 SHARED FEATURES (ATHLETE AND ANORECTIC)

DIETARY FADDISM

Controlled caloric consumption
Specific carbohydrate avoidance
Low body weight
Resting bradycardia and hypotension
Increased physical activity
Amenorrhea or oligomenorrhea
Anemia (may or may not be present)

DISTINGUISHED FEATURES

Athlete
   Purposeful training
   Increased exercise tolerance
   Good muscular development
   Accurate body image
   Body fat level within defined normal range
   Increased plasma volume
   Increased oxygen extraction from blood
   Efficient energy metabolism
   Increased high-density lipoprotein-2
Anorectic patient
   Aimless physical activity
   Poor or decreasing exercise performance
   Poor muscular development
   Flawed body image (believes herself to be overweight)
   Body fat below normal level
   Electrolyte abnormalities if abusing laxatives and/or diuretics
   Cold intolerance
   Dry skin
   Cardiac arrhythmias
   Lanugo hair
   Leukocyte dysfunction

Adapted from McSherry [152]; with permission.

Although anorexic individuals may be easier to identify because of their very low weights or precipitous weight drops, they often have a strong amount of denial, which makes them difficult to approach. Individuals with bulimia, on the other hand, may be more difficult to detect because their weight is at or above normal; however, once the right questions are asked, they often reach out for help because they feel so out of control of their eating patterns.

If a trainer, coach, teammate, roommate, or parent is concerned about an individual athlete, the first step is to openly discuss this concern with the athlete in a nonconfrontational manner. The athlete should understand that their position on the team is not threatened, and that the well-being and health of the athlete is the primary concern. Participation can often continue as long as the health of the athlete is not compromised, or as long as they are not at risk for significant injury with continued participation.

Treatment of disordered eating

Once an individual is identified, the treatment plan is multifaceted and involves three essential components: physician, psychologic counseling or psychiatric help, and nutrition counseling. Although the nutritionist is often the first person consulted, this is probably where help is needed last. Eating disorders are not food or nutrition problems, but merely the symptom of underlying problems. Too often the initial response of those working with an anorexic individual is "they just need to eat more," and concerned individuals may even make efforts such as baking cookies or taking them out to dinner. Primary treatment centers around psychotherapy, and although individuals may at first be wary of obtaining counseling, this step must be emphasized. Additional members of the treatment team can include the family, coach, and athletic trainer, as well as team members and a sports psychologist. Once the individual is starting to make progress, the nutritionist can be very helpful in further educating the athlete and helping her to make good nutritional decisions.

Eating disorders remain difficult to treat and are often very frustrating for the individual, their family, teammates, coaches, and anyone else involved. Treatment is a lengthy, difficult, and unfortunately often unsuccessful process. The consequences can be tragic, which is why education and prevention is so important. A referral pattern that is part of the Weight Control and Eating Disorder Policy at the

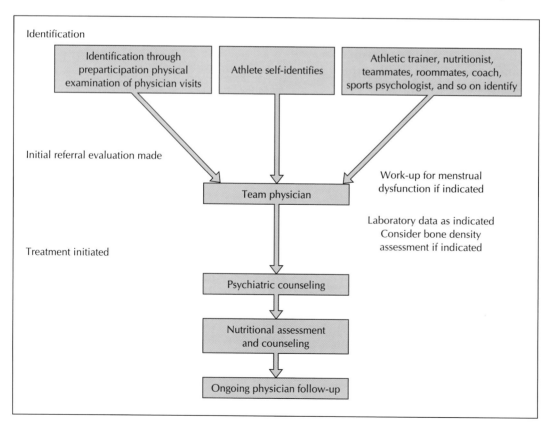

FIGURE 15.3
Follow-up should be coordinated with physician, psychiatrist, and nutritionist if possible. Input from coaches, athletic trainers, and sports psychologists is recommended if permissible and available. Disqualification and return to sport issues to be decided by team physician with input from all available resources.

Pennsylvania State University is shown in Figure 15.3. The female triad is a new concept, and exciting research is underway. It is hoped that as we continue to learn about the triggers of disordered eating, we can be better able to prevent girls and women from succumbing to these patterns and the consequences associated with them.

EXERCISE AND PREGNANCY

More women have made exercise an important part of their everyday life, and for those in childbearing years, the issue of how exercise affects pregnancy, as well as how pregnancy affects exercise performance, has been readdressed. The American College of Obstetricians and Gynecologists (ACOG) [99] published guidelines in 1985 for exercise during pregnancy, but some studies [109] questioned whether these recommendations were too conservative. More recently, the recommendations by ACOG have been updated (Table 15.6). The exercise recommendations during pregnancy given to a woman who exercises regularly and sometimes at high levels may differ significantly from those presented to a sedentary woman who decides to start exercising for the first time when she becomes pregnant. This area of study is exciting, and thus far the information appears to demonstrate that as long as certain precautions are

Table 15.6	AMERICAN COLLEGE OF OBSTETRICIANS AND GYNECOLOGISTS GUIDELINES FOR EXERCISE DURING PREGNANCY AND THE POSTPARTUM PERIOD*

Exercise guidelines: There are no data in humans to indicate that pregnant women should limit exercise intensity and lower target heart rates because of potential adverse effects. For women who do not have any additional risk factors for adverse maternal or perinatal outcome, the following recommendations may be made:

1. During pregnancy, women can continue to exercise and derive health benefits even from mild-to-moderate exercise routines. Regular exercise (at least three times per week) is preferable to intermittent activity.
2. Women should avoid exercise in the supine position after the first trimester. Such a position is associated with decreased cardiac output in most pregnant women: because the remaining cardiac output will be preferentially distributed away from splanchnic beds (including the uterus) during vigorous exercise, such regimens are best avoided during pregnancy. Prolonged periods of motionless standing should also be avoided.
3. Women should be aware of the decreased oxygen available for aerobic exercise during pregnancy. They should also be encouraged to modify the intensity of their exercise according to maternal symptoms. Pregnant women should stop exercising when fatigued and not exercise to exhaustion. Weight-bearing exercises may under some circumstances be continued at intensities similar to those prior to pregnancy throughout pregnancy. Non–weight-bearing exercises such as cycling or swimming will minimize the risk of injury and facilitate the continuation of exercise during pregnancy.
4. Morphologic changes in pregnancy should serve as a relative contraindication to types of exercise in which loss of balance could be detrimental to maternal or fetal well-being, especially in the third trimester. Further, any type of exercise involving the potential for even mild abdominal trauma should be avoided.
5. Pregnancy requires additional 300 kcal/d in order to maintain metabolic homeostasis. Thus, women who exercise during pregnancy should be particularly careful to ensure an adequate diet.
6. Pregnant women who exercise in the first trimester should augment heat dissipation by ensuring adequate hydration, appropriate clothing, and optimal environmental surroundings during exercise.
7. Many of the physiologic and morphologic changes of pregnancy persist 4-6 weeks postpartum. Thus, prepregnancy exercise routines should be resumed gradually based on a woman's physical capability.

Contraindications to exercise

The aforementioned recommendations are intended for women who do not have any additional risk factors for adverse maternal or perinatal outcome. A number of medical or obstetric conditions may lead the obstetrician to recommend modifications of these principles. The following conditions should be considered contraindications to exercise during pregnancy:

Pregnancy-induced hypertension
Preterm rupture of membranes
Preterm labor during the prior or current pregnancy or both
Incompetent cervix/cerclage
Persistent second or third trimester bleeding
Intrauterine growth retardation
In addition, women with certain other medical or obstetric conditions, including chronic hypertension or active thyroid, cardiac, vascular, or pulmonary disease, should be evaluated carefully in order to determine whether an exercise program is appropriate.

*Adapted from American College of Obstetricians and Gynecologists [108]; with permission.

taken, exercise during pregnancy is safe and beneficial to both the developing fetus and mother.

The risks and benefits of exercise in pregnancy may well differ in women who are fit and train at a competitive level prior to pregnancy, compared with sedentary women. A complete exercise history included as part of the prenatal evaluation will be useful in individualizing exercise recommendations. There are some precautions that should be taken, and certain situations in which exercise may place the fetus or mother at unwarranted risk, and in whom exercise should be limited. In considering exercise during pregnancy, it is helpful to assess both fetal risks and maternal risks as well as potential benefits [110–112], keeping in mind that recommendations must always be individualized.

Changes with pregnancy

Pregnancy causes an increase in heart rate, stroke volume, and cardiac output. Oxygen consumption (VO_2) during pregnancy increases by 10% during the course of pregnancy when walking and running speeds are kept constant [113], although these changes may not be significant when body weight is taken into account. Pregnancy does not appear to affect maximal VO_2, although this may depend somewhat on the exercise modality. For both cycle ergometry [114] and treadmill exercise [115], VO_{2max} is unaffected, whereas in swimming ergometry [116], VO_{2max} decreases as pregnancy progresses.

Cardiac output increases during pregnancy, due to both an increase in heart rate [115] and stroke volume [117], with both variables increasing throughout the course of pregnancy. Stroke volume may play the greater role as pregnancy progresses, with an increase in plasma volume being the primary cause for this increase.

Pregnancy causes a decrease in the expiratory reserve volume and a decrease in the functional reserve capacity, but vital capacity remains unchanged. Pregnancy increases the ventilatory response to exercise, both at submaximal as well as maximal exercise intensities. In both situations, this increase is possibly caused by a direct progesterone effect and an increased CO_2 sensitivity. The ventilation at maximal exercise is increased by 7% to 8% in both cycle ergometry as well as treadmill exercise [115].

The stress response of exercise in the pregnant woman is not clearly understood, and research examining the effects of cortisol, catecholamines, prolactin, glucagon, growth hormone, and insulin are underway [118]. The release of these substances in response to exercise may be altered during pregnancy, with a blunting of the overall stress response. Why and to what purpose these changes occur has not been fully elucidated.

Other changes that occur with pregnancy are related to anatomic alterations to accommodate the fetus, and these include an increase in lumbar lordosis, increased ligamentous laxity, and an increase in the anterior tilt of the pelvis. The center of gravity moves upward and anteriorly, with the increase in lumbar lordosis and rotation of the pelvis on the femur compensating for this. These changes often make exercise or activities requiring balance more challenging. Additionally, with an average increase in total body weight of 15% to 25% [119], there may be an increased potential for injury (a combined effect of increased load along with altered biomechanics) if there are difficulties with balance.

For these reasons, swimming is an excellent form of exercise for the pregnant woman. This exercise modality is also beneficial because it can help prevent the core temperature from increasing and the buoyant position may allow for better blood flow to the fetus. The mother does not have the balance control problems of land exercise, and the increased laxity that accompanies pregnancy may put the mother at more risk during land exercise compared with water exercise. Swimming may not be an available option for all women but should be considered in the exercise prescription.

Risks of exercise during pregnancy

The fetal risks during pregnancy can be thought of as any increase in fetal stress, assessed by changes in fetal heart rate, amniotic fluid volume, fetal movements and breathing, as well as muscular tone. The most common and easiest screen for fetal distress is a change in fetal heart rate or "biophysical profile." The range of normal fetal heart rates is approximately 120 to 160 beats per minute (bpm). Fetal tachycardia occurs if fetal heart rate is greater than 160 bpm for more than 10 minutes, and fetal bradycardia occurs if fetal heart rate is less than 120 bpm for greater than 1 minute [120].

The fetal heart rate increase in response to exercise is reported to average 10 to 30 bpm, with little alteration secondary to exercise intensity or age of gestation [118]. Mild or moderate exercise caused an increase in fetal heart rate that returned to normal within 15 minutes, whereas strenuous exercise required 30 minutes. Another study assessing women at 28 to 38 weeks of gestation who jogged 1.5 miles three times weekly found that there was no evidence for fetal distress with this regimen [121]. In another study of women at 32 to 39 weeks of gestation, swimming 30 to 45 minutes three times weekly did not demonstrate evidence for fetal distress [122]. Although the maternal heart rate in these women reached 80% of their predicted maximum, and increased fetal movement did occur, the fetal heart rate averaged 149 bpm, and there was no exercise-induced tachycardia or bradycardia noted. These studies demonstrate that although the maternal heart rate may increase with exercise, this may not unduly stress the fetus.

Another concern of exercise during pregnancy is that a relative hypoxemia may occur that may increase fetal risk. During the third trimester, exercise has been shown to cause a shunting of blood away from the uterus to increase the blood flow to muscles, which in turn may lead to fetal hypoxemia [123] There is some evidence that conditioning may blunt this response, which is believed to be due in part to an increase in catecholamine release [124]. Therefore, in a woman who is sedentary, the concern for hypoxia may be more valid than in the well-conditioned woman.

One of the most important concerns for the exercising woman during pregnancy is hyperthermia [119]. Animal studies have demonstrated that an increase in core temperature above 39° C can lead to an increase in neural defects. The critical core temperature above which defects occur appears to be 39°C. Hydration, proper clothing, and adequate thermoregulatory mechanisms need to be addressed when exercising, and this is of prime importance during pregnancy.

Exercise during pregnancy at different barometric pressures warrants special attention and may pose additional stress on both the maternal and fetal systems. Living at high altitude, or activities such as mountain climbing or mountain skiing, are examples of decreased barometric pressure. Above 2500 meters, an increase in the maternal ventilatory response to hypoxia exists and may represent an increased fetal risk [125]. It is important to consider other medical conditions that may alter a woman's ability to respond to environmental stresses. These include preeclampsia, anemia, or diabetes, and caution should be taken when contemplating exercise at higher elevations for pregnant woman with these problems.

Snorkeling and scuba diving are examples of activities that occur at increased barometric pressures. When divers rise from these pressures and return to atmospheric pressure, potential tissue damage can occur if ascent occurs too quickly. This condition is often referred to as "the bends," and is believed to be secondary to nitrogen escape from cells. It is unclear how this effects the developing fetus, and current recommendations are to avoid scuba diving or snorkeling below the surface during pregnancy.

The effects of exercise on fetal growth appear to show that strenuous exercise may lead to delivery of infants who are 300 to 500 g smaller and maternal weight gain is less than in non-exercising mothers [126]. Whether the lower birth weight is detrimental to the health of the mother or newborn has not been elucidated. If a mother is involved in hard labor, prolonged standing, or is nutritionally deficient, strenuous exercise may place an increased negative effect on fetal growth [127]. This same study also demonstrated that women who were physically active had a smaller chance of delivering prematurely. These studies demonstrate that the relationship between exercise and fetal growth needs to be studied further.

Benefits of exercise during pregnancy

There are several additional benefits of exercise during pregnancy. Exercise controls excessive weight gain, increases overall energy levels and sleep, and may shorten labor and decrease labor complications. In addition, exercise improves self-image and gives women some sense of control during what can at times be for many a difficult process. Gestational diabetes occurs in 4% to 7% of normal pregnancies, and although diet and insulin therapy have been used, exercise has been studied as an alternative method for treating these women. Diabetic and non-diabetic populations respond similarly to exercise during pregnancy [128,129]. These studies also demonstrate that carbohydrate tolerance is improved and the need for insulin is reduced when exercise is used therapeutically in gestational diabetics. Additionally, no adverse effects on the mother or fetus has been demonstrated in the exercise regimens used in these studies.

In conclusion, exercise certainly has beneficial effects for women, and these transcend pregnancy. Certain precautions should be taken, and the recommendations should be individualized, taking into account the level of fitness present prior to pregnancy. Various exercise modalities exist that will be an enjoyable part of the pregnancy process, and can enable a woman to have an active pregnancy, enjoy the positive effects of exercise, and perhaps improve the well-being of the newborn. As long as reasonable precautions are taken, inclusion of an exercise program is likely to be safe and beneficial for most women.

NUTRITION

The female athlete has some nutritional needs that are different than their male counterparts. Numerous studies have demonstrated the poor eating behavior of athletes, and especially in the female athlete. The main nutritional concerns in the female athlete include total caloric intake, as well as specific intake of protein, fat, calcium, and iron. Total caloric intake is often restricted in the female athlete, and this may well stem from societal influences as well as those discussed above that lead to disordered eating patterns. It is not uncommon for many women to be constantly dieting, and the intake of protein, fat, and calcium as well as total calories may well be limited. Additionally, with such a rage for supplementation, many athletes will use supplements in the hope they can obtain nutrients yet avoid calories.

In order to optimize athletic performance, adequate caloric intake, both in quality and quantity, is necessary. The ideal diet should consist of carbohydrate (6 to 10 g/kg/body weight) protein (0.8 g/kg) and the remainder from fat [130,131]. The breakdown can also be thought of as 60% to 70% carbohydrate, 10% to 15% protein, and 25% to 30% fat. Recently, the protein intake for athletic individuals has been increased to 1.0 to 1.2 g/kg, and ratio recommendations have increased the protein intake to 20% to 25%, with a decrease in the fat intake to 10% to 15%. According to Clark, "Theoretically, women who eat more than 1200–1500 calories from a variety of wholesome foods can obtain most nutrients necessary for top athletic performance (with the possible exception of iron)" [132]. The bottom line, therefore, is to emphasize proper food selection, not supplementation, when making recommendations to athletes.

Iron deficiency and anemia

Iron deficiency in athletes is a topic that has been well documented and reviewed [133,134] Anemia may or may not be present, but decreased iron stores have been reported in various studies in as many as 9.5% to 57% of young athletes [135–137]. Increases in plasma volume also occur as a result of

exercise, ranging from 6% to 25% [133]. Ferritin levels decrease during training [135,137], and girls, more so than boys, take in significantly less than the recommended daily allowance (RDA) of iron, putting women at an even higher risk for iron deficiency [136,137] . The cause of iron deficiency anemia in the athlete can be attributed to different mechanisms, including hemolysis with hemoglobinuria, gastrointestinal loss, and loss through sweat [138]. Athletes are not immune from other disorders that cause iron deficiency, such as ulcerative colitis, which underscores the need for a complete and systematic approach.

Female athletes are at increased risk of iron deficiency due to the increased iron loss that occurs with menses. In evaluating for iron deficiency, a complete blood count that includes erythrocyte indices is helpful. Additional studies include ferritin, which measures iron stores, as well as serum iron and total iron binding capacity, are helpful. Ferritin is also an acute phase reactant, increasing with infection or inflammation and decreasing with exercise, and therefore needs to be correlated with the clinical situation. Correction of anemia has been shown to improve performance [138]. Iron deficiency should be treated with supplementation as well as education on intake of iron-rich foods along with vitamin C, which increases absorption. Follow-up laboratory studies should be obtained 3 to 6 months after treatment. For the young athlete, screening hemoglobin as well as ferritin measurements may be a useful part of the preparticipation physical examination.

Calcium intake

Calcium intake is also important for the female athlete, and is of particular concern given the risks of the female triad discussed earlier. Female athletes take in less than two thirds of the RDA of calcium, and because peak bone mass is accumulated by the second decade, calcium intake is essential to ensure bone health. The NIH Consensus Conference has recommended a calcium intake of 1200 to 1500 mg/d [139]. The young athlete should understand the importance of consuming adequate calcium. A vitamin D intake of 400 to 800 IU/d is also important.

Fat and total caloric intake

Total caloric intake is also a concern for the female athlete, and many athletes do not consume adequate calories. Female athletes often exercise excessively, yet restrict their caloric intake. Many athletes underestimate what their caloric intake should be, and feel they can only eat if they have exercised. Additionally, many athletes restrict their fat intake, such that the fat-soluble vitamins, A, D, E, and K are also at risk for being deficient. The potential risks of consuming a diet that contains less than 10% fat include low energy intake and low levels of protein, iron, zinc, and vitamin E. Deficiencies have also been noted in zinc, magnesium, folate, and vitamins B_6, C, A, and B_{12}. How these deficiencies affect performance or injury remains to be more clearly discerned.

MUSCULOSKELETAL ISSUES

It is easy to recognize that menstrual dysfunction, eating disorders, and pregnancy are issues that relate specifically to the female athlete. In recent years, as girls and women increase their fitness levels and train harder and more intensely, there has been an increased understanding that there are musculoskeletal issues that are also specific to the female athlete. In the female athlete, there is an increased incidence of anterior cruciate ligament (ACL) injuries, patellofemoral dysfunction, and foot abnormalities. Flexibility issues, ligamentous laxity, and sport-specific risks of injury are important to address when assessing the female athlete. As more research is done in these areas, it may be possible to institute preventative rehabilitation to prevent injuries and possibly improve performance.

Alhough the absolute increase in muscle size and strength seen in response to strength training and conditioning is less in women than men, women respond the same to training. Women show the same strength gains in response to training as men when lean body mass is taken into account [140]. Strength training improves the ability of muscles, bones, ligaments and musculotendinous connections to withstand stress, and can increase power and endurance. A sport-specific strengthening program that is organized and supervised can optimize performance as well as avoid injury.

Specific clinical problems

Iliotibial friction syndrome, patellofemoral dysfunction (PFD), reflex sympathetic dystrophy, greater trochanteric bursitis, and possibly ankle and ACL sprains seem to appear more often in women than in men [141]. The cause of these differences remain unclear, but may include differences in biomechanics, muscle imbalances, or differences in biomechanics of jumping or running, from other sport-specific activities. It is essential that work continues to address the increased incidence of certain injuries in the female population. Prospective studies are also needed to consider the increased athleticism that female athletes have now compared with the past.

Patellofemoral dysfunction

Patellofemoral dysfunction is a patellar tracking problem that is potentiated by an increased Q angle, along with genu recurvatum and genu valgum. The tracking of the patella depends on the musculature of the extensor mechanism as well as the biomechanical alignment of the patellofemoral joint itself. Therefore, the development of the vastus obliquus and the vastus lateralis, as well as the tightness of the retinaculum and the iliotibial band attachments, are all important. Characteristically, PFD presents as anterior knee pain, made worse with climbing or descending stairs or sitting for a prolonged period of time. It is important to assess for the presence of an effusion, as this can decrease the strength of the quadriceps complex as measured by Cybex testing by as much as 10% to 40% [142]. In addition, although a sympathetic effusion can be seen in PFD, its presence should also expand the differential diagnosis to include meniscal lesions, ligamentous injury, articular surface defects, or osteochondral defects.

The main treatment goals for PFD include strengthening of the vastus medialis obliquus as well as correction of biomechanical problems, especially pronation, when possible. Taping techniques have been used to keep the patella in a more pain-free and functional position to facilitate the vastus medialis obliquus strengthening exercises. Closed-chain kinetic exercises, such as partial squats, are excellent rehabilitative exercises to use. Open-chain kinetic exercises, such as knee extensions or short arc exercises, have recently lost favor because they are not sport-specific, although they may play a role in sports such as soccer and karate.

Trochanteric bursitis

Another musculoskeletal problem commonly seen in the female athlete is greater trochanteric bursitis. This condition is made worse by varus at the hip, femoral neck anteversion, and tight iliotibial band (ITB) structures. In most situations, tight lateral structures compress the bursa and often irritate it with repetitive sliding over the greater trochanter. Occasionally, this can also cause "snapping hip" which is often not painful, and is due to the repetitive sliding of the ITB over the greater trochanter. On physical examination, trochanteric bursitis there presents with pain during both passive and active leg abduction, although there is usually no pain with resisted abduction in neutral (unless there is a concomitant tendinitis or strain). Treatment with conservative measures such as oral non-steroidal anti-inflammatory drugs , ice massage, ITB stretching, and modalities such as phonophoresis or iontophoresis is usually sufficient, along with consideration of biomechanical and training pattern alterations. If this is not successful, steroid injection into the bursa may be of benefit.

There has been some concern over muscle imbalances in female athletes that may put them at increased risk for injury. This may be of particular concern in sports that have a high incidence of lower extremity injuries. Knapik *et al.* [143] demonstrated a higher incidence of lower extremity injuries in female collegiate athletes with an imbalance in muscle strength and flexibility. A knee flexor to extensor ratio less than 0.75 at 180° per second was associated with a higher incidence of injury. Further research in this area is needed.

Anterior cruciate ligament injuries

Recent data for ACL injuries in female athletes raise significant concern [138,144–146]. For almost every sport tracked by the NCAA, there are more ACL injuries in women than men. A study of NCAA male and female soccer and basketball athletes looked at knee injuries and found a six-fold and two-fold increase in ACL injuries, respectively, in both sports for women compared with men [144]. The 4-year data have not yet been reviewed, but they appear to follow the same trend (Arendt and Dick, Personal communication). A recent study in Norwegian soccer players also found a two-fold increase in ACL injuries in the women compared with the men [145]. These statistics are alarming given the number of female participants involved in these sports, as well as the significant nature of this particular injury.

Although there were some early beliefs that the increase in ACL injuries was due to inferior strength and endurance training of female athlete, ACL injuries are also more common at the Olympic level in basketball [146]. In addition, the severity of the

injuries and the need for surgery was also higher in the female athletes. Other theories explaining the increased incidence of ACL injury include muscle imbalances, trochlear groove size or configuration, biomechanical differences in jumping and landing technique, and malalignment differences. This area of research is very important, and it is hoped that with continued interest in this area, we will soon understand the mechanisms and be able to incorporate preventative measures to decrease the incidence of ACL injuries.

Upper extremity injuries

There is no significant difference in upper extremity injuries in male and female athletes, except for possibly impingement syndrome (in swimmers) and thoracic outlet syndrome [147]. These entities are otherwise no different in presentation, physical examination, and treatment. A sport-specific strengthening program is again helpful in stabilizing the joint and providing additional power for performance as well as injury prevention.

PREVENTION

Strengthening and conditioning programs are important in preventing injuries and improving performance, and should be emphasized to ensure safe participation in sport. The better conditioned an athlete is, the less likely they will become injured. "Conditioning" includes aerobic and anaerobic conditioning as well as strengthening and flexibility work. Strength deficits and imbalances should be addressed during the pre-participation examination, and sport-specific strengthening programs can be provided. Each program should be designed specifically for the individual and the sport they are involved in, and the physician can work closely with the coach and trainer to identify the optimal conditioning and strengthening program.

CONCLUSIONS

Exercise is important not only for general health, positive lifestyle behaviors, and positive self-image, but also in learning skills such as goal-setting, teamwork, commitment, and self-reliance. It has been demonstrated that female athletes have a better and more positive body image than nonathletes [148]. These skills are hard to master, and sport allows the young individual to learn these life skills in a "game" situation. All of what young girls can learn from sport should not be overshadowed by the medical problems that can prevent them from participation. Additionally, some of the problems that a young female athlete may be at particular risk for, such as poor nutrition, eating disorders, and amenorrhea need to be understood and recognized early so that they can be treated early. Education is the cornerstone of understanding and identifying these issues early on so that prevention of irreversible consequences is possible.

Female athletes should be encouraged to understand how their body functions, how exercise effects it, and how proper nutrition and training can improve their performance. In addition, the preparticipation examination can be used to identify athletes at risk and to screen for musculoskeletal problems, strength deficits, or imbalances that may also affect their performance. The ultimate goal is to provide information such that the young female athlete can participate safely and establish healthy lifestyle behaviors that will remain a part of them throughout life.

REFERENCES AND RECOMMENDED READING

1. Harris SS, Caspersen CJ, DeFreise GH, Estes EH: Physical activity counseling for healthy adults as a primary preventive intervention in the clinical setting. *JAMA* 1989, 261:3590–3598.

2. Leon AS, Connett J, Jacobs DR, Rauramaa R: Leisure time physical activity levels and risk of coronary heart disease and death: the multiple risk factor intervention trial. *JAMA* 1987, 258:2388–2395.

3. Powell KE, Thompson PD, Casperson CJ, Kendrick JS: Physical activity and the incidence of coronary heart disease. *Ann Rev Public Health* 1987, 8:253–287.

4. Chalip L, Villige J, Duignan: Sex-role identity in a select sample of women field hockey players. *Int J Sports Psychology* 1980, 11:240–248.

5. Colton, Gore: Risk, resiliency, and resistance: current research on adolescent girls. MS Foundation: 1991.

6. Shangold MM, Mirkin G: *Women and Exercise: Physiology and Sports Medicine.* Philadelphia: F.A. Davis; 1988:279.

7. Tanner JM: *Growth at Adolescence,* ed 2. Oxford: Blackwell Scientific Publications; 1962.

8. Wells CL: *Women, Sport, and Performance,* ed 2. Champaign, IL: Human Kinetics Books; 1991.

9. Teitz CC (ed): *The Female Athlete.* Rosemont, IL: American Academy of Orthopedic Surgeons; 1997.

10. Sanborn CF, Jankowski CM: Physiologic considerations for women in sport. *Clin Sports Med* 1994, 13:315–328.

11. Komi PV (ed): *Strength and Power in Sport.* Oxford: Blackwell Scientific Publications; 1992.

12. Drinkwater BL: Physiological response of women to exercise. *Exerc Sports Rev* 1973, 1:125–153.

13. Wilmore JH, Brown CH: Physiological profiles of women distance runners. *Med Sci Sports Exerc* 1974, 6:178–181.

14. Cureton KJ, Collins MA, Hill DW, McElhannon FM: Muscle hypertrophy in men and women. *Med Sci Sports Exerc* 1988, 20:338–344.

15. Berg K: Aerobic function in female athletes. *Clin Sports Med* 1984, 3:779–789.

16. Griffin LY: The Female as a Sports Participant. *J Med Assoc Ga* 1992, 81:285–287.

17. Astrand P, Rodahl K: *Textbook of Work Physiology,* ed 2. New York: McGraw-Hill; 1977.

18. DeVries J: *Physiology of Exercise for Physical Education and Athletics,* ed 3. Dubuque, IA: William C. Brown; 1980.

19. Blair SN, Kohl HW, Paffenbarger RS, *et al.*: Physical fitness and all-cause mortality. *JAMA* 1989, 262:2395–2401.

20. Doody KM, Carr BR: Amenorrhea. *Obstet Gynecol Clin North Am* 1990, 17:361–387.

21. Pattison J: Hormone replacement therapy. In *Medical and Orthopedic Issues of Active and Athletic Women.* Edited by Agostini R. Philadelphia: Hanley & Belfus; 1994:183–190.

22. Dombovy ML, Bonekat HW, Williams TJ, *et al.*: Exercise performance and ventilatory response in the menstrual cycle. *Med Sci Sports Exerc* 1987, 19:111–117.

23. Vellar OD: Changes in hemoglobin concentration and hematocrit during the menstrual cycle. *Acta Obstet Gynecol Scand* 1974, 53:243–246.

24. Lebrun CM, McKenzie DC, Prior JC, *et al.*: Effects of menstrual cycle phase on athletic performance. *Med Sci Sports Exerc* 1995, 27:437–444.

25. Hessemer V, Bruck K: Influence of menstrual cycle on thermoregulatory, metabolic, and heart rate responses to exercise at night. *J Appl Physiol* 1985, 59:1911–1917.

26. Horvath SM, Drinkwater BL: Thermoregulation and the menstrual cycle. *Aviat Space Environ Med* 1982, 53:790–794.

27. DeSouza MJ, Maguire MS, Rubin K, *et al.*: Effects of menstrual phase and amenorrhea on exercise reponses in runners. *Med Sci Sports Exerc* 1990, 22:575–580.

28. Littler WA, Bojorges-Bueno R, Banks J: Cardiovascular dynamics in women during the menstrual cycle and oral contraceptive therapy. *Thorax* 1974, 29:567–570.

29. Lehtovirta P, Kuikka J, Pyorala T: Hemodynamic effects of oral contraceptives during exercise. *Int J Gynaecol Obstet* 1977, 15:35–37.

30. Lebrun CM: Effect of the different phases of the menstrual cycle and oral contraceptives on athletic performance. *Sports Med* 1993, 16:400–430.

31. Schoene RB, Robertson HT, Pierson DJ, Peterson AP: Respiratory drives and exercise in menstrual cycles of athletic and nonathletic women. *J Appl Physiol* 1981, 50:1300–1305.

32. Dombovy ML, Bonekat HW, Williams TJ, *et al.*: Exercise performance and ventilatory response in the menstrual cycle. *Med Sci Sports Exerc* 1987, 19:111–117.

33. Bonekat HW, Dombovy ML, Staats BA: Progesterone-induced changes in exercise performance and ventilatory response. *Med Sci Sports Exerc* 1987, 19:118–123.

34. Dibrezzo R, Fort IL, Brown B: Relationships among strength, endurance, weight and body fat during three phases of the menstrual cycle. *J Sports Med Phys Fitness* 1991, 31:89–94.

35. Quadagno D, Faquin L, Lim G-N, *et al*.: The menstrual cycle: does it affect athletic performance? *Phys Sports Med* 1991, 19:121–124.

36. Wirth JC, Lohman TG: The relationship of static muscle function to use of oral contraceptives. *Med Sci Sports Exerc* 1982, 14:16–20.

37. Carpenter AJ, Nunnely SA: Endogenous hormones subtly alter women's response to heat stress. *J Appl Physiol* 1989, 65:2313–2317.

38. Pivarnik JM, Lee W, Miller JF: Physiological and perceptual responses to cycle and treadmill exercise during pregnancy. *Med Sci Sports Exerc* 1991, 23:470–475.

39. Hessemer V, Bruck K: Influence of menstrual cycle on thermoregulatory, metabolic, and heart rate responses to exercise at night. *J App Physiol* 1985, 59:1911–1917.

40. Hessemer V, Bruck K: Influence of menstrual cycle on shivering skin blood flow and sweating responses measured at night. *J Appl Physiol* 1985, 59:1902–1910.

41. Bunt JC: Metabolic actions of estradiol: significance for acute and chronic exercise responses. *Med Sci Sports Exerc* 1990, 22:286–290.

42. Hatta H, Atomi Y, Shinohara S, *et al*.: The effects of ovarian hormones on glucose and fatty acid oxidation during exercise in female ovariectomized rats. *Horm Metab Res* 1988, 20:609–611.

43. Jurkowski JEH, Jones NL, Toews CJ: Effects of menstrual cycle on blood lactate, O_2 delivery and performance during exercise. *J Appl Physiol* 1981, 51:1493–1499.

44. Tarnopolsky LJ, MacDougall JD, Atkinson SA: Gender differences in substrate for endurance exercise. *J Appl Physiol* 1990, 68:302–308.

45. Bemenn DA, Boileau RA, Bahr JM, *et al*.: Effects of oral contraceptives on hormonal and metabolic responses during exercise. *Med Sci Sports Exerc* 1992, 24:434–441.

46. Bale P, Nelson G: The effects of menstruation on performance of swimmers. *Aust J Sci Med Sport* 1985, 17:19–22.

47. Flint MM, Drinkwater BL, Horvath SM: Effects of training on women's response to sub maximal exercise. *Med Sci Sports Exerc* 1974, 6:89.

48. Nicklas BJ, Hackney AC, Sharp RL: The menstrual cycle and exercise: performance, muscle glycogen and substrate responses. *Int J Sports Med* 1989, 10:264–269.

49. Robertson LA, Higgs LS: Menstrual cycle variations in physical work capacity, post-exercise blood lactate, and perceived exertion. *Can J Appl Sports Sci* 1983, 8:220.

50. DeSouza MJ, Maguire MS, Rubin K, *et al*.: Effects of menstrual phase and amenorrhea on exercise reponses in runners. *Med Sci Sports Exerc* 1990, 22:575–580.

51. Dombovy ML, Bonekat HW, Williams TJ, *et al*.: Exercise performance and ventilatory response in the menstrual cycle. *Med Sci Sports Exerc* 1987, 19:111–117.

52. DeBruyn-Prevost P, Masset C, Sturbois X: Physiological response from 18-25 years women to aerobic and anaerobic physical fitness tests at different periods during the menstrual cycle. J Sports Med 1984, 24:144–148.

53. Huisveld IA, Hospers JEH, Bernink MJ, *et al*.: The effect of oral contraceptives and exercise on hemostatic and fibrinolytic mechanisms in trained women. *Int J Sports Med* 1983, 4:97–103.

54. Notelovitz M, Zauner C, McKenzie L, *et al*.: The effect of low-dose contraceptives on cardiorespiratory function, coagulation, and lipids in exercising young women: a preliminary report. *Am J Obstet Gynecol* 1987, 156:591–598.

55. Moller-Nielsen J, Hammar M: Women's soccer injuries in relation to the menstrual cycle and oral contraceptive use. *Med Sci Sports Exerc* 1989, 21:126–129.

56. Kaiserauer S, Snyder AC, Sleeper M, *et al*.: Nutritional, physiological, and menstrual status of distance runners. *Med Sci Sports Exerc* 1989, 21:120–125.

57. Frisch RE, Gotz-Welbergen AV, McArthur JW, *et al*.: Delayed menarche and amenorrhea of college athletes in relation to age of onset of training. *JAMA* 1981, 246:1559–1563.

58. Mansfield MJ, Emans SJ: Anorexia nervosa, athletics, and amenorrhea. *Pediatr Clin North Am* 1989, 36:533–549.

59. Dink JH, Scheckter CB, Drinkwater BL, *et al*.: Higher serum cortisol levels in exercise associated amenorrhea. *Ann Intern Med* 1988, 108:530.

60. Boyden TW, Pamenter RS, Grosso D: Prolactin responses, menstrual cycles, and body composition of women runners. *J Clin Endocrinol Metab* 1982, 54:711.

61. Bunt JC: Metabolic actions of estradiol: significance for acute and chronic exercise responses. *Med Sci Sports Exerc* 1990, 22:286–290.

62. Hawlett TA, Tomlin S, Ngahfoong L, *et al*.: Release of B-endorphin and metenkephalin during exercise in normal women: response to training. *Br Med J* 1984, 288:1950.

63. Cummings DC, Vickovic MM, Wall SR, *et al*.: Defects in pulsatile LH release in normally menstruating runners. *J Clin Endocrinol Metab* 1985, 60:810–812.

64. McArthur JW, Bullen BA, Beitins IZ, *et al*.: Hypothalamic amenorrhea in runners of normal body composition. *Endocrinol Res Commun* 1980, 7:13.

65. Frisch RE, McArthur JW: Menstrual cycles: fatness as a determinant of minimum weight and height necessary for their maintenance or onset. *Science* 1974, 185:849.

66. Marcus R, Cann C, Madvig P, *et al*.: Menstrual function and bone mass in elite women distance runners: endocrine and metabolic features. *Ann Intern Med* 1985, 102:158–163.

67. Prior JC, *et al*.: Spinal bone loss and ovulatory disturbances. *N Engl J Med* 1990, 323:1221.

68. Schwartz B, Cumming DC, Riordan E, *et al*.: Exercise-associated amenorrhea: a distinct entity? *Am J Obstet Gynecol* 1981, 141:662.

69. Lutter JM, Suchman S: Menstrual patterns in female runners. *Phys Sports Med* 1982, 10:60.

70. Bonen A, Keizer HA: Athletic menstrual cycle irregularity: endocrine response to exercise and training. *Phys Sports Med* 1984, 12:78.22

71. Loucks AB, Horvath SM: Athletic amenorrhea: a review. *Med Sci Sports Exerc* 1985, 17:45.

72. Prior JC, Cameron K, Yuen BH, *et al*.: Menstrual cycle changes with marathon training: anovulation and short luteal phase. *Can J Appl Sports Sci* 1982, 7:173–177.

73. Schwartz B, Cumming DC, Riordan E, *et al*.: Exercise-associated amenorrhea: a distinct entity? *Am J Obstet Gynecol* 1981, 141:662.

74. Frisch RE, Hall GH, Aoki TT, *et al*.: Metabolic, endocrine and reproductive changes of a woman channel swimmer. *Metabolism* 1984, 33:1106.

75. Prior JC, *et al.*: Spinal bone loss and ovulatory disturbances. New Engl J Med 1990, 323:1221.

76. Shangold MM, Levine HS: The effect of marathon training upon menstrual function. *Am J Obstet Gynecol* 1982, 143:862–869.

77. White CM, Hergenroeder AC: Amenorrhea, osteopenia, and the female athlete. *Pediatr Clin North Am* 1990, 37:1125.

78. Gonzalez ER: Chronic anovulation may increase post menopausal breast cancer risk. *JAMA* 1983, 249:445–446.

79. Otis CL: Exercise-associated amenorrhea. *Clin Sports Med* 1992, 11:351.

80. Marcus R, Cann C, Madvig P, *et al.*: Menstrual function and bone mass in elite women distance runners: endocrine and metabolic features. *Ann Intern Med* 1985, 102:158–163.

81. Drinkwater BL, Nilson K, Chestnut CH III, *et al.*: Bone mineral content of amenorrheic and eumenorrheic athletes. *N Engl J Med* 1984, 311:277.

82. Cann CE, Martin MC, Genant, *et al.*: Decreased spinal mineral content in amenorrheic women. *JAMA* 1984, 251:626–629.

83. Lamon-Fava S, Fisher EC, Nelson ME: Effects of exercise and menstrual cycle status on plasma lipids, low density lipoprotein particle size and apolipoproteins. *J Clin Encocrinol Metab* 1989, 68:17–21.

84. Smith EL, Gilligan: Mechanical forces and bone. *Bone Miner Res* 1989, 6:1399.

85. Marcus R, Carter DR: The role of physical activity in bone mass regulation. *Adv Sports Med Fitness* 1988, 1:63–82.

86. Dalsky GP: The role of exercise in the prevention of osteoporosis. *Compr Ther* 1989, 15:30–37.

87. Drinkwater BL, Nilson K, Ott S, *et al.*: Bone mineral density after resumption of menses in amenorrheic athletes. *JAMA* 1986, 256:380.

88. Drinkwater BL, Bruemmer B, Chestnut CH III: Menstrual history as a determinant of current bone density in young athletes. *JAMA* 1990, 263:545.

89. Myburgh KH, Hutchins J, Fataar AB, *et al.*: Low bone density is an etiologic factor for stress fractures in athletes. *Ann Intern Med* 1990, 113:754–759.

90. Kadel NJ, Teitz CC, Kronmal RA: Stress fractures in ballet dancers. *Am J Sports Med* 1992, 20:445–449.

91. Licata AA: Stress fractures in young athletic women: case reports of unsuspected cortisol-induced osteoporosis. *Med Sci Sports Exerc* 1992, 24:955–957.

92. Lindberg JS, Fears WB, Hunt MM, *et al.*: Exercise-induced amenorrhea and bone density. *Ann Intern Med* 1984, 101:647–648.

93. Riffee JM: Osteoporosis: prevention and management. *Am Pharm* 1992, 321:61–71.

94. Emans SJ, Grace E, Hoffer FA, *et al.*: Estrogen deficiency in adolescents and young adults: impact on bone mineral content and effects of estrogen replacement therapy. *Obstet Gynecol* 1990, 76:585–592.

95. Yeager KK, Agostini R, Nattiv A, Drinkwater B: The female athlete triad: disordered eating, amenorrhea, osteoporosis [commentary]. *Med Sci Sports Exerc* 1993, 25:775.

96. Putukian M: The female triad. In *Sports Medicine and Arthroscopy Review*, vol 3. 1995.

97. Putukian M: The female triad: eating disorders, amenorrhea, and osteoporosis. *Med Clin North Am* 1994, 78:345–356.

98. American College of Sports Medicine: Position stand on the female athlete triad. *Med Sci Sports Exerc* 1997, 29:i–ix.

99. Ettinger B, Miller P, McClung MR: Use of bone densitometry results for decisions about therapy for osteoporosis. *Ann Intern Med* 1996, 125:623.

100. Gilchrist NL: Bone density estimation. *N Z Med J* 1988, 101:260.

101. Cummings SR, Kelsey JL, Nevitt MC, *et al.*: Epidemiology of osteoporosis and osteoporotic fractures. *Epidemiol Rev* 1985, 7:178.

102. NIH concensus conference: Optimal calcium intake. *JAMA* 1994, 272:1942–1948.

103. Chow R, Harrison JE, Notarius C: Effect of two randomized exercise programs on bone mass of healthy post menopausal women. *BMJ* 1987, 295:1441–1444.

104. Ettinger B, Genant HK, Cann CE: Postmenopausal bone loss is prevented by treatment with low-dosage estrogen with calcium. *Ann Intern Med* 1987, 106:40–45.

105. Smith EL Jr, Reddan W, Smith PE: Physical activity and calcium modalities for bone mineral increase in aged women. *Med Sci Sports Exerc* 1981, 13:60–64.

106. Snow CM: Exercise and bone mass in young and premenopausal women. *Bone* 1996, 18:51S–55S.

107. Felson DT, Zhang Y, Hannan MT, *et al.*: The effect of postmenopausal estrogen therapy on bone density in elderly women. *N Engl J Med* 1993, 329:1141–1146.

108. American College of Obstetricians and Gynecologists (ACOG): Technical Bulletin: exercise during pregnancy and the postnatal period. Washington, DC: American College of Obstetricians and Gynecologists; 1985.

109. Wolfe LA, Hall P, Webb KA, *et al.*: Prescription of aerobic exercise during pregnancy. *Sports Med* 1989, 8:273–301.

110. Jarski RW, Trippett DL: The risks and benefits of exercise during pregnancy. *J Fam Pract* 1990, 30:185–189.

111. McMurray RG, Mottola MF, Wolfe LA, *et al.*: Recent advances in understanding maternal and fetal responses to exercise. *Med Sci Sports Exerc* 1993, 25:1305–1321.

112. White J: Exercising for two: what's safe for the active pregnant woman? *Phys Sports Med* 1992, 20:179–186.

113. Pivarnik JM, Lee W, Miller JF: Physiological and perceptual responses to cycle and treadmill exercise during pregnancy. *Med Sci Sports Exerc* 1991, 23:470–475.

114. Sady MA, Haydon BB, Sady SP, *et al.*: Cardiovascular response to maximal exercise during pregnancy and at two and seven months postpartum. *Am J Obstet Gynecol* 1990, 162:1181–1185.

115. Lotgering FK, Van Doorn MB, Struijk PC, *et al.*: Maximal aerobic exercise in pregnant women: heart rate, O_2 consumption, CO_2 production, and ventilation. *J Appl Physiol* 1991, 70:1016–1023.

116. McMurray RG, Hackney AC, Katz VL, *et al.*: Pregnancy induced changes in maximal oxygen uptake during swimming. *J Appl Physiol* 1991, 71:1454–1459.

117. Pivarnik JM, Lee W, Miller JF, *et al.*: Alterations in plasma volume and protein during cycle exercise throughout pregnancy. *Med Sci Sports Exerc* 1990, 22:751–755.

118. McMurray RG, Mottola MF, Wolfe LA, *et al.*: Recent advances in understanding maternal and fetal responses to exercise. *Med Sci Sports Exerc* 1993, 25:1305–1321.

119. Artal R: Exercise and pregnancy. *Clin Sports Med* 1992, 11:363–376.

120. McMurray RG, Hackney ACM, Jatz VKM, *et al.*: Pregnancy induced changes in maximal oxygen uptake during swimming. *J Appl Physiol* 1991, 71:1454–1459.

121. Hauth JC, Gilstrap LC, Widmer M: Fetal heart rate reactivity before and during the third semester. *Am J Obstet and Gynecol* 1982, 142:545–547.

122. Dressendorfer RH, Goodlin RC: Fetal heart rate reponse to maternal exercise testing. *Phys Sports Med* 1980, 8:91–94.

123. Anderson TD: Exercise and sport in pregnancy. *Midwife Health Visit Commun Nurse* 1986, 22:275–278.

124. Morton MJ, Paul MS, Metcalfe J: Exercise during pregnancy. *Med Clin North Am* 1985, 69:97–108.

125. Moore LG, McCullouogh RE, Weil JV: Increased hypoxic ventilatory response in pregnancy: relationship to hormonal and metabolic changes. *J Appl Physiol* 1987, 62:158–163.

126. Clapp JF III, Capeless EL: Neonatal morphometrics after endurance exercise during pregnancy. *Am J Obstet Gynecol* 1990, 163:1805–1811.

127. Tafari N, Naeye RL, Gobzie A: Effects of maternal undernutrition and heavy physical work during pregnancy on birth weight. *Br J Obstet Gynecol* 1980, 87:222–226.

128. Jojanovic-Peterson L, Durak EP, Peterson CM: Randomized trial of diet versus diet plus cardiovascular conditioning on glucose levels in gestational diabetes. *Am J Obstet Gynecol* 1989, 161:415–419.

129. Artal R, Masaki D: Exercise in gestational diabetes. *Practical Diabetology* 1989, 8:7–14.

130. Costill D: Carbohydrates for exercise; dietary demands for optimal performance. *Int J Sports Med* 1988, 9:1–18.

131. Friedman J, Lemon P: Effect of chronic endurance exercise on retention of dietary protein. *Int J Sports Med* 1989, 10:118–123.

132. Clark N: Nutritional problems and training intensity, activity level, and athletic performance. In *The Athletic Female*. Edited by Pearl AJ. 1993:165–168.

133. Balaban EP: Sports anemia. *Clin Sports Med* 1992, 11:313–325.

134. Rauniker RA, Sabio H: Anemia in adolescent athletes. *Am J Dis Child* 1992, 146:1201–1205.

135. Risser WL Lee EJ, Poindexter HBW, *et al.*: Iron deficiency in female athletes: its prevalence and impact on performance. *Med Sci Sports Exerc* 1988, 20:116–121.

136. Nickerson HJ, Holubets MC, Weiler BR, *et al.*: Causes of iron deficiency in adolescent athletes. *J Pediatr* 1989, 114:657–663.

137. Zelisko JA, Noble HB, Porter M: A comparison of men's and women's professional basketball injuries. *Am J Sports Med* 1982, 10:297–299.

138. Rowland TW: Iron deficiency in the young athlete. *Pediatr Clin North Am* 1990, 37:1153–1163.

139. NIH consensus conference: Optimal calcium intake. JAMA 1994, 272:1942–1948.

140. Malone TR, Sanders B: Strength training and the athletic female. Edited by Pearl AJ. In *The Athletic Woman*. Champaign, IL: Human Kinetics Publishers; 1993:169–184.

141. Ciullo JV: Pearl AJ (ed): Lower extremity injuries. In *The Athletic Woman*. Champaign, IL: Human Kinetics Publishers; 1993.

142. Wood L, Ferrell WR, Baxendale RH: Pressures in normal and acutely distended knee joints and effects on quadriceps maximal voluntary contractions. *J Exp Physiol* 1988, 73:305–314.

143. Knapik JJ, Bauman CL, Jones BH, *et al.*: Preseason strength and flexibility imbalances associated with athletic injuries in female collegiate athletes. *Am J Sports Med* 1991, 19:76–81.

144. Arendt EA, Dick RW: Gender specific knee injury patterns in collegiate basketball and soccer athletes: NCAA data and review of literature. *Am J Sports Med* 1995, 23:694–701.

145. Bjordal JM, Arnoy F, Hannestad B, Strand T: Epidemiology of anterior cruciate ligament injuries in soccer. *Am J Sports Med* 1997, 25:341–345.

146. Ireland ML, Wall C: Epidemiology and comparison of knee injuries in elite male and female United States basketball athletes. *Med Sci Sports Exerc* 1990, 22:592.

147. Teitz CC (ed): The upper extremities. In *The Female Athlete*. Rosemont, IL: American Academy of Orthopedic Surgeons; 1997:39–43.

148. Chalip L, Villiger J, Duigan P: Sex role identity in a select sample of women field hockey players. *Int J Sports Psychol* 1980, 11:240–248.

149. Carr BR, Wilson JD: Disorders of the ovary and female reproductive tract. In *Harrison's Principles of Internal Medicine*, ed 11. Edited by Braunwald E, Isselbacher KJ, *et al.* New York: McGraw-Hill; 1987:1818–1836.

150. Pearl AJ (ed): *The Female Athlete*. Champaign, IL: Human Kinetics Publishers; 1993.

151. Task Force on the *Diagnostic and Statistical Manual of Mental Disorders-IV*: DSM-IV draft criteria. Washington, DC: American Psychiatric Association; 1993:1–2.

152. McSherry JA: The diagnostic challenge of anorexia nervosa. *Am Fam Phys* 1984, 29:144.

153. Putukian M: The athletic woman. In *Office Sports Medicine*. Edited by Mellion M. Philadelphia: Hanley and Belfus; 1996:81–101.

16

MEDICOLEGAL ISSUES

Matthew J. Mitten

Legal issues continue to be a concern of the sports medicine practitioner, and important recent medicolegal developments are covered in this chapter [1•]. Although several lawsuits have been brought against sports medicine physicians alleging malpractice, little legal precedent has been established, because most cases settle before the merits of asserted claims are judicially resolved. Nevertheless, a review of these cases identifies potential areas of legal liability in connection with the provision of sports medicine care. This chapter also discusses recent cases upholding the team physician's legal authority to medically disqualify a physically impaired athlete from competition. In addition, a discussion of legal challenges by athletes to mandatory testing for use of performance-enhancing or recreational drugs is included in this chapter.

MALPRACTICE LITIGATION

While providing medical care to an athlete, a physician has a legal obligation to have and use the knowledge, skill, and care ordinarily possessed and used by members of his or her specialty in good standing (depending on the state of medical science at the time such care is rendered) [2•]. The law allows the medical profession to collectively determine the parameters of appropriate sports medicine care and to establish proper medical practices and treatment that should be followed within those boundaries. In other words, a physician must adhere to customary or accepted sports medicine practices within his or her specialty.

The medical standard of care, which must be established by physician expert testimony, is the legal standard of care in a malpractice case. For example, in *Gardner v Holifield* (693 So2d 652 [FL App 1994]), the court held that the testimony of two cardiologists that another cardiologist had negligently treated a college basketball player's heart condition was evidence of malpractice. This expert testimony established that the defendant physician failed to implement an appropriate course of treatment for the player's condition (diagnosed as Marfan syndrome) and had medically cleared him to engage in weight training and other activities inappropriate for his condition.

In the past, courts did not recognize sports medicine as a separate medical specialty for the purpose of determining the legal standard of care in malpractice litigation, presumably because there existed no national medical specialty board certification or standardized sports medicine training. This judicial view will probably change as sports medicine evolves and becomes recognized as a separate area of specialization by the medical profession. The American Osteopathic Association now provides board certification for sports medicine. Although the American Board of Medical Specialties does not currently have a separate certification board for sports medicine, a consortium of its member boards offers a certificate of added qualification to board-certified physicians who pass a competency examination in sports medicine. In the future, courts likely will hold physicians certified in sports medicine (or those espousing to be specialists in sports medicine) to a higher standard of care within their respective specialties when treating athletes. For example, a family practice physician may be held to the standard of care of a family practitioner with expertise and experience in sports medicine in treating an athlete.

Recent lawsuits arising out of the deaths of college basketball players Hank Gathers and Earnest Killum illustrate areas of potential legal liability in connection with the provision of sports medicine care to athletes. In *Gathers v Loyola-Marymount University* (13 No. C795027 [CA Super Ct 1990]) Gathers' heirs asserted that Gathers' physicians did not fully inform him of the seriousness of having ventricular tachycardia and should not have medically cleared him to continue playing college basketball with his condition. Gathers' heirs alleged that the physicians providing such clearance acted negligently according to the 16th Bethesda Conference guidelines regarding competitive athletics participation with cardiovascular abnormalities. These guidelines, which were in effect at the time of treatment, recommend that athletes with ventricular tachycardia should not participate in competitive sports [3]. The heirs also claimed that Gathers was given a nontherapeutic dosage of heart medication to enable him to perform well in upcoming intercol-

legiate basketball tournament games. This negligent medical treatment allegedly caused Gathers to collapse and die during a March 1990 basketball game at Loyola-Marymount University.

In *Lillard v State of Oregon* (14 No. BC2941 [CA Super Ct 1993]), Earnest Killum's mother alleged that her son's death was caused by his physicians' failure to inform him of the material medical risks of continuing to play basketball at Oregon State University with an impaired vascular condition caused by two prior strokes. After these strokes, Killum experienced numbness and slurred speech during a recreational basketball game; tests determined that he had peripheral vascular disease. Physicians prescribed anticoagulant agents, and he was initially advised to withdraw from competitive basketball. Thereafter, his medications were reduced, and he was cleared by the defendant physicians to resume playing college basketball, despite recommendations to the contrary by a consultant. He died one month later, apparently of a massive cerebral infarction, in an off-court incident.

Killum's mother claimed that his physicians negligently treated him. More specifically, she contended that they breached their legal duty to Killum by 1) prescribing a nontherapeutic dosage of medication, 2) medically clearing him to return to college basketball, which subjected him to an increased risk of death or serious bodily harm, and 3) compromising his medical care to advance a university's economic interests in his athletic ability.

The *Gathers* and *Killum* cases illustrate that reducing medically necessary drugs to nontherapeutic levels, prescribing improper performance-enhancing drugs (*eg*, steroids), or providing other medically inappropriate treatment to enable or enhance athletic performance may constitute malpractice. Physicians must carefully consider the parameters of the acceptable medical risks of athletic participation with an illness, injury, or physical abnormality as well as when or if a return to play is appropriate. Those practicing sports medicine should always adhere to their paramount obligation to protect an athlete's health.

It is a serious violation of a physician's ethical and legal duties to 1) allow nonmedical factors to impair his or her best medical judgment when making clearance recommendations for an athlete or 2) withhold information from an athlete concerning the health risks of athletic participation with a certain condition. Courts have held that a team physician can be liable for negligence or fraud if he or she fails to provide an athlete with full disclosure of material information about playing with a medical condition or the potential consequences of a proposed treatment. In *Krueger v San Francisco Forty Niners* (234 Cal Rptr 579 [Ct App 1987]), a California court held that a professional football team's conscious failure to inform a player that he risked a permanent knee injury by continuing to play was fraudulent concealment. The court found that the plaintiff was not informed by team physicians of the true nature and extent of his knee injuries (the consequences of steroid-injection treatment) or the long-term dangers associated with playing professional football with his medical condition. The court found that the purpose of this nondisclosure was to induce the plaintiff to continue playing football despite his injuries, thereby constituting fraud.

The important lesson to be learned from the *Gathers*, *Killum*, and *Krueger* cases is that a physician should refuse to clear an athlete to participate in a sport if there is a significant medical risk of harm from playing, regardless of the team's needs or a player's willingness to take medically unwarranted risks. In formulating a participation recommendation, a physician should only consider the athlete's medical best interests. In cases in which there is an uncertain potential for life-threatening or permanently disabling harm to a medically impaired athlete, the best means to avoid malpractice liability is to err on the side of caution and recommend against athletic participation.

Various groups of physicians and sports medicine societies recently have been formulating guidelines suggesting the appropriate parameters of preparticipation screening for certain medical conditions and recommendations concerning athletic participation for physically impaired athletes or returning to play after an injury [4–6]. As the *Gathers* case demonstrates, it is likely that, in litigation, a physician's noncompliance with applicable guidelines will be alleged to constitute malpractice.

In a malpractice suit, guidelines regarding the care of athletes are admissible evidence of proper medical practice if they have a valid scientific or clinical basis and reflect the current state of the medical art. Standing alone, such guidelines do not conclusively establish the legal standard of care with which physicians must comply when providing care and treatment to athletes. The current legal standard of care is accepted or customary medical practice within a physician's specialty, but state-of-the-art medical guidelines are relevant in determining what constitutes good medical practice under the circumstances [1•].

In some states, generally applicable Good Samaritan statutes or specific laws regarding those volunteering to serve as team physicians may provide immunity to malpractice claims brought by athletes. This statutory immunity generally protects only physicians who provide negligent emergency medical care in good faith and without compensation to an athlete with an apparent life-threatening condition or serious injury. Willful or wanton emergency treatment or gross negligence by a physician is not immune from tort liability.

Some jurisdictions provide broader tort immunity for team physicians found to be employees (rather than independent contractors or consultants) of a public institution or professional team within the state that extends beyond the provision of emergency medical care to an athlete. In *Gardner v Holifield*, the Florida court ruled that the alleged negligent medical care provided to a college basketball player by a physician in his capacity as director of a public university's student health center was encompassed within the scope of tort immunity under Florida law. State employees, including physicians, are immune from liability for negligence committed within the scope and course of their state employment, the court said. However, any negligent medical care provided to a player by a physician while acting in his capacity as a private physician is not immunized from liability.

In California, professional athletes cannot sue team physicians for negligent medical care. In *Hendy v Losse* (819 P2d 1 [CA 1992]), a professional football player sued team physicians for negligently diagnosing and treating a knee injury suffered during a game and advising him to continue playing football. In dismissing these claims, the California Supreme Court held that California's workmen's compensation law bars tort suits between coemployees for injuries caused within the scope of employment. The court found that the player and physician were both employed by the San Diego Chargers and that the physician acted within the scope of his employment in treating the player. Thus, the player's exclusive remedy for his harm was workmen's compensation.

These judicial interpretations of specific state laws notwithstanding, physicians providing negligent nonemergency medical care to athletes are not normally immune from malpractice liability. Preparticipation physical examinations, general nonemergency medical care rendered to athletes, and physician decisions regarding whether an athlete may return to a game are not usually subject to immunity.

LITIGATION BY ATHLETES DENIED MEDICAL CLEARANCE TO PLAY SPORTS

Federal laws such as the Americans With Disabilities Act and the Rehabilitation Act of 1973 prohibit unjustified discrimination against people who have physical abnormalities and impairments. Athletes have relied on these statutes in support of claims that their exclusion from a sport by team officials based on the team physician's recommendation is illegal [7•]. Recent judicial precedent, however, has upheld the legal authority of the team physician to medically disqualify an athlete whose physical condition exposes him or her to an enhanced risk of death or serious injury during athletics competition.

In *Knapp v Northwestern University* (101 F3d 473 [7th Cir 1996]), a federal appellate court held that Northwestern University did not violate the Rehabilitation Act in following its team physician's recommendation that an athlete with idiopathic ventricular fibrillation not play intercollegiate basketball. As a high school senior, Nicholas Knapp suffered sudden cardiac arrest while playing recreational basketball and required cardiopulmonary resuscitation and defibrillation to restart his heart. Thereafter, he had an internal cardioverter–defibrillator implanted in his abdomen. He subsequently has played competitive recreational basketball without any incidents of cardiac arrest and has received medical clearance to play college basketball from three cardiologists who examined him. The court, however, explained that Knapp's exclusion from Northwestern's basketball team was legally justified:

[M]edical determinations of this sort are best left to team doctors and universities as long as they are made with reason and rationality and with full regard to possible and reasonable accommodations. In such cases as ours, where Northwestern has examined both Knapp and his medical records, has considered his medical history and the relation between his prior sudden cardiac death and the possibility of future occurrences, has considered the severity of the potential injury, and has rationally and reasonably reviewed consensus medical opinions and recommendations in the pertinent field— regardless whether conflicting medical opinions exist— the university has the right to determine that an individual is not otherwise medically qualified to play without violating the Rehabilitation Act. The place of the court in such cases is to make sure that the decision-maker has reasonably considered and relied on sufficient evidence specific to the individual and the potential injury, not to determine on its own which evidence it believes is more persuasive.

Instead, in the midst of conflicting expert testimony regarding the degree of serious risk of harm or death, the court's place is to ensure that the exclusion or disqualification of an individual was individualized, reasonably made, and based on competent medical evidence. So long as these factors exist, it will be the rare case regarding participation in athletics where a court may substitute its judgment for that of the school's team physicians. . . .

In closing, we wish to make care that we are not saying Northwestern's decision necessarily is the right decision. We say only that it is not an illegal one under the Rehabilitation Act. On the same facts, another team physician at another university, reviewing the same medical history, physical evaluation, and medical recommendations, might reasonably decide that Knapp met the physical qualifications for playing on an intercollegiate basketball team. Simply put, all universities need not evaluate risk the same way. What we say in this case is that if substantial evidence supports the decision-maker—here Northwestern— that decision must be respected.

It is important to note that the *Knapp* case holds that it is legally appropriate for physicians to follow consensus medical guidelines in making participation recommendations for athletes with physical abnormalities. This judicial view is consistent with the essential requirement of both the Americans With Disabilities Act and the Rehabilitation Act that there be a reasonable medical basis for excluding an athlete from a sport. Thus, consensus guidelines and recommendations probably will play an important role in future athletics-participation disputes, both in preventing and resolving litigation.

Similarly, in *Pahulu v University of Kansas* (897 FSupp 1387 [D KS 1995]), a federal district court upheld the team physician's "conservative" medical disqualification of a college football player with an abnormally narrow cervical canal after an episode of transient quadriplegia during a scrimmage. After consulting with a neurosurgeon, the team physician concluded that the athlete was at extremely high risk for sustaining permanent, severe neurologic injury including quadriplegia if he resumed football. The athlete wanted to resume playing because three other medical specialists concluded that he was at no greater risk of permanent paralysis than any other player.

ATHLETE LEGAL CHALLENGES TO MANDATORY DRUG TESTING

The legality of mandatory drug testing of professional athletes is governed by the terms of the collective bargaining agreement (CBA) negotiated by the players' union and representatives of the team owners. The CBA determines the scope of permissible drug testing and procedures regarding the methods of obtaining samples of body fluids from players for testing. It also establishes notification requirements and confidentiality safeguards as well as required player treatment and potential disciplinary action for positive test results. Rather than litigation in a court, the CBA generally requires arbitration of player challenges to drug testing procedures and results.

In a 1995 case, *Vernonia School District 47J v Acton* (115 SCt 2386 [1985]), the U.S. Supreme Court held that mandatory testing of elementary and high school athletes for recreational drug usage by a public school district is constitutional. The Court concluded that the school district's legitimate interests in preventing drug use, protecting athletes' health and safety, and providing drug users with assistance programs outweighed any invasion of tested athletes' privacy interests. There is a custodial relationship between a school district and minor children, and athletes have a lesser expectation of privacy than other students regarding medical examinations and procedures. The Court relied on evidence that drug use increases the risk of sports-related injury and on expert testimony concerning the deleterious effects of drugs on motivation, memory, judgment, reaction, coordination, and performance. The Court noted that test results were disclosed only to a limited class of school personnel (*eg*, superintendents, principals, and athletic directors) who have a need to know this information.

In *Hill v National Collegiate Athletic Association* (NCAA) (26 Cal Rptr 2d 834 [CA 1994]) the California supreme court held that the NCAA's testing of randomly selected athletes competing in postseason championships and football bowl games for certain designated performance-enhancing and recreational drugs does not violate the California constitution. As a private entity, the NCAA is not subject to the constraints of the U.S. Constitution in conducting drug testing. The court determined that the NCAA's interests in preserving the integrity of intercollegiate athletic competition and protecting the health and safety of athletes justified the limited infringement of adult athletes' privacy interests. Appropriate procedures were used to safeguard the integrity of the testing process and ensure confidentiality of test results. The court stated that testing for the use of illegal and dangerous drugs as well as those that may potentially affect athletic performance in either a positive or negative manner is permissible despite some scientific controversy about the effects of particular drugs.

In *Brennan v Board of Trustees for University of Louisiana Systems* (691 So2d 324 [LA Ct App 1997]), a Louisiana appellate court recently held that a public university's suspension of an athlete who tested positive for steroid use from intercollegiate athletic competition is not unconstitutional. The university took this action based on the results of drug tests administered by the NCAA. Applying the same analysis as the court that heard the *Hill* case, the Louisiana court found that a university shares the NCAA's interests in ensuring fair intercollegiate sports competition and protecting the health and safety of athletes, which outweigh invasion of an athlete's privacy interests by drug testing. The court relied on the expert medical testimony that test results established a pattern of impermissible testosterone use by the athlete. The court noted with approval that the university's director of sports medicine previously had fully explained the NCAA's drug testing program to the athlete and warned him about taking any drugs or other substances without consulting a member of the university's medical staff.

However, in *University of Colorado v Derdeyn* (863 P2d 929 [CO 1993]), the Colorado supreme court held that a public university's random urinalysis drug testing of its athletes violated both the federal and Colorado constitutions. The court noted that one of the intrusive aspects of the drug testing program is that it sometimes creates untrusting and confrontational relations between athletes and team medical personnel. Although the court found that a university's interest in protecting the health and safety of its athletes is valid, the court concluded that the university's interests did not outweigh what it characterized as the significant intrusion that the drug testing program imposed on the privacy of college athletes. This case establishes precedent only in Colorado and is contrary to the developing judicial trend to uphold the legality of drug testing of college athletes as long as appropriate testing procedures and confidentiality safeguards are used.

REFERENCES AND RECOMMENDED READING

Recently published papers of particular interest have been highlighted as:

•   Of special interest

••   Of outstanding interest

1.•   Herbert DL, Herbert WG (eds): *The Sports Medicine Standards and Malpractice Reporter*. Canton, OH: PRC Publishing.
Quarterly update of important legal issues in sports medicine.

2.•   Mitten MJ: Team physicians and competitive athletes: allocating legal responsibility for athletic injuries. *U Pitt L Rev* 1993, 55:129–169.
In-depth discussion of sports medicine malpractice liability issues.

3.   Mitchell JH, Maron BJ, Epstein SJ: 16th Bethesda Conference: cardiovascular abnormalities in the athlete: recommendations regarding eligibility for competition. *J Am Coll Cardiol* 1985, 6:1186–1232.

4.   American Academy of Family Physicians, American Academy of Pediatrics, American Medical Society for Sports Medicine, American Othropaedic Society for Sports Medicine, American Osteopathic Academy of Sports Medicine: *Preparticipation Physical Evaluation*, ed 2. Minneapolis, MN: McGraw-Hill; 1997.

5.   Mason BJ, Thompson PD, Puffer JC, *et al.*: Cardiovascular preparticipation screening of competitive athletes with cardiovascular abnormalities. *Circulation* 1996, 94:850–856.

6.   26th Bethesda Conference: recommendations for determining eligibility for competition in athletes with cardiovascular abnormalities. *J Am Coll Cardiol* 1994, 24:845–899.

7.•   Mitten MJ: When is disqualification from sports justified?: medical judgment vs. patients' rights. *Phy and Sportsmed* 1996, 24:75–78.
Overview of recent litigation by physically impaired athletes.

INDEX

Page numbers followed by f and t indicate figures and tables, respectively.

A

Abrasion arthroplasty, 145
Achilles tendon
    allograft in knee injuries of, 78, 80–81
    injury of, 107, 107f
Acromegaly, 165–166
Acute medial elbow rupture, 33f–34f, 33–34
Adductor muscle injury, 61
Adjustment disorders
    in performance psychology, 184
Adolescence
    mechanical back pain in, 14–15
    osteochondral defects in, 144
    scoliosis in, 15
    spinal injury in, 9, 10t, 11–12
    spinal variants in, 4
Aerobic exercise
    after spinal injury, 12
    in conditioning, 189–190
Aggrecans
    cartilage, 138f–139f, 139
Aging
    coronary artery disease and, 152
    hip fracture and, 58
    osteoarthritis *versus*, 144
    periosteal and perichondrial grafting and, 145
Airway restriction in asthma, 159–161, 160t
Alcohol consumption, 159, 170
    anabolic steroid use and, 165
Allografting
    in anterior cruciate ligament repair, 72–73
    HIV transmission in, 89–90
    in lateral collateral ligament repair, 81
    in meniscal repair, 89–90, 90f
    in osteochondral knee lesions, 93–95, 94f
    in posterior cruciate ligament repair, 78, 80
Altitude
    fetal risks of, 223
Amenorrhea, 211, 213
    in eating disorders, 183
    exercise-induced, 213–214
    stress fractures and, 63, 104–105, 214
American Board of Medical Specialties, 232
American College of Obstetricians and Gynecologists
    exercise guidelines of, 221, 221t
American College of Sports Medicine
    conditioning guidelines of, 193
    exercise testing guidelines of, 152, 157, 190t, 191
American Medical Association
    amphetamines studied by, 169
American Osteopathic Association certification, 232
American Psychological Association
    sport psychology in, 176
American Sports Medicine Institute
    curve ball pitching contraindicated by, 28
Americans with Disabilities Act, 234
Amphetamines, 169
Anabolic steroids, 164–165, 166f, 167t
    testing for, 172
Anaerobic fitness, 190
Anemia, 224
Angiotensin converting enzyme inhibitors, 159
Ankle and foot injury, 103–116
    arthroscopy in, 112f–113f, 112–114
    exertional compartment syndrome in, 103–104, 104f–105f
    fractures in, 114f, 114–115
        stress, 104–106
    great toe, 115, 115f
    instability in, 111f, 111–112
    nerve entrapment in, 107–110, 108f
    os trigonum, 110f–111f, 110–111
    plantar fasciitis in, 110
    tendon injuries in, 106–107, 107f
Anorexia nervosa, 183, 217–221, 218t–219t, 220f
Anovulation, 213
Anterior cruciate ligament injury, 71–77, 72f–76f, 126–130
    meniscal repair and, 89
    in women, 226
Anterior interosseus nerve injury, 39

Anterior slide test, 22, 22f
Anterior talofibular ligament injury, 111–112
Anterior tibialis tendon injury, 107
Antibiotics
    in postarthroscopic infection, 92
Antiglide plate
    in ankle fracture, 114f, 115
Anxiety disorders
    in performance psychology, 183
Aortic valve stenosis, 157, 191t
Arm injury
    forearm, 25–41, 27f–28f, 30f–38f
    upper, 19–24, 20f–23f
Arousal control
    in performance psychology, 179–181, 180f
Arrhythmias
    cardiac, 154f–156f, 154–156, 191t
Arthritis
    after hip dislocation, 57
    spinal, 15, 15f
Arthrography
    in ulnar collateral injury, 35–36, 36f
Arthropathy
    facet, 15
Arthroplasty
    abrasion, 145
Arthroscopy
    in ankle and foot injuries, 112f–113f, 112–114
    in elbow flexion contracture, 26
    in knee injury
        in anterior cruciate ligament repair, 73, 73f
        complications of, 92–93
        in meniscal repair, 86f–87f, 86–87
        pain management in, 93
    in refractory lateral epicondylitis, 26
    in shoulder injury, 19–23, 20f, 23f
    in triceps tendinitis and olecranon tip injury, 31, 31f
    in ulnar collateral injury, 36–37, 37f
    in valgus extension overload syndrome, 32, 33f
Articular cartilage, 133–147
    chondrocyte-matrix interactions in, 141–142
    composition of, 134f–139f, 134–140
    defect in knee of, 93–95, 94f
    matrix of see Cartilage matrix
    repair and regeneration of, 144–146
    response to injury of, 142f–143f, 142–144
    structure of, 134f–135f, 140–141
Articular cartilage defect
    knee, 93–95, 94f
Aspiration
    of knee joint effusion, 70
Association for the Advancement of Sport Psychology, 176
Asthma, 159–161, 160t
Asymmetry of rotation
    cervical spinal, 2, 2f
Athletic heart syndrome, 153
Atrioventricular block, 155
Attentional control
    in performance psychology, 181f–182f, 181–182
Autografting
    in anterior cruciate ligament repair, 72
    in meniscal repair, 89
    in posterior cruciate ligament repair, 78, 80
Avascular necrosis
    in hip dislocation, 56–57
Avulsion
    flexor digitorum profundus, 52f, 53
    labral, 20
Avulsion fracture
    hip, 56t, 57–58, 58f

B

Back pain, 1–15 *see also* specific disorders; Spine
Ballet dancers
    scoliosis in, 15
    spondylolysis in, 12–13
    stress fractures in, 105t, 105–106
Bankart shoulder lesion, 20–21

Barometric pressure
    fetal risks of, 223
Baseball players
    chest wall injury in, 7–8
    elbow flexion contracture in, 26
    olecranon physeal fracture nonunion in, 29
    Panner's disease in, 27–28
    safety devices for, 7–8
    tobacco use by, 171
    ulnar collateral injury in, 35–36, 38
    valgus extension overload syndrome in, 32
Basketball players
    litigation by and on behalf of, 232–234
    os trigonum fracture in, 110f–111f, 110–111
Beer, 170
Bennett's fracture dislocation, 49
Berndt and Hardy classification of talus osteochondral lesions, 112f, 113
Beta-blockers, 159, 171
Bicyclists see Cyclists
Biglycan
    cartilage, 139–140
Blatt capsulodesis, 45, 45f
Bleeding disorder
    in knee, 97–98
Blood flow
    in ligament healing, 125–126, 126f
Blood hyperviscosity
    from erythropoietin, 167
Body composition, 208–209, 213
Body weight
    creatine and, 164
    in eating disorders, 218, 218t, 220
    in hypertension, 159
    menstrual dysfunction and, 216
    in pregnancy, 222–223
Bodybuilders
    distal biceps tendon rupture in, 26
Bone density measurement, 216, 217t
Bone patellar tendon bone graft
    in anterior cruciate ligament repair, 72, 74–77
    in posterior cruciate ligament repair, 78, 80
Bone scanning
    in hip and thigh stress fracture, 63f, 63–64
    in os trigonum fracture, 110f–111f, 110–111
Boutonniere deformity, 51–52
Boxer's fracture, 50–51
Boxing
    cardiac contusion in, 7
Brachial plexus neuropathy
    in contact sports, 3, 5
Bracing
    after knee injuries, 77, 80
    in scoliosis, 15
    in spinal fracture, 9
    in ulnar collateral injury, 38
Bradycardia, 153–155
Breathing
    in performance psychology, 180
Brennan v Board of Trustees for University of Louisiana Systems, 235
Broström procedure, 112, 116
Bulimia nervosa, 183, 217–221, 218t, 220f
Bundle branch block, 156
Bupivacaine
    postarthroscopic, 93
Burner injury, 3, 5
Burning hand syndrome, 5
Bursitis
    trochanteric, 65, 225–226

C

Caffeine, 169, 169t
Calcium channel antagonists, 159
Calcium intake in women, 215, 217, 224
California malpractice laws, 233
Capitellar fracture, 29
Capsular release arthroscopy
    in elbow flexion contracture, 26

Cardiac arrhythmias, 154f–156f, 154–156, 191t
Cardiac contusion, 7
Cardiac disorders see Cardiopulmonary disorders; specific disorders
Cardiomyopathy, 153
Cardiopulmonary disorders, 151–161
    from anabolic steroids, 167t
    anomalous coronary arteries as, 154
    arrhythmic, 154f–156f, 154–156
    asthma as, 159–161, 160t
    cardiomyopathy as, 153
    coronary arterial, 157t, 157–158
    hypertension as, 158t, 158–159
    malpractice in, 232
    in Marfan syndrome, 157
    murmurs in, 152, 156–157
    myocarditis as, 154
    normal physiology versus, 153
    pericarditis as, 154
    screening for, 151–152, 152f, 152t, 191t, 191–192
    sudden death from, 153
    symptoms of, 191t
    valvular, 156–157
    vocal cord dysfunction versus, 161
Cardiovascular system
    stimulants and, 168, 168t
    in women, 209, 211–212, 222
Carpal instability, 44f–46f, 44–46
Carpometacarpal joint dislocation, 49
Cartilage see Articular cartilage
Cartilage matrix
    artificial, 146
    chondrocyte interaction with, 141–142
    injury to, 142
    regions of, 135f, 138f, 141
    structure and function of, 134f–139f, 135–136, 138–140
Cell transplantation
    cartilage repair and, 145–146
Centers for Disease Control
    on sedentary Americans, 187
Central nervous system stimulants, 168t
Cervical spinal injury, 1–7
    evaluation after, 2f, 2t, 2–3
    incidence of, 6f
    on-field evaluation of, 2–3
    prevention of, 6–7
    return to play after, 5–6
    treatment of, 3–6, 4f
Chest protector
    for baseball players, 8
Chest wall injury, 7–9
Childhood
    spinal variants in, 3–4, 4f
Cholesterol, 213
Chondrocytes
    injury to, 142f, 142–143
    matrix interaction with, 141–142
    structure and function of, 134f–138f, 134–135, 140–141
    transplantation of, 95, 145–146
Chondromalacia
    in valgus extension overload syndrome, 32
Chondroplasty
    in osteochondral knee lesions, 94
Cigarette smoking, 159
Cimaterol, 169
Clenbuterol, 168–169
Cocaine, 170
Coffee, 169, 169t
Cognitive strategies
    in performance psychology, 181
Collagen
    cartilage, 135f–138f, 136, 138–140
    ligament, 124, 126, 126f, 129
Collateral ligament injury
    thumb, 49–50, 50f
Comminuted fracture
    olecranon, 30
Compartment syndrome
    ankle and foot, 103–104, 104f–105f
    postarthroscopic, 92–93
    thigh, 60–61
Competitive seasons
    training cycles and, 195–197
Compliance in training, 189
Compression test
    in iliotibial band-friction syndrome, 99
Computed tomographic arthrography
    in ulnar collateral injury, 35–36, 36f
Computed tomography

in ankle and foot injury, 105
    in hip and thigh injury, 56, 63, 63f
    in spinal injury, 4, 9, 12
Concentration
    in performance psychology, 181f–182f, 181–182
Conditioning, 187–204 see also Training
    basic, 193t, 193–200, 194f–196f, 195t
    skill training and, 189–191
    in women, 209
Congenital aortic valve stenosis, 157
Consumer Product Safety Commission
    baseball-related injury reported by, 7
Contact sports see also specific sports
    spinal injury in, 3, 5–10
Contracture
    elbow flexion, 26
Contusion
    cardiac, 7
    spinal, 9–10, 10t
    thigh, 59, 61
Coronary artery anomaly, 154
    sudden death from, 153
Coronary artery disease, 157t, 157–158
Coronoid fracture, 29
Corpus luteum, 210, 210f
Corticosteroids
    in disc herniation, 12, 15
    in iliotibial-band friction syndrome, 65
    in osteitis pubis, 61
    in postarthroscopic infection, 92–93
    in snapping hip syndrome, 65
Coxsackie virus
    heart disease from, 154
Crank test
    in shoulder injury, 22f, 22–23
Creatine, 163–164
Creep
    in ligament biomechanics, 122, 123f
Cross-training, 198–199
Cyclists
    exertional compartment syndrome in, 104
    Guyon's canal nerve compression in, 49
    iliotibial-band friction syndrome in, 65
    possible erythropoietin abuse in, 168
    sport psychology studies in, 176
    training of, 198
Cylert, 171
Cytokines
    in chondrocyte-matrix interactions, 141–142
    in osteochondral injury, 143

D

Decorin
    cartilage, 139–140
Denis method of fracture assessment, 10
Depression
    in performance psychology, 182–183
deQuervain's tenosynovitis, 47
Diabetes
    gestational, 223
Diagnostic and Statistical Manual
    on eating disorders, 218
Diet
    amenorrhea and, 213
    creatine sources in, 164
    in women athletes, 224–225
Dilated cardiomyopathy, 153
Disc injury
    arthritis in, 15
    cervical, 6
    lumbar, 11f, 11–13
    thoracic, 8
Dislocation
    ankle and foot tendon, 106–107
    elbow, 28–29
        in coronoid fractures, 29
        in radial fractures, 29
    hip, 55–57, 56t, 57f
    interphalangeal joint, 51–52
    shoulder, 19–21
    thumb, 49
    wrist, 44, 44f
Dissociative carpal instability, 44
Distal biceps tendon rupture, 26
Distal interphalangeal joint dislocation, 52
Distal radial fracture
    wheel-related, 31

Diuretics
    abuse of, 171
    in hypertension, 159
Dorsal impaction syndrome, 47
Dorsal intercalary segment instability, 44–46, 45f
Drug use, 163–172 see also specific drugs
    antihypertensive, 159
    beta-blockers in, 171
    diuretics in, 171
    in eating disorders, 218, 218t
    ergogenic, 163–170
        anabolic steroids in, 164–165, 166f, 167t
        creatine in, 163–164
        erythropoietin in, 167–168
        growth hormone in, 156–167
        stimulants in, 168t–169t, 168–170
    malpractice in, 232–233
    probenecid in, 171
    recreational, 170–171
    Ritalin and Cylert in, 171
    testing for, 171–172, 235
    war against, 163
Duke lesion, 114
Dynamic exercise
    spine-strengthening, 2
Dynasplint
    in elbow flexion contracture, 26
Dyspnea
    in heart disease, 153–154

E

Eating disorders
    causes of, 219
    classification of, 217–218, 218t
    diagnosis of, 219t, 219–220
    in performance psychology, 183
    risks of, 218–219
    treatment of, 220f, 220–221
Echocardiography, 152–154, 156–157
Elbow and forearm injury, 25–41
    acute medial elbow rupture in, 33f–34f, 33–34
    dislocations in, 28–29
    distal biceps tendon ruptures in, 26
    flexion contracture in, 26
    flexor-pronator sprain in, 32–33
    fractures in
        capitellar, 29
        coronoid, 29
        olecranon, 30
        physeal nonunion of olecranon, 29–30, 30f
        radial head, 29
        ulnar fatigue, 31
        wheel-related, 31
    neuropathies in, 38–40
    osteochondrosis and osteochondritis dissecans in, 27f–28f, 27–28
    posterior rotatory instability in, 26–27, 27f
    refractory lateral epicondylitis in, 26
    triceps tendon and olecranon tip in, 31, 31f
    ulnar collateral ligament overload in, 34–38, 35f–38f
    valgus extension overload in, 32, 32f–33
Electrocardiography, 154f–156f, 154–156
Endobutton graft fixation, 73
Endocrine system
    anabolic steroids and, 167t
    stimulants and, 168t
Endoscopy
    in meniscal repair, 88
Endurance training, 197–199
Ephedrine, 169–170
Epicondylitis
    refractory lateral, 26
Epitestosterone, 165
Ergogenic drug use, 163–170 see also Drug use; specific agents
Erythropoietin, 167–168, 171
Essex-Lopresti injury, 29
Estradiol, 210, 210f, 212–214
Estrogen, 211–217, 215f, 216t
Ethanol, 170–171
Exercise see also Training
    after hip dislocation, 56
    after knee injuries, 77, 80
    after spinal injury, 2, 7, 12
    after thigh stress fracture, 64
    after ulnar nerve injury, 40
    amenorrhea induced by, 213–214

asthma in, 159–161
basic conditioning, 193
ergogenic drug use and, 164–170, 166*f*
in hypertension, 159
in pregnancy, 221*t*, 221–224
in ulnar collateral injury, 36
Exercise testing guidelines, 190*t*, 191
Exertional compartment syndrome
ankle and foot, 103–104, 104*f*–105*f*
Extracellular matrix
cartilage *see* Cartilage matrix

F

Facet arthropathy, 15
Fasciitis
plantar, 110
Fatigue fracture *see* Stress fracture
Female athlete triad
disordered eating in, 217–221, 218*t*–219*t*, 220*f*
osteoporosis in, 216*t*–217*t*, 216–217
Femoral stress fracture, 63*f*, 63–65, 65*f*
Fetal risks of exercise, 222–223
Fibrin clot
in meniscal repair, 88, 88*f*
in osteochondral knee lesions, 93
Fibromodulin
cartilage, 139–140
Fibular fracture, 114*f*
Figure skaters
spondylolysis in, 11*f*
Finger
jersey, 52*f*, 53
mallet, 52, 52*f*
First aid
in cervical spinal injuries, 2–3
Fisher modification of Berndt and Hardy classification, 112*f*, 113
Fitness conditioning, 193
Flak jacket
in spinal injury, 9
Flexion contracture
elbow, 26
Flexor digitorum profundus avulsion, 52*f*, 53
Flexor-pronator sprain, 32–33
Fluid irrigation systems
in postarthroscopic infection, 92
Follicle-stimulating hormone, 210*f*, 210–211
Foot injury, 103–116 *see also* Ankle and foot injury
Football players
ankle and foot injuries in, 105*t*, 114–115, 115*f*
finger injuries in, 52*f*, 52–53
malpractice in, 233
shoulder injury in, 23
spinal injuries in, 3, 5–7
Forearm and elbow injury, 25–41 *see also* Elbow and forearm injury; specific injuries
Forefoot fracture, 106
Fracture
ankle and foot, 104–106, 114*f*, 114–115
capitellar, 29
coronoid, 29
fatigue *see* Stress fracture
hip and thigh, 56*t*, 57–58, 58*f*, 62–65, 63*f*, 65*f*
interphalangeal joint, 51
metacarpal, 50–51
thumb, 49
olecranon, 30
nonunion of, 29–30, 30*f*
osteoporotic, 215–216
phalangeal, 51–52
radial head, 29
rib, 7
spinal, 3, 5, 6*f*, 7–12, 8, 10*t*
stress *see* Stress fracture
ulnar fatigue, 31
wheel-related forearm, 31
wrist, 47–48, 48*f*
Fulcrum test
in femoral stress fractures, 64
Fulkerson's technique, 95

G

Gait
in hip and thigh stress fracture, 62
Game keeper's thumb, 49

Gardner v Holifield, 231–233
Gathers v Loyola-Marymount University, 232–233
Gender differences
in body composition, 208–209
in skeletal maturity, 208
in stress fractures, 105
Gene therapy
in ligament healing, 129
Gestational diabetes, 223
Gigantism, 165
Glutamine
in overtraining, 203
Glycosaminoglycans
cartilage, 137*f*, 139
Goal setting
in performance psychology, 178–179
in training, 188–189
Gonadotropin hormone-releasing hormone, 210
Gore Smoother
in posterior cruciate ligament repair, 80
Grafting
HIV transmission in, 89–90
in ligament repair
anterior cruciate, 72*f*–76*f*, 72–77, 129–130
lateral collateral, 81
medial collateral, 129
posterior cruciate, 78–80
in meniscal repair, 89–91, 90*f*
periosteal and perichondrial, 145
Great toe injury, 115, 115*f*
Greater trochanter avulsion fracture, 58
Gretzky
Wayne, 8
Griffith
Coleman, 176
Growth factors
cartilage and, 141–143, 146
in ligament healing, 128–129
Growth hormone, 156–167, 171
Guyon's canal nerve compression, 48–49
Gymnasts
arthritis in, 15, 15*f*
Panner's disease in, 27–28
spinal injury in, 11–14
wrist injuries in, 47

H

Hahn-Steinthal capitellar fracture, 29
Halo vest stabilization
in cervical spinal injury, 6
Hamate hook fracture, 48
Hamstring graft
in anterior cruciate ligament repair, 72*f*, 72–77, 75*f*
Hamstring injury, 61–62, 62*f*
Hand and wrist injury, 43–53
diagnosis of, 43–44
dislocations in
carpometacarpal, 49
wrist, 44, 44*f*
fractures in
hamate hook, 48
metacarpal, 50–51
phalangeal, 51
wrist, 47–48, 48*f*
interphalangeal joint, 51–52
jersey finger in, 52*f*, 53
mallet finger in, 52*f*, 52–53
nerve compression in, 48–49
thumb, 49–50
wrist tendinitis in, 47
Healing
articular cartilage in, 133–134, 142*f*–143*f*, 142–146
Healthy People 2000 goals, 193
Heart disease *see* Cardiopulmonary disorders; specific
disorders
Helmets
in cervical spinal injuries, 3, 6
Hemarthrosis
knee, 97
Hematoma
in osteochondral injury, 143
Hemophilia
knee surgery in, 97–98
Hendy v Losse, 233
Heparin
in asthma, 161
Hepatic disorders
from anabolic steroids, 167*t*

Heterotopic ossification
thigh, 60, 60*f*
Hill v National Collegiate Athletic Association, 235
Hindfoot fracture, 106
Hip and thigh injury, 55–66
fractures in
avulsion, 56*t*, 57–58, 58*f*
hip, 56*t*, 58
stress, 56*t*, 62–65, 63*f*, 65*f*
hamstring, 61–62, 62*f*
heterotropic ossification in, 60, 60*f*
hip dislocation and subluxation in, 55–57, 56*t*, 57*f*
hip pointer in, 59
osteitis pubis in, 61
thigh compartment syndrome in, 60–61
thigh contusion in, 59, 61
Hip pointer, 59
Hockey players, 8, 171
Human growth hormone, 165–167, 171
Human immunodeficiency virus
transmission by allograft of, 89–90
Hypertension, 158*t*, 158–159, 191*t*
Hyperthermia in pregnancy, 222
Hypertrophic cardiomyopathy, 153
Hyperviscosity syndrome
from erythropoietin, 167
Hypoxemia
fetal, 223

I

Ice hockey players
chest injury in, 8
tobacco use by, 171
Idiopathic dilated cardiomyopathy, 153
Iliac spine avulsion fracture, 57–58
Iliopsoas tendon
in snapping hip syndrome, 65
Iliotibial band-friction syndrome, 65–66, 99
Imagery
in performance psychology, 180–181
Imaging techniques *see also* specific techniques
in knee injuries, 70–71, 71*f*, 91–92, 96, 98
Immobilization
after knee injuries, 77, 80, 128
chondrocyte activity and, 135
Infection
heart disease from, 154
postarthroscopic, 92
spinal, 15
Inflammation
in ligament healing, 125–126
Injury *see* specific injuries and structures; Trauma
In-line skaters
forearm fractures in, 31
Inside-out meniscal repair technique, 86–87, 87*f*
Instability
ankle, 111*f*, 111–112
carpal, 44*f*–46*f*, 44–46
elbow posterior rotatory, 26–27, 27*f*
knee
ligament healing and, 128
patellar, 95*f*, 95–96
shoulder, 20*f*, 21–21
spinal, 3–4, 4*f*
Interdigital nerve entrapment, 109–110
Interleukin-6
in overtraining, 203
International Olympic Committee
substances banned by, 165, 167–171
in war against drugs, 163
Intersection syndrome, 47
Inverted-U theory of arousal regulation, 180, 180*f*
Iron deficiency, 224
Ischial tuberosity avulsion fracture, 58, 58*f*
Isometric exercise
spine-strengthening, 2

J

Jersey finger, 52*f*, 53
Jewett extension brace
in spinal fracture, 9
Jogger's foot, 109
Joints *see also* Ligaments; specific joints
articular cartilage in, 133–147
forces in stability of, 122, 122*f*
laxity of shoulder, 24

Journal of Sport Psychology, 176–177
Jumpers
    training of, 190, 199

K

Killum
    Earnest, 232–233
Kissing lesion
    in valgus extension overload syndrome, 32
Knapp v Northwestern University, 234
Knee
    arthroscopy of, 92–93
    bleeding disorders of, 97–98
    cartilage repair in, 145–146
    iliotibial band-friction syndrome of, 65–66, 99
    ligament injuries of, 69–82
        anterior cruciate, 71–77, 72f–76f, 125–130, 226
        healing of, 125–127, 126f, 127t
        history and examination in, 69–70, 70f
        imaging in, 70–71, 71f
        lateral collateral, 81
        medial collateral, 77, 125–129, 126f, 128f
        posterior cruciate, 77–81, 79f
        treatment of, 127–130, 128f
    ligament stability of, 69
    meniscal injuries of, 85–92, 86f–88f, 90f–91f
    Osgood-Schlatter disease of, 97, 97f
    osteochondral lesions of, 93–95, 94f
    patellar injuries of, 95f, 95–97
    patellofemoral dysfunction in, 225
    pigmented villonodular synovitis of, 98–99
    in quadriceps contusion, 59–60
Kocher-Lorenz capitellar fracture, 29
Korean martial arts
    chest injury in, 8
Krueger v San Francisco Forty Niners, 233
Kyphosis, 9, 9f, 14, 14f

L

Labral injury, 22f, 22–23
Lachman anterior laxity testing, 70, 70f, 76
Lacrosse
    chest injury in, 7–8
Lactate
    training and, 198
Lateral antebrachial nerve injury, 39–40
Lateral collateral ligament injury, 81
Lateral epicondylitis, 26
Lateral malleolar fracture, 114f, 115
Laxity
    shoulder, 24
Leg injury
    ankle and foot, 103–116 *see also* Ankle and foot injury
    hip and thigh, 55–66 *see also* Hip and thigh injury
Legal issues, 231–235
Lesser trochanter avulsion fracture, 58
Lifestyle modification
    in hypertension, 159
Lift-off test
    in shoulder injury, 21f, 21–22
Ligaments
    biology of, 124, 124f
    biomechanics of, 122, 122f, 123
    function of, 121f, 121–122
    injury to *see also* specific ligaments
        ankle, 111–112
        healing of, 125–127, 126f, 127t
        knee, 69–82, 125–130, 126t
        mechanisms of, 124–125, 125t
        reconstruction in, 129–130
        treatment of, 127–129, 128f
Lillard v State of Oregon, 232–233
Lipoproteins, 213
Litigation
    for denial of medical clearance, 234
    for drug testing challenges, 235
    malpractice, 231–233
Load-*versus*-elongation curve
    in ligament biomechanics, 122, 123f
Lumbar spinal injury, 9–15, 10t, 11f, 14f–15f
Lunate dislocation, 44, 44f
Lung disease, 159–161, 160t
Lunotriquetral ligament injury, 44, 46, 46f
Luteinizing hormone, 210, 210f, 213

M

Macrocycles in training, 195, 196f
Madelung's deformity, 47
Magnetic resonance arthrography
    in ulnar collateral injury, 36
Magnetic resonance imaging
    in ankle and foot injury, 103, 107, 115
    in hip and thigh injury, 61–63
    in knee injury, 70–71, 71f, 78, 91–92, 96, 98
    in shoulder injury, 21–22
    in spinal injury, 4, 8, 11, 13–14
Malleolar fracture, 114f, 115
Mallet finger, 52, 52f
Malpractice litigation, 231–233
Marfan syndrome, 157, 232
Marijuana, 170
Mason radial head fractures
    treatment of, 29
Matrix
    cartilage *see* Cartilage matrix
    ligament, 124, 126
Maximal mechanical power output training, 199
Mechanical low-back pain, 14–15
Medial collateral ligament injury, 77, 127–129
    healing of, 125–127, 126f, 127t, 128f
Medial plantar nerve entrapment, 109
Median nerve injury, 38–39
Medical history
    in training assessment, 191–192
Medicolegal issues, 231–235
Menarche, 208, 213
Meniscal injury
    allografts in, 89–91, 90–91
    in anterior cruciate ligament-deficient knees, 88–89
    imaging in, 91–92
    indications for repair of, 85–86
    meniscal replacement in, 89
    meniscectomy in, 85–88, 86f–88f
    synovial fluid analysis in, 85
    synovitis *versus*, 98
Meniscectomy, 85–88, 86f–88f
    osteoarthritis after, 85, 88–89
Menopause, 208, 211, 215
Menstrual cycle
    dysfunctional, 213–216, 215f
    normal, 210f, 210–211
    oral contraceptives and, 211–213
    stress fractures and, 63, 104–105
Mental skills
    in performance psychology, 176–177
Mesocycles in training, 195–197
Metabolism
    menstrual cycle and, 212
Metacarpal fracture, 50–51
    thumb, 49
Metacarpophalangeal joint dislocation, 49
Metatarsal fracture, 106
Metatarsophalangeal joint injury, 115, 115t
Methylprednisolone
    in cervical spinal injury, 6
Methylxanthines, 169, 169t
Microcycles in training, 195–197
Microtrauma
    spinal, 10t, 13
Military recruit training, 200
Mitral valve disorders, 156–157
Mood disorders
    in performance psychology, 183
Morton's neuroma, 109–110
Motion
    in ligament healing, 128
Murmurs
    cardiac, 152, 156–157
Muscle injury
    in hip avulsion fractures, 57
    overuse, 200–201
    quadriceps contusion in, 59–60
Muscle relaxation
    in performance psychology, 180
Muscle splitting
    in rotator cuff repair, 23
    in ulnar collateral injury repair, 37f, 37–38
Musculotendinous strain
    in spinal injury, 8, 10, 10t
    thigh, 61
Myocarditis, 154
Myositis ossificans traumatica
    in thigh injury, 60

N

National Collegiate Athletic Association
    litigation against, 235
    spearing banned by, 6f
    substances banned by, 165, 167–171
National Federation of High School Athletic Associations
    spearing banned by, 6f
National Football League
    anabolic steroid use in, 164
National Institutes of Health
    asthma guidelines of, 159–160, 160t
Neck injury, 1–7, 2f, 2t, 4f, 6f
Necrosis
    in hip dislocation, 56–57
Neoplasm
    spinal, 15
Nerve compression
    wrist, 48–49
Nerve entrapment
    ankle and foot, 107–110, 108f
Neuropathy *see also* Nerve compression; specific nerves
    anterior interosseus, 39
    cervical spinal, 3, 5
    lateral antebrachial cutaneous, 39–40
    median, 38–39
    radial, 39
    ulnar, 40
New Zealand rugby rules
    cervical spinal injuries and, 7
Nicotine, 171
Nondissociative carpal instability, 44, 46
Nonsteroidal anti-inflammatory drugs
    postarthroscopic, 93
    in ulnar collateral injury, 36
Notchplasty
    in anterior cruciate ligament repair, 73, 73f
Nutrition in women, 224–225
    in eating disorders, 220

O

O'Brien test
    in shoulder injury, 23
Ohio State University Sports Medicine Center, 175, 183–185
Olecranon fracture, 30
    nonunion of, 29–30, 30f
    in skateboard elbow, 31
Olecranon tip injury
    triceps tendon and, 31, 31f
Oligomenorrhea, 211
Olympics
    sport psychology in, 176
On-field assessment
    of cervical spinal injuries, 2–3
Oral contraceptives, 211–215
Orthosis
    in ankle instability, 112
    in spinal injury, 9–10, 14
Os trigonum injury, 110f–111f, 110–111
Osgood-Schlatter disease, 97, 97f
Osteitis pubis, 61
Osteoarthritis
    after meniscectomy, 85, 88–89
    age-related changes *versus*, 144
    growth factors in, 146
Osteochondral lesion
    ankle, 112f–113f, 112–113
    cartilage response to, 143f, 143–144
    knee, 93–95, 94f
Osteochondritis dissecans
    knee, 95
    lateral elbow, 27–28, 28f
Osteochondrosis
    lateral elbow, 27f, 27–28
Osteophyte
    in valgus extension overload syndrome, 32, 32f
Osteoporosis
    amenorrhea and, 105, 214
    in eating disorders, 183
    menopause and, 211, 216–217
    risks factors for, 217t
Outside-in meniscal repair technique, 86f, 86–87
Overload
    ulnar collateral ligament injuries from, 34–38, 35f–38f
    valgus extension, 32, 32f–33f
Overtraining, 202t, 202–203

Overuse injury *see also* other injuries; Stress fracture
 hip and thigh, 56t, 62–66, 63f, 65f
 iliotibial band-friction syndrome as, 99
 spinal, 11, 13–14
 training and, 200–203, 202t
Ovulation, 210, 210f

P

Pahulu v University of Kansas, 234
Pain management
 postarthroscopic, 93
Palpitations
 in cardiac arrhythmias, 155
Panner's disease, 27f, 27–28
Patella
 instability of, 95f, 95–96
 tendinitis of, 96–97
Patellofemoral dysfunction, 225
Peak flow meters
 in asthma, 159–160
Pelvic obliquity
 overuse injury in, 201
Pennsylvania State University eating disorder policy, 220f, 220–221
Performance in sports *see also* Training
 oral contraceptives and menstrual cycle in, 211–213
 psychology of *see* Performance psychology
Performance psychology, 175–185
 arousal control in, 179–181, 180f
 attentional control in, 181f–182f, 181–182
 clinical issues in, 182–184
 credentials in, 177
 goal setting in, 178–179
 history of, 176–177
 mental skills in, 177–178
 sport psychology *versus*, 175
 in sports medicine setting, 184–185
Pericarditis, 154
Perichondrial grafting, 145
Periodization in training, 194–197, 195f–196f, 195t
Periosteal grafting, 145
Peroneal nerve entrapment, 107–109, 108f
Peroneal tendon injury, 106
Phalangeal fracture, 51–52
Phenylephrine, 169–170
Phenylpropanolamine, 169–170
Physical examination
 in training assessment, 191t–192t, 191–192
Physical therapy
 in spinal fracture, 9
Pigmented villonodular synovitis
 of knee, 98–99
Plantar fasciitis, 110
Pneumothorax, 7
Posterior cruciate ligament injury, 77–81, 79f
Posterior rotatory instability
 elbow, 26–27, 27f
Posterior tibialis tendon injury, 106–107
Posterolateral complex injury, 81
Posterolateral rotatory instability maneuver, 26–27, 27f
Posture
 in kyphosis, 9
Pre-excitation
 ventricular, 154f, 155
Pregnancy, 221t, 221–224
Premature ventricular contractions, 155–156, 156f
Pressure
 barometric, 223
 in exertional compartment syndrome, 103–104
Probenecid, 171
Progesterone, 210, 210f, 212–215, 215f
Progressive resistive exercise
 in disc herniation, 12
Pronation, 201, 208
Prosthesis
 meniscal, 89
Protein
 dietary, 224
 noncollagenous cartilage, 136, 139–140
Proteoglycans
 cartilage, 135f–136f, 136, 139–140
Pseudarthrosis
 spinal, 15, 15f
Pseudo-Boutonniere deformity, 52
Pseudoephedrine, 169–170
Psychology
 anabolic steroids and, 165, 167t

of eating disorders, 218t, 218–219
 performance, 175–185 *see also* Performance psychology
Puberty, 208, 213
Pulmonary disease, 159–161, 160t

Q

Quadriceps active test, 70
Quadriceps femoris contusion, 59–60

R

Radial collateral ligament injury, 50
Radial fracture, 31
Radial head fracture, 29
Radial nerve injury, 39
Radiation therapy
 in pigmented villonodular synovitis, 98
Radiography
 after spinal injury, 2–4, 4f, 8–10
 in hip and thigh injury, 55–56, 57f–58f, 60f, 60–64, 62f–63f
 in knee injury, 70
 in valgus extension overload syndrome, 32
Radionuclide scanning
 in hip and thigh stress fracture, 63
Range-of-motion exercise
 after hip dislocation, 56
 after spinal injury, 2, 2f, 12
 after thigh injury, 61, 64
Reconstruction
 ligament, 129–130
Recreational drug use, 170–171
Refractory lateral epicondylitis, 26
Rehabilitation
 after knee injuries, 77, 80–81
 in training programs, 201–202
Rehabilitation Act, 234
Remodeling
 in ligament healing, 126
Renal disorders
 from anabolic steroids, 167t
 in lumbar contusion, 10
Rheumatic heart disease, 156
Rib injury, 7–8
Rib-tip syndrome, 7
Ritalin, 171
Rolando's fracture, 49
Rotator cuff injury, 23f, 23–24
Rotator interval repair, 20f–21f, 20–21
Rotatory instability
 elbow, 26–27, 27f
Rowers
 training of, 198–199
Rugby players
 spinal injuries in, 6–7
Runners
 amenorrheic, 213–214
 exertional compartment syndrome in, 104
 iliotibial-band friction syndrome in, 65
 stress fractures in, 63, 104–105, 105t
 training of, 198–199
Rupture
 acute medial elbow, 33f–34f, 33–34
 ankle and foot tendon, 106–107, 107f
 distal biceps, 26
 subscapularis, 21f, 21–22

S

Salbutamol, 169
Saphenous nerve entrapment, 108–109
Scaphoid fracture, 47–48, 48f
Scapholunate advanced collapse wrist deformity, 45–46
Scapholunate ligament disruption, 45
Scar
 in ligament healing, 125–126, 128
Scheuermann's kyphosis, 9, 9f, 14, 14f
Schmorl's node, 11, 14f
Scoliosis, 15
Scrum
 cervical spinal injuries in, 7
Self-talk
 in performance psychology, 181
Shoulder injury, 19–24
 Bankart lesions in, 20–21

dislocation in, 19–21
 instability in, 20f, 20–21
 labral, 22f, 22–23
 laxity in, 23
 rotator cuff repair in, 23f, 23–24
 rotator interval repair in, 20f–21f, 20–21
 subscapularis rupture in, 21f, 21–22
Silicone rubber splint
 in scaphoid fracture, 48, 48f
Single-photon emission computed tomography
 in spinal arthritis, 15
 in spinal injury, 11, 13
Sinus arrhythmia, 154f, 154–155
Skateboard elbow, 31
Skateboarders
 forearm fractures in, 31
Skeletal maturity, 208
Skiers
 hip fracture in, 58
 thumb injuries in, 49–50
Smoking, 159, 171
Snapping hip syndrome, 65
Soccer players
 oral contraceptives in, 212–213
Sodium intake
 in hypertension, 159
Soft drinks, 169, 169t
Softball pitchers
 ulnar fatigue fractures in, 31
Somatotropin, 165–167
Spina bifida occulta, 12
Spine
 fusion of, 6
 infection of, 15
 injury of, 1–15
  cervical, 1–7, 2f, 2t, 4f, 6f
  lumbar, 9–15, 10t, 11f, 14f–15f
  thoracic, 7–9, 9f
 neoplasms of, 15
 radiographic variations of, 3–4, 4f
 scoliosis of, 15
 stenosis of, 5
Splinting
 in ulnar collateral injury, 38
 for wrist fractures, 48, 48f
Spondylolysis, 11f, 11–13
Spondylolysthesis, 12–13
Sport medicine facility
 performance psychology in, 184–185
Sport psychology *see also* Performance psychology
 performance psychology *versus*, 175
Sport-specific conditioning and training, 194, 194f, 197–198
Sprain
 ankle, 111f, 111–112
 flexor-pronator, 32–33
Squat lifts, 199
Squeeze test, 111, 111f
Stener's lesion, 50
Stenosis
 aortic valve, 157, 191t
 mitral valve, 156
 spinal, 5
Sternal injury, 7–8
Steroids
 anabolic, 164–165, 166f, 167t
Stimulants, 168t–169t, 168–170
Stinger injury, 3, 5
Strain
 thigh, 61
Strength
 menstrual cycle and, 212
 training for, 199
Strengthening exercise
 after thigh injury, 61–62
 cervical spinal, 2, 7
 in women, 209
Stress fracture
 amenorrhea and, 63
 ankle and foot, 104–106
 hip and thigh, 56t, 62–65, 63f, 65f
 prevention of recurrent, 63
 spinal, 12
 tibial, 105f, 105–106
 ulnar, 31
Stress testing
 in cardiopulmonary screening, 152
Stress-relaxation
 in ligament biomechanics, 122, 123f

Stress-*versus*-strain curve
  in ligament biomechanics, 122, 123f, 124
Suave-Kapandji procedure, 47
Subchondral bone penetration
  cartilage repair in, 145
Subluxation
  ankle and foot tendon, 106
  hip, 56t, 57
  interphalangeal joint, 51
Subscapularis rupture, 21f, 21–22
Sudden death, 153–154
Supraventricular tachycardia, 154f–155f, 155
Sural nerve entrapment, 109
Surgical treatment *see also* Arthroscopy
  of acute medial elbow rupture, 33–34, 34f
  of ankle and foot injuries, 106–107, 107f, 109–111, 110f,
    114f, 114–115
  of anterior cruciate ligament injuries, 71–77, 72f–76f
  of carpal instability, 45f–46f, 45–46
  of elbow and forearm fractures, 29–30, 30f
  of hand injuries, 49–51
  of hip and thigh injuries, 56, 58, 60–62, 64–65
  of lateral collateral ligament injuries, 81
  of medial collateral ligament injuries, 77
  of meniscal injuries, 85–91, 86f–87f, 90f–91f
  of osteochondral knee lesions, 93–95, 94f
  of patellar injuries, 95–97
  of pigmented villonodular synovitis, 98–99
  of posterior cruciate ligament injuries, 78–80, 79f
  of shoulder injuries, 20f–21f, 20–24, 23f
  of spinal injuries, 6, 12
  of ulnar nerve injuries, 40
  of wrist fractures, 48
Suture repair
  of ligament injuries, 127
Swan neck deformity, 52
Swimmers
  pregnant, 222
  training of, 198–199
Syncope
  in hypertrophic cardiomyopathy, 153
Syndesmosis injury, 111, 111f
Synovectomy
  knee, 98
Synovial fluid analysis
  in meniscal injury, 85
Synovial impingement
  ankle, 114
Synovial joint
  articular cartilage in, 133–147
  ligament healing in, 122f, 125
Synovitis
  pigmented villonodular, 98–99

T

Tachycardia, 154f–156f, 155–156
Taekwon-do, 8
Talus *see also* Ankle and foot injury
  osteochondral lesions of, 112f–113f, 113
Taping
  in ankle instability, 112
Tarsal navicular fracture, 106
Tarsal tunnel nerve entrapment, 109
Tea, 169, 169t
Team physicians
  in training programs, 189
Tear
  meniscal, 85–86 *see also* Meniscal injury
  triangular fibrocartilage complex, 46–47
Telos radiography
  in ulnar collateral injury, 35, 35f

Tendinitis
  ankle and foot, 106
  patellar, 96–97
  triceps, 31
  wrist, 47
Tendon injury
  ankle and foot, 106–107, 107f
Tennis elbow, 26
Tennis players
  disc herniation in, 12f
  tennis elbow in, 26
  ulnar fatigue fractures in, 31
Tenosynovitis
  ankle and foot, 106
  deQuervain's, 47
  iliopsoas tendon, 65
Tension pneumothorax, 7
Testosterone derivatives, 164–165, 171
Testosterone/cortisol ratio
  in overtraining, 203
T-Fix suture device
  in meniscal repair, 88
Thermoregulation
  menstrual cycle and, 212
Thigh injury, 55–66 *see also* Hip and thigh injury
Thompson test, 107
Thoracic spinal injury, 7–9, 9f
Tibial fracture, 105f, 105–106
Tibiotalar spur, 114
Tinel's sign
  in ulnar collateral injury, 35
Tissue fluid
  in cartilage matrix, 136, 136f–137f
Tobacco, 159, 171
Toe injury, 115, 115f
Track athletes *see also* Runners
  stress fractures in, 105
Traction
  in cervical spinal injury, 6
Traction apophysitis of the tibial tubercle, 97
Traction palsy
  in contact sports, 3
Training, 187–204
  basic conditioning in, 193t, 193–200, 194f–196f, 195t
  needs assessment in, 187–191, 188f, 188t
  optimal, 187
  overuse injuries in, 200–203, 202t
  physical assessment in, 190t–192t, 191–192
Trauma *see also* specific injuries and structures
  ankle and foot, 103–116
  elbow and forearm, 25–41
  hand and wrist, 43–53
  hip and thigh, 55–66
  knee, 69–82, 85–99
  ligament, 124–125
  in performance psychology, 184
  prevention in women of, 226
  response of cartilage to, 142f–143f, 142–144
  risk factors in, 192, 192t
  shoulder and upper arm, 19–24
  spinal and chest wall, 1–15
  in training assessment, 192
Triangular fibrocartilage complex tear, 46–47
Triceps tendon injury
  olecranon tip and, 31, 31f
Triplett
  Norman, 176
Trochanteric bursitis, 65, 225–226
T-sign
  in ulnar collateral injury, 36, 36f
Turf toe, 115, 115f

U

Ulnar collateral ligament injury
  in acute medial elbow rupture, 34
  from repetitive overload, 34–38, 35–38
  thumb, 49–50, 50f
  in valgus extension overload syndrome, 32
Ulnar fatigue fracture, 31
Ulnar nerve injury, 40
Ulnocarpal impaction syndrome, 47
United States Olympic Committee
  marijuana banned by, 170
  sport psychologist hired by, 176
Urine drug testing, 172

V

Valgus extension overload syndrome, 32, 32f–33f
Valgus knee displacement, 69
Valgus stress test
  in knee injury, 70
  in ulnar collateral injury, 36
Valvular heart disease, 156–157, 191t
Varus knee displacement, 69
Varus stress test
  in knee injury, 70
Ventricular pre-excitation, 154f, 155
Vernonia School District 47J v Acton, 235
Vertebral body-neurocanal ratio
  in cervical spinal injury, 5
Viral infection
  heart disease from, 154
Viscoelasticity
  in ligament biomechanics, 122, 123f, 124
Vitamin D intake, 217
Vocal cord dysfunction, 161
Volar intercalary segment instability, 46, 46f
Volar plate injury, 52

W

Wandering atrial pacemaker, 155
Water running, 201–202
Water ski jumpers
  kyphosis in, 9
Watson's maneuver, 45
Weight *see* Body weight
Weightlifters
  distal biceps tendon rupture in, 26
  training in, 190, 194, 199
Wheel-related fracture
  forearm, 31
Wilkinson's sign, 12
Wolff-Parkinson-White syndrome, 154f, 155
Women in sports, 207–227
  eating disorders in, 216–221 *see also* Eating disorders
  female athlete triad in, 216t–219t, 216–221, 220f
  injury prevention in, 226
  menstrual cycle in, 209–216 *see also* Menstrual cycle
  musculoskeletal issues in, 225–226
  nutrition in, 224–225
  physiologic variables in, 207–209
  pregnancy in, 221t, 221–224
  stress fractures in, 63, 105
Wrist and hand injury, 43–53 *see also* Hand and wrist
  injury

Z

Zileuton
  in asthma, 161